Management of Emergency Cases in the Field

Editor

ISABELLE KILCOYNE

VETERINARY CLINICS OF NORTH AMERICA: EQUINE PRACTICE

www.vetequine.theclinics.com

Consulting Editor
THOMAS J. DIVERS

August 2021 • Volume 37 • Number 2

ELSEVIER

1600 John F. Kennedy Boulevard • Suite 1800 • Philadelphia, Pennsylvania, 19103-2899

http://www.vetequine.theclinics.com

VETERINARY CLINICS OF NORTH AMERICA: EQUINE PRACTICE Volume 37, Number 2
August 2021 ISSN 0749-0739, ISBN-13: 978-0-323-79186-1

Editor: Katerina Heidhausen
Developmental Editor: Ann Gielou Posedio

Veterinary Clinics of North America: Equine Practice (ISSN 0749-0739) is published in April, August, and December by Elsevier Inc., 360 Park Avenue South, New York, NY 10010-1710. Business and Editorial Offices: 1600 John F. Kennedy Blvd., Suite 1800, Philadelphia, PA 19103-2899. Subscription prices are $293.00 per year (domestic individuals), $766.00 per year (domestic institutions), $100.00 per year (domestic students/residents), $334.00 per year (Canadian individuals), $820.00 per year (Canadian institutions), $820.00 per year (international individuals), $365.00 per year (international institutions), $100.00 per year (Canadian students/residents), and $180.00 per year (international students/residents). To receive student/resident rate, orders must be accompanied by name of affiliated institution, date of term, and the signature of program/residency coordinator on institution letterhead. Orders will be billed at individual rate until proof of status is received. Foreign air speed delivery is included in all *Clinics* subscription prices. All prices are subject to change without notice. **POSTMASTER:** Send address changes to *Veterinary Clinics of North America: Equine Practice*, 3251 Riverport Lane, Maryland Heights, MO 63043. Customer Service (orders, claims, online, change of address): Elsevier Health Sciences Division, Subscription **Customer Service, 3251 Riverport Lane, Maryland Heights, MO 63043. Tel: 1-800-654-2452 (U.S. and Canada); 314-447-8871 (outside U.S. and Canada). Fax: 314-447-8029. E-mail: journalscustomerservice-usa@elsevier.com (for print support);** E-mail: **journalsonlinesupport-usa@ elsevier.com (for online support).**

Reprints. For copies of 100 or more of articles in this publication, please contact the Commercial Reprints Department, Elsevier Inc., 360 Park Avenue South, New York, NY 10010-1710. Tel.: 212-633-3874; Fax: 212-633-3820; E-mail: reprints@elsevier.com.

Veterinary Clinics of North America: Equine Practice is covered in *MEDLINE/PubMed (Index Medicus), Excerpta Medica, Current Contents/Agriculture, Biology and Environmental Sciences,* and *ISI.*

Contributors

CONSULTING EDITOR

THOMAS J. DIVERS, DVM
Diplomate, American College of Veterinary Internal Medicine; Diplomate, American College of Veterinary Emergency and Critical Care; Steffen Professor of Veterinary Medicine, Department of Clinical Sciences, Section of Large Animal Medicine, College of Veterinary Medicine, Cornell University, Ithaca, New York, USA

EDITOR

ISABELLE KILCOYNE, MVB
Diplomate, American College of Veterinary Surgeons; Assistant Professor of Equine Emergency and Critical Care, Department of Surgical and Radiological Sciences, UC Davis School of Veterinary Medicine, Davis, California, USA

AUTHORS

DEBRA C. ARCHER, BVMS, PhD
CertES, Diplomate, European College of Veterinary Surgeons FRCVS; Professor of Equine Surgery, Department of Equine Clinical Studies, University of Liverpool, Leahurst Campus, Wirral, United Kingdom

ASHLEY G. BOYLE, DVM
Diplomate, American College of Veterinary Internal Medicine; Associate Professor, Department of Clinical Studies New Bolton Center, University of Pennsylvania School of Veterinary Medicine, Kennett Square, Pennsylvania, USA

JULIE E. DECHANT, DVM, MS
Diplomate, American College of Veterinary Surgeons; Diplomate, American College of Veterinary Emergency and Critical Care; Professor of Clinical Equine Surgical Emergency and Critical Care, Department of Surgical and Radiological Sciences, School of Veterinary Medicine, University of California, Davis, Davis, California, USA

ANN E. DWYER, DVM
Genesee Valley Equine Clinic, Scottsville, New York, USA

KRISTA ESTELL, DVM
Diplomate, American College of Veterinary Internal Medicine; Clinical Assistant Professor, Virginia Tech's Marion duPont Scott Equine Medical Center, Leesburg, Virginia, USA

LARRY D. GALUPPO, DVM
Diplomate, American College of Veterinary Surgeons; Professor Equine Surgery, Department of Surgical and Radiological Sciences, UC Davis School of Veterinary Medicine, The William R. Pritchard Veterinary Medical Teaching Hospital, University of California, Davis, Davis, California, USA

ISABELLE KILCOYNE, MVB
Diplomate, American College of Veterinary Surgeons; Assistant Professor of Equine Emergency and Critical Care, Department of Surgical and Radiological Sciences, UC Davis School of Veterinary Medicine, Davis, California, USA

KRISTINA G. LU, VMD
Diplomate, American College of Theriogenologists; Hagyard Equine Medical Institute, Lexington, Kentucky, USA

RODOLFO MADRIGAL, DVM
Diplomate, American College of Veterinary Internal Medicine; Equine Sports Medicine and Surgery, Weatherford, Texas, USA

K. GARY MAGDESIAN, DVM
Diplomate, American College of Veterinary Internal Medicine; Diplomate, American College of Veterinary Emergency Critical Care; Diplomate American College of Veterinary Clinical Pharmacology; Certificate in Veterinary Acupuncture; Professor and Roberta A. and Carla Henry Endowed Chair in Emergency Medicine and Critical Care, Department of Medicine and Epidemiology (VM: VME), School of Veterinary Medicine, University of California, Davis, Davis, California, USA

JESSICA M. MORGAN, PhD, DVM
Diplomate, American College of Veterinary Sports Medicine and Rehabilitation; Assistant Professor, Equine Field Service, Department of Medicine and Epidemiology, UC Davis School of Veterinary Medicine, The William R. Pritchard Veterinary Medical Teaching Hospital, University of California, Davis, Davis, California, USA

JORGE E. NIETO, MVZ, PhD
Diplomate, American College of Veterinary Surgeons; Diplomate, American College Veterinary Sport Medicine and Rehabilitation; Department of Surgical and Radiological Sciences, UC Davis School of Veterinary Medicine, Davis, California, USA

DIANE M. RHODES, DVM
Diplomate, American College of Veterinary Internal Medicine; Loomis Basin Equine Medical Center, Penryn, California, USA

KAREN RICKARDS, BVSc, PhD
MRCVS, Deputy Director of Veterinary Services, Veterinary Department, The Donkey Sanctuary, Honiton, Devon, United Kingdom

SHARON J. SPIER, DVM, PhD
Diplomate, American College of Veterinary Internal Medicine; Department of Medicine and Epidemiology, UC Davis School of Veterinary Medicine, Davis, California, USA

KIM A. SPRAYBERRY, DVM
Diplomate, American College of Veterinary Internal Medicine, Diplomate, American College of Veterinary Emergency and Critical Care; Professor, Department of Animal Sciences, Cal Poly University San Luis Obispo, San Luis Obispo, California, USA

REBEKAH J.E. SULLIVAN, BVSc
Cert AVP (EM), MRCVS, Veterinary surgeon, Veterinary Department, The Donkey Sanctuary, Honiton, Devon, United Kingdom

ELSBETH A. SWAIN O'FALLON, DVM
Diplomate, American College of Veterinary Internal Medicine; Department of Clinical Sciences, James L. Voss Veterinary Teaching Hospital, Colorado State University, Fort Collins, Colorado, USA

TRACY A. TURNER, DVM, MS
Diplomate, American College of Veterinary Surgeons; Diplomate, American College Veterinary Sport Medicine and Rehabilitation; Turner Equine Sports Medicine and Surgery, Stillwater, Minnesota, USA

W. DAVID WILSON, BVMS, MS
Hon Diplomate, American College of Veterinary Internal Medicine, Professor Emeritus, Department of Medicine and Epidemiology (VM: VME), School of Veterinary Medicine, University of California, Davis, Davis, California, USA

Contents

Acute Central Nervous System Trauma in the Field   245

Krista Estell

> Acute central nervous system (CNS) trauma in the field is best approached by a systematic and thorough physical and neurologic examination that allows the practitioner to localize the brain or spinal cord injury. The skull and vertebral canal are complex 3-dimensional structures, and orthogonal radiographic views are necessary for an accurate diagnosis. Therapeutics aimed at decreasing pain, inflammation, and edema or increased intracranial pressure in the case of traumatic brain injury should be administered. Survival and return to athleticism can be achieved even in moderate-to-severe traumatic CNS injury with appropriate medical management.

Castration Complications: A Review of Castration Techniques and How to Manage Complications   259

Isabelle Kilcoyne and Sharon J. Spier

> Castration is one of the most common surgical procedures performed in equine practice. Open, closed, and semiclosed techniques are described for castration of horses, and the procedure may be performed in a standing, sedated animal or in a recumbent animal under general anesthesia. Although a relatively routine procedure, complications can occur, with reported complication rates ranging from 10.2% to 60%. Most complications are mild and resolve rapidly with appropriate treatment, but more serious or life-threatening complications can also occur. A thorough knowledge of male reproductive anatomy combined with good surgical technique is imperative to help reduce the rate of complications.

Orthopedic Infections—Clinical Applications of Intravenous Regional Limb Perfusion in the Field   275

Isabelle Kilcoyne and Jorge E. Nieto

> For the equine veterinarian, orthopedic emergencies are a common occurrence in clinical practice, with traumatic wounds of the distal limb and penetrating injuries of the hoof being some of the most common medical conditions to affect horses. Intravenous regional limb perfusion is a technique widely used for the treatment of orthopedic infections in horses. The objectives of this review are to discuss some of the clinical applications for this treatment modality in the field and to review the technique for the practitioner.

placentitis, hydropsic conditions, prepubic tendon and abdominal wall compromise, and uterine torsion are included. Clinical recognition of the problem, diagnostic procedures, and treatments are summarized.

Selected conditions affecting broodmares are discussed, including arterial rupture, dystocia, foal support with ex utero intrapartum treatment, uterine prolapse, postpartum colic, the metritis/sepsis/systemic inflammatory response syndrome complex, and retained fetal membranes. Postpartum colic beyond third-stage labor contractions should prompt comprehensive examination for direct injuries to the reproductive tract or indirect injury of the intestinal tract. Perforation or rupture of the uterus is typically recognized 1 to 3 days after foaling, with depression, fever, and leukopenia; laminitis and progression to founder can be fulminant. The same concerns are relevant in mares with retention of fetal membranes.

Foal emergencies can be intimidating to manage in the field, yet many conditions will respond well to the supportive care possible on the farm. Triage of the foal targets focused supportive care to stabilize the foal before referral to a hospital or to facilitate the management in the field. There are many diagnostic and therapeutic options available in the field setting to support a successful outcome on the farm.

Colic is one of the most frequent emergencies necessitating veterinary attention. Referral is not an option in many cases; therefore, the ability to diagnose and treat colic in an ambulatory setting is paramount. Portable imaging and point-of-care testing has improved the ability to identify lesions and assess the patient's status. In cases when field management is the only option, practitioners should be aware of the various treatment options available.

Ophthalmic problems account for up to 20% of emergencies in equine practice. Presenting problems may involve the periocular region, adnexa, or globe. Practitioners must have the experience to restrain horses with painful ocular conditions and the knowledge of how to perform a thorough eye examination. A range of clinical skills is required for the necessary diagnostic tests such as corneal cytology, ultrasound and tonometry, and common standing surgical procedures such as eyelid repair or instillation of a subpalpebral lavage system. Therapy, which may involve frequent administration of multiple medications, must be targeted to the specific diagnosis.

VETERINARY CLINICS OF NORTH AMERICA: EQUINE PRACTICE

RELATED SERIES

Veterinary Clinics of North America: Food Animal Practice
https://www.vetfood.theclinics.com/

THE CLINICS ARE NOW AVAILABLE ONLINE!
Access your subscription at:
www.theclinics.com

Preface

Advances in Equine Ambulatory Medicine and Surgery

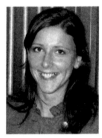

Isabelle Kilcoyne, MVB, DipACVS
Editor

Major advancements have been made in recent years that have increased the diagnostic and therapeutic capabilities of the ambulatory practitioner. Point-of-care ultrasound and digital radiology are now widely available in addition to stall-side blood analyzers, which allow a more efficient diagnosis to expedite treatment in the field, or referral, resulting in better outcomes and survival.

The goal of this issue is to summarize current knowledge across a variety of topics with an emphasis on the management of emergency cases in the field. It has been a privilege and an honor to have been invited by Dr Divers to edit and contribute to the current issue. These articles represent some of the advances that have been made in the past few decades as well as the current thinking of some esteemed individuals who have been engaged in the science and practice of equine medicine and surgery. I would like to thank each author for their hard work and outstanding contributions to this issue, and I trust it will act as a valuable resource to the ambulatory veterinarian. I would additionally like to thank the team at Elsevier, particularly Donald Mumford, for their guidance and hard work collating this issue.

Finally, I would like to dedicate this issue to my mother, Roisin, and my father, Thomas B. Kilcoyne, MVB, MRCVS (1941-2019), who was the first of many practitioners to enkindle and nurture a passion in me for veterinary medicine. I am very proud

Vet Clin Equine 37 (2021) xiii–xiv
https://doi.org/10.1016/j.cveq.2021.05.001
0749-0739/21/© 2021 Published by Elsevier Inc.

to be part of this ever-evolving profession, and I am excited to see what further advancements are made in the fields of equine medicine and surgery in the coming years.

Isabelle Kilcoyne, MVB, DipACVS
Assistant Professor of Equine Emergency and Critical Care
Department of Surgical and
Radiological Sciences
UC Davis School of Veterinary Medicine
One Shields Avenue
Davis, CA 95616, USA

E-mail address:
ikilcoyne@ucdavis.edu

Acute Central Nervous System Trauma in the Field

Krista Estell, DVM

KEYWORDS

- Spinal cord • Central nervous system • Trauma • Traumatic brain injury
- Traumatic spinal cord injury

KEY POINTS

- A thorough neurologic examination should be performed in cases of trauma and should include systematic evaluation of the cranial nerves, palpation, and a dynamic examination if possible.
- Many fractures of the cranium and vertebrae are difficult to identify radiographically. Orthogonal views are always recommended in cases where fracture is suspected.
- Treatment is targeted to reduce pain, inflammation, and edema associated with traumatic brain and spinal cord injury.
- Clinical signs and response to treatment are the most important indicators of prognosis.

TRAUMATIC BRAIN AND SPINAL CORD INJURY

Introduction

The central nervous system (CNS) is composed of the brain and spinal cord, two relatively soft organs cushioned by the cerebrospinal fluid (CSF) and surrounded by the bony calvarium and vertebrae. A history of flipping over backwards, high-speed collision, and falls are often reported in horses presenting with traumatic CNS injury. Fortunately, traumatic CNS injuries occur relatively infrequently. In a study reviewing fatal musculoskeletal injuries in racing Quarter Horses, vertebral injuries occurred in just 10% of cases.[1] A study documenting fatal injuries in racehorses over a 2-year period documented that only 1/478 horses died as a result of trauma to the CNS.[2] Jumping seems to increase the risk of traumatic spinal cord injury, as 29/125 track fatalities were the result of vertebral fractures in a study that included steeple chase and hurdling horses.[3] Traumatic brain and spinal cord injuries may also occur in the field and can be associated with handling. Although traumatic CNS injury is a relatively uncommon emergency facing the equine practitioner compared with colic or laceration, CNS injury can result in dramatic clinical signs, and the field practitioner should be prepared to effectively diagnose, develop a treatment plan, and provide

Virginia Tech's Marion duPont Scott Equine Medical Center, 17690 Old Waterford Rd, Leesburg, VA 20176, USA
E-mail address: bishopk@vt.edu

Vet Clin Equine 37 (2021) 245–258
https://doi.org/10.1016/j.cveq.2021.04.001
0749-0739/21/© 2021 Elsevier Inc. All rights reserved.

vetequine.theclinics.com

prognostic information for horses with neurologic disease as a result of traumatic injury.

There are relatively few studies that are specific to equine traumatic brain and spinal cord injury; most of the information available on pathophysiology, treatment, and prognosis is extrapolated from human or small animal literature. Traumatic brain injury (TBI) occurs when a traumatic event causes the brain to move rapidly within the bony calvarium, resulting in damage to the brain parenchyma and/or tearing or rupture of the blood vessels within the skull. The brain parenchyma can also be injured by skull fragments or foreign objects. The initial injury to parenchyma and blood vessels is classified as primary injury. In cases of collision with a fixed object, there are often two areas of injury—the coup and contrecoup. The coup injury occurs on the side of the trauma, and the contrecoup injury occurs opposite the side of trauma as a result of brain displacement. Traumatic brain injury is a result of direct primary injury and indirect secondary injury. The initial primary injury and associated hemorrhage causes hypoperfusion, ischemia, and an increase in intracranial pressure, resulting in a cascade of events classified as secondary injury. Secondary injury is characterized by hypoxia and ischemia, brain edema and increased intracranial pressure, altered cellular energy metabolism and signaling, and the production of reactive oxygen species.[4] Although it can be devastating, secondary injury occurs gradually and represents an opportunity for the veterinarian to interrupt the cascade of events with treatments targeted to decrease edema and inflammation and prevent further oxidative damage. Traumatic spinal cord injury follows a similar primary and secondary injury pattern as TBI. Although we commonly think of spinal cord injury causing neurologic deficits to the limbs only, it is important to remember that cervical spinal cord injury may cause respiratory failure if the descending motor pathways are injured, and damage to the cervicothoracic spinal cord can result in lack of sympathetic innervation and hypotension.

PHYSICAL AND NEUROLOGIC EVALUATION

Examination of a horse that has suffered trauma to the CNS should be systematic and as thorough as possible. Start with a physical examination with special attention paid to palpation of pulse quality, capillary refill time, and hydration status. In cases of TBI, hypotension can worsen secondary injury and subsequent brain damage. Hypotension is a negative prognostic indicator in humans with TBI.[5] Gentle palpation of the head, neck, topline, and extremities should be performed to assess for areas of pain, heat, swelling, or crepitus. The external ear canals should be checked for evidence of hemorrhage or CSF leakage. Patchy, asymmetric sweating of the neck is an indicator of spinal nerve compression and can help localize the area of trauma.

Next, a systematic neurologic examination should be performed with the goal of localizing the neurologic lesion and grading the severity of the resulting ataxia. Mentation assessment can be difficult in horses that have undergone a traumatic event, as clinical signs of pain can mimic those of mental obtundation, and a horse may be distressed if they have an acute loss of conscious proprioception or motor function. In addition to mentation changes, horses with TBI may display circling, seizures, lack of sensory perception, or recumbency. A full evaluation of the cranial nerves should be performed as outlined in **Table 1**. If cranial nerve deficits are found, the next step is to determine if the deficits are a result of central injury to the brain or brainstem or if they are due to injury to the nerves after they exit the skull. Multiple cranial nerve deficits point to a central lesion in the brain or brainstem, particularly if the occur on both sides of the head or if they are accompanied by mentation change. Assessment

Table 1 Basic cranial nerve examination	
Menace Response	Evaluates CN II, visual pathways, visual and motor cortex, cerebellum, CN VII.
Pupillary Light Reflex	Evaluates CN II, CN III.
Eye Position	CN VIII—sensory to the position of the head. CN III, IV, VI—motor to extraocular muscles.
Oculocephalic Reflex—Gently Move the Head Laterally and Vertically	CN VIII provides information on position of the head in space to the extraocular muscles that are controlled by CN III, IV, and VI. The eye should rotate ventrally when the head is lifted. When the head is rotated laterally, the fast phase of physiologic nystagmus should be in the direction that the head is moving.
Dazzle Reflex	Light is perceived by CN II and travels to the contralateral rostral colliculus of the midbrain; CN VII causes blink response.
Palpebral Reflex and Facial Sensation	Evaluates sensory fibers of CN V and motor function of CN VII as touch stimulates a blink.
Facial Symmetry	CN VII—motor to the muscles of facial expression including the lip and eyelid. CN V—motor to the muscles of mastication including the temporalis and masseter muscles.
Prehension, Mastication, and Swallowing	CN VII—prehension, salivation. CN V—jaw tone and mastication. CN XII—tongue tone. CN IX, X, XI—pharyngeal sensation, protect the airway, and swallow.

Abbreviation: CN, cranial nerve.

of the visual pathway and pupillary light reflex is also helpful in differentiating between visual cortex and peripheral neurologic damage and localization of the traumatic injury (**Figs. 1** and **2**). In cases of severe TBI, the optic nerves may be torn from their attachments to the cerebral hemispheres, resulting in blindness. Acute vestibular disease secondary to TBI in the horse can be particularly alarming if clinical signs are severe. Horses with unilateral vestibular disease present with base-wide ataxia, head tilt, lean, and circling. Circling may also occur with damage to the cerebrum, although this is generally a propulsive, forward circling, whereas damage to the vestibular system results in a more lateral or falling type of circling. In addition, horses with vestibular disease also often have nystagmus and/or strabismus. The vestibular system can be separated into three parts—the peripheral vestibulocochlear nerve (cranial nerve [CN] VIII), the central vestibulocochlear nucleus in the brainstem, and the portion of the vestibular system located within the cerebellum. The direction of the clinical signs and presence of conscious proprioceptive or motor deficits can be used to localize the damage and are outlined in **Table 2**. When describing the direction of head tilt, the direction that the poll is tilted toward should be used. The facial nerve (CN VII) and vestibulocochlear nerve (CN VIII) exit the skull in close proximity to each other, and facial nerve paresis often accompanies peripheral vestibular disease. Vestibular signs may also occur secondary to fracture of the paracondylar process (**Fig. 3**) or trauma to the cranial cervical spine either as a result of swelling and damage to the vestibular nerve or as a result of damage to the spinal nerves that communicate to the vestibular

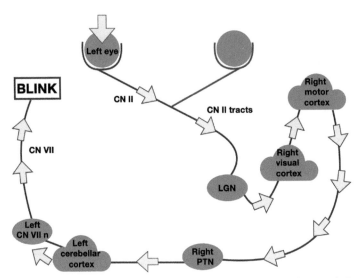

Fig. 1. This simplified diagram outlines the rather complicated pathway of the menace response. The left eye is stimulated, and the information is carried via the left optic nerve (CN II) where it decussates across the optic chiasma and travels through the ventral brain to the right lateral geniculate nucleus (LGN) and then to the right visual cortex and motor cortex in the brain. Then it travels to the right pretectal nucleus (PTN) after which there is decussation of the pathway to the left cerebellar cortex and CN VII nucleus in the brainstem. The left facial nerve (CN VII) travels to the muscles of the eyelid and the lid closes. The horse may also move their head away from the visual stimulus. Although most of the retinal fibers decussate and travel to the contralateral optical cortex, the temporal retinal fibers remain ipsilateral. Close evaluation of the menace response may disclose deficits in the nasal or temporal visual fields.

system regarding the position of the head and neck.[6] Horner syndrome is caused by disruption of sympathetic innervation and can occur as a result of trauma to the cranial neck or sympathetic trunk in the jugular groove. In horses, Horner syndrome is characterized by a constricted pupil, a drooped eyelid and visible third eyelid, and patchy sweating at the base of the ear.

Next, assessment of cutaneous reflexes of the neck, trunk, and gluteal region should be performed with a pen or capped needle. In cases of trauma, spinal nerve damage or discomfort may prevent the normal skin twitch response. Anal tone and tail tone should be assessed if this was not done with the temperature check. Lateral flexibility of the entire vertebral column can be assessed by holding the tail and gently rocking the hip; normal horses display an easy oscillating motion and do not resent manipulation. Flexibility of the cervical vertebral column should be assessed first manually with gentle traction and then while using an incentive. In general, horses with cervical trauma hold their heads and necks extended and may be reluctant or unable to raise or lower their head.

A dynamic neurologic examination should be performed next with the goal of localizing the lesion to a spinal cord segment (**Fig. 4**) and grading the neurologic deficits based on severity. The modified Mayhew scale is the most widely used grading scale for ataxia; horses are graded 1 to 5 as follows. Grade 1: intermittent or subtle abnormalities are seen during special circumstances or tests; grade 2: consistent mild deficits during all tests and on the straight line; grade 3: consistent moderate deficits easily seen by an untrained eye; grade 4: consistent severe deficits with risk of falling

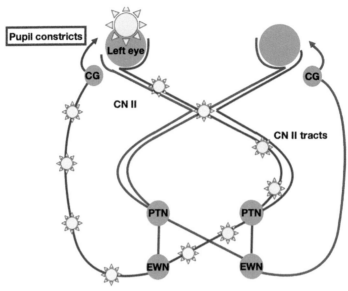

Fig. 2. This diagram outlines the pathway of the direct pupillary light reflex (PLR). The direct and consensual PLR should be evaluated. Light signal travels via the optic nerve fibers, most of which decussate at the optic chiasma to the contralateral pretectal nucleus (PTN). The PLR tracts decussate again at the ipsilateral Edinger-Westphal nucleus (EWN) and travels via CN III to the ciliary ganglion and cause constriction of the pupil. Although the optic nerve tracts run through the ventral aspect of the brain, there is no visual cortex involvement.

and difficulty rising from recumbency; and grade 5: recumbency, unable to rise under own power.[7] The thoroughness of the dynamic neurologic examination should be tailored to the severity of the neurologic disease. A typical dynamic examination includes walking in a straight line, navigating over obstacles and a hill, and tight turns in both direction in addition to reversing, walking while the head is elevated, and a

Table 2			
Localizing vestibular disease			
	Peripheral	**Central**	**Paradoxic**
Head Tilt	Toward lesion	Toward lesion	Away from lesion
Lean/Circle	Toward lesion	Toward lesion	Away from lesion
Nystagmus	Horizontal, rotary Fast phase away from lesion	Horizontal, rotary, vertical Fast phase away from lesion	Variable nystagmus Fast phase toward lesion
Ataxia	Base wide, staggering. May have extensor rigidity opposite the lesion	Conscious proprioceptive deficits	Hypermetria with conscious proprioceptive deficits on the same side as the lesion
Mentation, Other CN Signs	Normal to anxious mentation; CN VII signs may be present	Mentation may be altered with multiple CNs effected	Variable

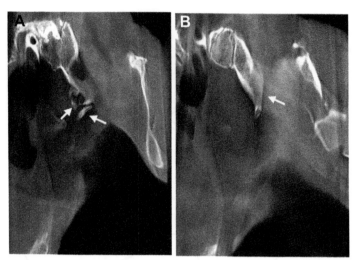

Fig. 3. (*A*) This is a sagittal cone beam CT image performed on a standing, sedated horse. Cranial is to the left side of the image. There are multiple osseus fragments arising from the caudoventral margin of the left paracondylar process highlighted by arrows. (*B*) This sagittal view taken at a slightly different plane shows the intact, right paracondylar process in the same horse.

tail pull to assess strength of the pelvic limbs. Neurologic deficits associated with spinal cord trauma vary and mild-to-moderate ataxia does not preclude the presence of vertebral fracture and spinal cord damage.

A horse that is recumbent as a result of traumatic CNS injury is difficult to evaluate and treat. Safety of the client, veterinary team, and horse is of the utmost concern during the examination and treatment process. In general, the safest place to be is along the dorsal aspect of the horse with a clear path of exit. Recumbency may make the

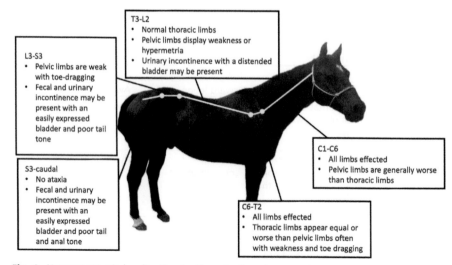

Fig. 4. Neuroanatomic localization to the spinal cord segments.

mental status of the affected horse difficult to evaluate, particularly as the horse be-comes exhausted. Conversely, horses that are frantically trying to rise may seem as if they are having seizures or are not mentally appropriate. If mentation and cranial nerves are normal, then the lesion is caudal to the first cervical vertebrae. A recumbent horse can be encouraged to stand by rocking it into sternal recumbency and then placing its thoracic limbs in an extended posture and applying steady traction to the halter forward and away from the side that it was lying on. If this effort is unsuc-cessful, the horse should be turned so the opposite side is down and allowed to rest before a second attempt is made. If the horse is unable to rise but able to dog-sit and has normal thoracic limb tone and placement, it likely has a spinal cord lesion caudal to T2. Deficits in both the thoracic and pelvic limbs suggest a lesion in the cer-vical spine. Rigid thoracic limbs and flaccid paralysis of the hindlimbs is diagnostic for Schiff-Sherrington posture and is caused by severe damage to the spinal cord be-tween T2 and L4.

If the horse is unable to stand, cutaneous reflexes and spinal reflexes can be assessed, although they are difficult to perform and interpret in the adult horse. The withdrawal, or flexor reflex, can be assessed by applying a hemostat to the distal limb. Flexion shows normal sensory function of the spinal nerves, function of the cor-responding spinal cord segments, and normal motor function. Spinal cord damage, peripheral nerve trauma, and exhaustion may blunt the withdrawal reflex. Although spinal reflexes can be difficult to perform and evaluate, they can be attempted. Ballot-ing the triceps muscle with force assesses the radial nerve and C7-T1 spinal seg-ments, whereas balloting the biceps assesses the musculocutaneous nerve and C6-C7 spinal cord segments. A hoof tester handle can be used to assess the patellar reflex that corresponds to the femoral nerve and L4-5 spinal cord segments. Ideally the limbs are held in flexion during assessment of the spinal reflexes; this is difficult to perform safely in the recumbent horse. Spasticity or hyperreflexia after stimulation indicates trauma and damage to the upper motor neuron (neurons within the brain or spinal cord), whereas hyporeflexia indicates damage to the lower motor neuron in the corresponding spinal cord segments or the peripheral nerve.

Regardless of the cause, prolonged recumbency in the horse is a negative prog-nostic indicator.[8,9] Myopathy and peripheral nerve damage serve to complicate the underlying neurologic disease, making it more difficult for the horse to rise. If referral to a tertiary facility for management in a sling is an option, the horse should be sent within the first few hours of recumbency for the best chance for a good outcome.

DIAGNOSTICS

A complete blood cell count and chemistry is indicated in all cases of traumatic brain and spinal cord injury. Once the neurologic lesion is localized, diagnostic imaging should be performed to determine if any fractures can be identified. Imaging the skull and vertebral column can be challenging in the field under normal circumstances. Because of the complex 3-dimensional nature of the skull and vertebral column, mul-tiple orthogonal views should be acquired. The benefits of acquiring diagnostic im-ages should be balanced with the risk of sedation and handling a neurologic horse. The administration of sedatives to a horse that has suffered brain or spinal cord injury may result in profound ataxia. In addition, acepromazine or other sedatives that cause hypotension may worsen secondary injury to the brain and spinal cord and should be avoided.

The complex occipitoatlantoaxial region is quite susceptible to trauma resulting in spinal cord injury, and catastrophic fracture may occur with little or no plain

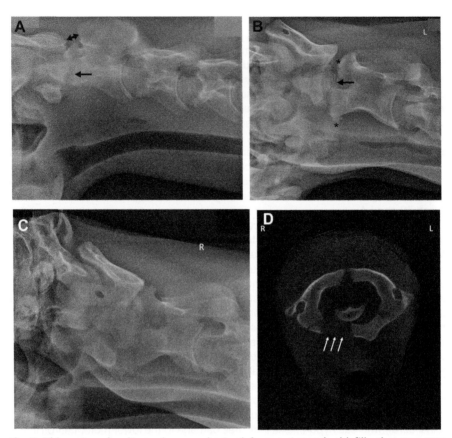

Fig. 5. This series of radiographs was obtained from a 4-month-old filly that was seen running into the side of a barn after which she developed acute neurologic signs. At presentation, the filly had grade 4/5 ataxia and swelling in the cranial cervical spine that was worse on the right side of the neck. (A) The lateral radiograph was relatively normal with the exception of subjective narrowing of the C1-C2 space (*double-sided arrow*) and widening of the ventral aspect of the physis associated with the separate ossification center of the dens of C2 (*arrow*). (B) The left dorsal to right ventral oblique reveals displacement of the dens (*arrow*) and a vertically oriented fracture of the right body of C1 with 2 displaced fragments visible (*). (C) The right dorsal to left ventral oblique is shown for comparison. (D) CT performed in the immediate postmortem period shows fracture of the right C1 body with considerable distraction along the fracture line (*arrows*).

radiographical evidence.[10] Basilar factures, often sustained after a horse rears and flips over backward, are similarly difficult to diagnose radiographically.[9] **Fig. 5** shows a 4-month-old Thoroughbred filly who was presented for evaluation after the owner witnessed a high-speed collision with a fixed object. At presentation, the filly had an extended head and neck posture and was unable to nurse. She was grade 4/5 ataxic at the walk. There was asymmetric swelling of the C1-C2 region, and the filly resented palpation of the area. Orthogonal radiographs of the cervical spine were obtained. Radiographic interpretation is complicated in this case by the presence of ossification centers. The lateral radiograph is fairly normal with the exception of subjective narrowing of the C1-C2 space and widening of the ventral aspect of the physis associated with the separate ossification center of the dens of C2. However, oblique radiographs of the area reveal a complete comminuted fracture of C1 and displacement of the C2 dens. The filly was subsequently euthanized due to a guarded prognosis for racing and the client's financial constraints. Computed tomography performed in the immediate postmortem period illustrates clearly the effects of the explosive force of a high-speed collision on the atlas and how complex fractures can be difficult to identify radiographically. Although this filly was euthanized, case reports describe survival after surgical stabilization of fractures in the atlantoaxial area.[11–13]

CSF collection should be carefully considered before it is performed and should ideally be restricted to cases in which trauma was not witnessed and other causes of neurologic disease need to be eliminated. The exception is if fever is present or if neurologic decompensation occurs, in which case CSF centesis should be performed to determine if bacterial meningitis is present. Cerebrospinal fluid changes that are collected from the atlantooccipital space, the C1-C2 space, or from the lumbosacral space; all collection techniques will require some degree of sedation or anesthesia, which will result in increased ataxia and exacerbation of neurologic signs. In cases of TBI with increased intracranial pressure, CSF collection may result in herniation of the brain through the foramen magnum as a result of a rapid decrease in intracranial pressure. CSF changes that are consistent with trauma include increased red blood cells and increased protein in the acute stage and xanthochromia in the chronic stage. Other biomarkers, including creatine kinase (CK) may be increased with traumatic injury, but CK elevation is not specific to trauma.[14,15] Bacterial meningitis is characterized by a neutrophilic pleocytosis (total nucleated cell count > 5/μL) and elevated protein. In cases of suspected bacterial meningitis, a culture of the CSF should be performed.

THERAPEUTIC OPTIONS

Therapeutics for traumatic brain and spinal cord disease are directed against the cascade of events that occurs after injury: pain, inflammation, edema, and the generation of oxygen free radicals. Drug categories, doses, and adverse effects are listed in **Table 3**.

Antiinflammatory and analgesic therapy with flunixin meglumine is a mainstay of treatment of traumatic brain and spinal cord injury. If additional analgesic therapy is needed, gabapentin or acetaminophen can be added. Gabapentin, an anticonvulsant drug that is also used for neuropathic pain, may be neuroprotective in cases of TBI although sedation is seen with higher doses. Gabapentin is used in humans with TBI and is recommended by the Brain Injury Association of America. Seizures, if they occur should be treated immediately with diazepam or midazolam. Recurrent seizures require treatment with anticonvulsants such as phenobarbital, gabapentin, or levetiracetam. Seizures that increase in frequency or severity in spite of treatment indicate a poor prognosis for recovery.

In cases of TBI, special attention should be paid to perfusion parameters with a goal of decreasing intracranial pressure while maintaining adequate cerebral blood flow. If fluid therapy is needed, fluids should be administered judiciously, with close monitoring of hydration status. Overhydration should be avoided, as it will worsen tissue edema and in cases of TBI may increase intracranial pressure.

Treatment to reduce edema and intracranial pressure is indicated in cases of TBI that present with obtundation or other evidence of brain dysfunction. Brain and spinal cord edema and surrounding soft tissue swelling can be treated with osmotic agents including hypertonic saline and mannitol.[16] Hypertonic saline has the added benefit of

Table 3
Therapeutics for acute traumatic brain and spinal cord injury management in the field

	Dose	Use	Adverse Effects
Flunixin Meglumine	1.1 mg/kg IV or PO q 12h	Analgesic, antiinflammatory	Nephrotoxic, right dorsal colitis
Acetaminophen	10–20 mg/kg PO q 12–24h	Analgesic, antiinflammatory	Potentially hepatotoxic with chronic use
Gabapentin	15–60 mg/kg PO q 8–12h	Analgesic, anticonvulsant	Sedation and lethargy at high doses
Hypertonic Saline	1 L/450–650 kg horse IV	Osmotic diuretic	Hypernatremia, hyperchloremia with repeat doses. Dehydration if unable to drink
Mannitol	0.5–1 g/kg IV	Osmotic diuretic	Hyperosmolality with repeated use. Dehydration if unable to drink
DMSO	0.1–1 g/kg as a 10% solution in saline or LRS IV q24h	Osmotic diuretic, antioxidant	Hemolysis if administered undiluted. Dehydration if unable to drink.
Diazepam	0.05–0.1 mg/kg IV	Anticonvulsant	Respiratory depression, excitability. Use for acute management of seizures
Levetiracetam	32 mg/kg PO q 12h	Anticonvulsant	Sedation
Phenobarbital	2–10 mg/kg PO q 12h 5–15 mg/kg IV slowly	Anticonvulsant	Sedation, respiratory depression, hepatotoxicity
Vitamin E	10–20 IU/kg PO q 24h	Antioxidant	Potential platelet dysfunction with high doses

Abbreviations: DMSO, Di-methyl sulfoxide; IV, intravenous; LRS, lactated Ringer solution.

assisting with volume resuscitation and increasing cerebral perfusion pressure while at the same time establishing a sodium gradient between the intravascular space and the interstitium, reducing intracranial pressure. Di-methyl sulfoxide (DMSO, administered as a 10% solution) is a potent diuretic and is also purported to have antioxidant capabilities that may help with edema as well as the inflammatory cascade that occurs in secondary injury. Antioxidant treatment with oral water-soluble vitamin E is generally recommended, although treatment is empiric with no evidence that vitamin E administration improves outcome in humans or horses.[17]

Antimicrobial administration should be considered in horses that have sustained severe traumatic injury to the head and neck, even in the absence of visible open wounds. In a study reviewing meningitis in horses, it was found that 32% of horses with a diagnosis of meningitis had a previous history of trauma.[18] A broad-spectrum antimicrobial such as oxytetracycline (6.6 mg/kg IV q12h), minocycline (4 mg/kg PO q12h) or chloramphenicol (40–60 mg/kg PO q6-8h) is a good choice for traumatic CNS injury.

The use of corticosteroids is controversial in cases of traumatic brain and spinal cord injury. No equine studies have been performed to determine the risk or benefit of corticosteroids after CNS trauma. Several human medical studies of TBI and spinal cord injury show no benefit of corticosteroids, and in some studies, increased mortality is reported in cases that received corticosteroids.[19,20] Steroids are generally not recommended in the management of human traumatic CNS injuries.[19,21] The prudent approach to corticosteroid administration in horses with CNS trauma is to withhold steroids from cases that are responding to medical management, particularly horses prone to laminitis as a result of equine metabolic syndrome or pars pituitary intermedia dysfunction. The author generally does not administer corticosteroids unless the horse does not respond to initial treatment with flunixin, osmotic agents, and gabapentin.

Good husbandry and nursing care should be provided to horses with a history or traumatic CNS injury. If possible, horses should be housed alone in a small flat paddock or large stall to allow the horse and handlers to move easily and safely. Feed and water should be elevated to a comfortable level. Keeping the head elevated at the level of the chest or above is particularly important in horses with TBI who are at risk of elevated intracranial pressure.

Surgical stabilization of fractured vertebrae has been described in several case reports, and a positive outcome may be achieved even in fractures involving the vertebral canal.[12,13] Surgical approaches to relieve spinal cord compression in cases of atlantoaxial subluxation have also been described.[22] Because horses have to stand and recover from anesthesia safely, the best surgical candidate is a horse with a vertebral fracture that displays only mild neurologic deficits. Horses should be stabilized medically if possible before referral for surgical evaluation of a vertebral fracture and should be shipped without being tied to the trailer to decrease risk of further injury.

Traumatic CNS injury that results in recumbency is difficult to treat. Horses are not physiologically equipped to spend a prolonged time in recumbency and are prone to self-trauma, myopathy, neuropathy, and respiratory distress. Horses with prolonged recumbency often require urinary catheterization and manual rectal evacuation. Support in a sling may improve clinical outcomes in horses unable to rise on their own after neurologic injury, but horses must be able to support their own weight in the sling once they are lifted. Referral should be facilitated within a few hours of onset of recumbency for the best chance of recovery.

CLINICAL OUTCOMES

A clinical axiom to remember when managing horses with neurologic injury is *"Treat the patient, not the radiograph."*[10] Clinical presentation is primarily influenced by the anatomic site of the fracture and degree of spinal cord compression. There are several case reports that describe survival and even return to athleticism after vertebral fracture that seem radiographically remarkable with both conservative and surgical management.[11,23] Similarly, horses with what seems to be severe skull trauma can recover, even when depressed fractures penetrate brain parenchyma or the brain is visible as a result of skull fracture (**Fig. 6**). A retrospective study evaluating survival after TBI in horses shipped to a referral center for treatment showed that 62% (21/34) horses survived to discharge.[9]

However, there are some clinical and clinicopathologic findings that carry a poor prognosis for recovery. If a horse becomes recumbent as a result of neurologic injury, the prognosis for survival is poor. A retrospective describing factors associated with survival in horses that are recumbent showed that out of 148 horses who were unable to rise on their own due to any underlying condition, 109 (74%) were subjected to

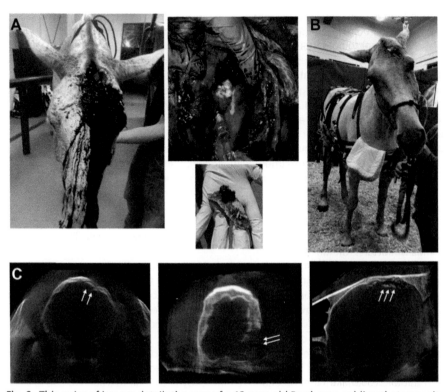

Fig. 6. This series of images details the case of a 12-year-old Percheron gelding that was witnessed colliding into a metal roof at speed. (*A*) The injury resulted in an L-shaped laceration of the temporalis muscle and a frontal bone fracture, part of which was sheared off in the collision. Brain parenchyma with apparently intact meninges is visible. (*B*) The gelding developed a fever and progressive neurologic signs in the following 24 hours as a result of the coup-contrecoup TBI. The gelding was moderately obtunded with an absent right-sided menace, a normal PLR, and mild grade 3/5 ataxia in all limbs with mild conscious proprioceptive deficits. These deficits were localized to the frontal cortex, left visual cortex, and motor cortex, respectively. Additionally, there was a right-sided head tilt that was exacerbated with blindfolding and light sedation that was localized to the right brainstem. It was presumed that a cranial-to-caudal left-to-right diagonal coup-contrecoup injury resulted in the neurologic abnormalities. (*C*) This is a series of standing, cone beam CT images. There is some image distortion due to movement. In the coronal, axial, and sagittal images a depressed comminuted fracture of the frontal bone is seen, with some fragments embedded in the brain parenchyma. This horse responded excellently to care in a sling with oxytetracycline, hypertonic saline, judicious fluid therapy, flunixin meglumine, and gabapentin. He was discharged 7 days after hospital admission. Vision slowly returned to the right eye. One year after TBI, the gelding is currently in work with no overt neurologic deficits.

euthanasia or died.[8] Horses that were able to be managed in a sling had an improved survival rate when compared with those recumbent horses that were not amenable to sling placement.[8] A study reviewing cases of TBI specifically corroborated that finding, with recumbency of more than 4 hours duration identified as a risk factor for nonsurvival.[9] This study also found that horses with basilar bone fractures were 7.5 times as likely not to survive as horses without.[9] A fracture of the bones of the skull or vertebrae may predispose to the introduction of bacteria into the CNS. The reported mortality rate is high in horses with meningitis as a result of traumatic injury, with one study reporting that 96.4% (27/28) of horses failed to survive.[18]

It is important to note that the healing process after a traumatic brain or spinal cord injury can span years; horses may show signs of improvement or, in some cases, may show progressive deterioration. After an intervertebral fracture has healed and developed an immovable articulation between two cervical vertebrae, the spinal cord cranial and caudal to the fracture site is susceptible to compression as a result of vertebral instability, arthritis, or misalignment: the so-called domino effect. Neurologic signs may occur as a result of the domino effect months to years after the initial trauma as remodeling of the fracture continues.[10]

CLINICS CARE POINTS

- A systematic neurologic evaluation and careful physical examination is the first step to diagnosing and treating a horse that has suffered CNS trauma.
- Many fractures of the skull and vertebrae are difficult to identify radiographically. Orthogonal views are always recommended in cases where fracture is suspected.
- Treatment is targeted to reduce pain, inflammation, and edema associated with traumatic brain and spinal cord injury.
- Clinical signs and response to treatment are the most important indicators of prognosis.

ACKNOWLEDGMENTS

The author would like to thank Drs Norrie Adams, Carin Stevens, Jairo Perez, and Emily Mangan for their help with the cases described in the manuscript. The author would also like to acknowledge Nation William Crow for their considerable help with **Fig. 4**.

DISCLOSURE

The author has no commercial or financial conflicts of interest to disclose.

REFERENCES

1. Sarrafian TL, Case JT, Kinde H, et al. Fatal musculoskeletal injuries of Quarter Horse racehorses: 314 cases (1990-2007). J Am Vet Med Assoc 2012;241(7): 935–42.
2. Johnson BJ, Stover SM, Daft BM, et al. Causes of death in racehorses over a 2 year period. Equine Vet J 1994;26(4):327–30.
3. Vaughan LC, Mason BJE. A clinical-pathological study of racing accidents in horses. Surgery department of Royal Veterinary College, Hawkshead Ln, North Mymms, Hatfield, Herts, England. London: RVC; 1976.
4. Prins M, Greco T, Giza CC. The pathophysiology of traumatic brain injury at a glance. Dis Models Mech 2013;6:1307–15.
5. Manley G, Damron S. Hypotension, hypoxia and head injury. Arch Surg 2001; 1(136):1118–23.
6. Lischer CJ, Walliser U, Witzmann P, et al. Fracture of the paracondylar process in four horses: advantages of CT imaging. Equine Vet J 2005;37(5):483–7.
7. Lunn DP, Mayhew IG. The neurological evaluation of horses. Equine Vet Educ 1989;1:94–101.

8. Winfield LS, Kass PH, Magdesian KG, et al. Factors associated with survival in 148 recumbent horses. Equine Vet J 2014;46:575–8.

9. Feary DJ, Magdesian KG, Aleman MA, et al. Traumatic brain injury in horses: 34 cases (1994-2004). J Am Vet Med Assoc 2007;231(2):259–66.

10. Mayhew IGJ. Cervical vertebral fractures. Equine Vet Educ 2009;21(10):536–9.

11. Gygax D, Furst A, Picek S, et al. Internal fixation of a fractured axis in an adult horse. Vet Surg 2011;40:636–40.

12. Rossignol F, Brandenberger O, Mespoulhes-Riviere C. Internal fixation of cervical fractures in three horses. Vet Surg 2016;45:104–9.

13. Barnes HG, Tucker RL, Grant BD, et al. Lag screw stabilization of a cervical vertebral fracture by use of computed tomography in a horse. J Am Vet Med Assoc 1995;206(2):221–3.

14. Jackson C, de Lahunta A, Divers T, et al. The diagnostic utility of cerebrospinal fluid creatine kinase activity in the horse. J Vet Intern Med 1996;10:246–51.

15. Furr MO, Tyler RD. Cerebrospinal fluid creatine kinase activity in horses with central nervous system disease: 69 cases (1984-1989). J Am Vet Med Assoc 1990; 197(2):245–8.

16. Gu J, Huang H, Huang Y, et al. Hypertonic saline or mannitol for treating elevated intracranial pressure in traumatic brain injury: a meta-analysis of randomized controlled trials. Neurosurg Rev 2019;42:499–509.

17. Finno CJ, Valberg SJ. A comparative review of Vitamin E and associated equine disorders. J Vet Intern Med 2012;26:1251–66.

18. Toth B, Aleman MA, Nogradi N, et al. Meningitis and meningoencephalomyelitis in horses: 28 cases (1985-2010). J Am Vet Med Assoc 2012;240:580–7.

19. Vos P, Diaz-Arrastia R. Traumatic brain injury. West Sussex, UK: Wiley Blackwell; 2015.

20. Hoshide R, Cheung V, Marshall L, et al. Do corticosteroids play a role in the management of traumatic brain injury? Surg Neurol Int 2016;7:84.

21. Bullock MR, Povlishock JT, editors. Guidelines for the management of severe traumatic brain injury. 3rd edition. New York: Mary Ann Liebert, Inc.; 2007.

22. Nixon AJ, Stashak TS. Laminectomy for relief of atlantoaxial subluxation in four horses. J Am Vet Med Assoc 1988;193:677–82.

23. Pinchbeck G, Murphy D. Cervical vertebral fracture in three foals. Equine Vet Educ 2001;13(1):8–12.

Castration Complications
A Review of Castration Techniques and How to Manage Complications

Isabelle Kilcoyne, MVB[a],*, Sharon J. Spier, DVM, PhD[b]

KEYWORDS

• Equine • Castration • Complications • Surgery • Hemorrhage

KEY POINTS

- The incidence of complications associated with castration is considered low and the mortality associated with the procedure very low, with rare fatalities occurring.
- Appropriate knowledge of technique and surgical procedure are imperative to aid in preventing complications, in addition to well-maintained equipment.
- Prompt recognition and management of any complications encountered should be instituted to prevent further morbidity, death, or malpractice claims, and the importance of client communications cannot be overemphasized when dealing with complications to help prevent misunderstandings and lawsuits.
- Although most complications encountered are mild and can be resolved quickly with appropriate therapy, eventration, hemorrhage, or infection should be considered emergencies and strong candidates for referral.

INTRODUCTION

Castration is one of the most common surgical procedures performed in equine practice. Open, closed, and semiclosed techniques are described for castration of horses, and the procedure may be performed in a standing, sedated animal or in a recumbent animal under general anesthesia.[1–3] Although a relatively routine procedure, complications can ccur, with reported complication rates ranging from 10.2% to 60%.[1,4–6] Most complications are mild and resolve rapidly with appropriate treatment, but more serious or life-threatening complications can also occur. A thorough knowledge of male reproductive anatomy and physiology combined with good surgical technique is imperative to help reduce the rate of complications.

---

[a] Department of Surgical and Radiological Sciences, UC Davis School of Veterinary Medicine, One Shields Avenue, Davis, CA 95616, USA; [b] Department of Medicine and Epidemiology, UC Davis School of Veterinary Medicine, One Shields Avenue, Davis, CA 95616, USA
* Corresponding author.
E-mail address: ikilcoyne@ucdavis.edu

Vet Clin Equine 37 (2021) 259–273
https://doi.org/10.1016/j.cveq.2021.04.002
0749-0739/21/© 2021 Elsevier Inc. All rights reserved.

PROCEDURE AND TECHNIQUES
Preoperative Assessment and Perioperative Care

All equids to be castrated should undergo a full physical examination before surgery, including palpation of the testicles and inguinal rings to rule out the presence of a possible cryptorchid or inguinal hernia, which may influence the surgical plan. At the author's institution, horses to be castrated under injectable general anesthesia generally have a short-term intravenous (IV) catheter placed in a jugular vein via aseptic technique before surgery. To facilitate catheter placement and palpation of the testicles before castration, animals in our practice are generally administered a combination of xylazine hydrochloride (0.5 mg/kg) and butorphanol tartrate (0.01 mg/kg IV) for sedation.

All equids undergoing any surgical procedure should be current on tetanus prophylaxis. If a tetanus toxoid vaccine has not been administered in the preceding 6 months, a booster vaccination is administered. If the tetanus status is unknown at the time of castration, a tetanus toxoid vaccine is administered and a booster vaccination is administered in 3 to 4 weeks.

The use of antimicrobials to prevent postoperative infections is debatable and generally based on clinician preference. In a 1995 survey involving more than 23,000 castrations, Moll and colleagues[7] showed that infectious/inflammatory complications were the most commonly encountered complications, and as part of that study they showed that horses administered antimicrobials were significantly less likely to develop infection compared with those that were not (2.9% vs 4% respectively). More recently, a survey from an Australian group[8] showed that only 10% of respondents (n = 115 veterinarians) did not administer any perioperative antimicrobials, with most (74%) of respondents administering 1 dose of procaine penicillin preoperatively and 1 dose 12 hours postoperatively. Another 2019 survey[5] performed in the United Kingdom found that almost all (97%; 460 out of 475) horses undergoing castration received a preoperative dose of antimicrobials, with procaine penicillin being the mostly used antimicrobial. One randomized clinical trial[9] has shown that administration of perioperative penicillin (25,000 U/kg) intramuscularly (IM) and a nonsteroidal antiinflammatory drug (NSAID) to horses undergoing standing castration once daily on the day of surgery and the following 2 days significantly reduced serum amyloid A (SAA) concentrations on day 8 after castration compared with horses that were only administered an NSAID.

Similarly, with regard to NSAID administration, there is much variation with regard to protocols in the literature. Preoperative use of nonsteroidal antiinflammatories (phenylbutazone 2.2 mg/kg; flunixin meglumine 1.1 mg/kg) is recommended in most instances, with 98% of 466 patients in a recent UK-based survey[5] on castration complications having been administered an NSAID preoperatively. In that study, phenylbutazone was the most commonly used NSAID, and postoperative administration was prescribed in only 39% of horses.

In general, at the authors' institution, horses receive 1 preoperative dose (22,000 U/kg) of IM procaine penicillin and a preoperative dose of flunixin meglumine (1.1 mg/kg) IV. In more mature horses with larger scrotums, a postoperative protocol of oral phenylbutazone (typically 2.2 mg/kg twice daily for 2–3 days) may be recommended.

Anesthetic Protocols and Surgical Techniques

Horses to be castrated under general anesthesia are premedicated with xylazine hydrochloride (1.1 mg/kg, IV), and, when sedation is deemed adequate, anesthesia is induced with ketamine hydrochloride (2.2 mg/kg IV) and diazepam (0.05 mg/kg, IV) or midazolam (0.05 mg/kg IV). At the authors' institution, the horses are placed in lateral recumbency with the hind limbs restrained to facilitate surgery. Anesthetic depth is monitored by heart rate, respiratory rate, movement (twitching of the ear, movement of the limbs), palpebral reflex, and presence of nystagmus. The clinician should note that, under total intravenous anesthesia, horses retain a palpebral reflex and show some degree of nystagmus. When an additional dose of anesthetic agent is deemed necessary to maintain an adequate plane of anesthesia, the authors typically administer half the induction doses of ketamine and xylazine (ie, ketamine 1.1 mg/kg IV and xylazine hydrochloride 0.5 mg/kg IV). Anesthetic management of donkeys and mules is similar to horses but with subtle differences.[10]

The scrotal area is routinely prepared for surgery with dilute povidone-iodine followed by intratesticular injection of 2% lidocaine hydrochloride, the dose of which may vary according to the size of the horse (typically 10–15 mL per testicle). A recent study[11] showed that intratesticular injection of mepivacaine (10 mL) resulted in improved cremaster muscle relaxation and fewer horses requiring additional doses of ketamine compared with the same intratesticular volume of lidocaine in 34 stallions undergoing castration using the Henderson Equine Castration Instrument (HECI).

For horses castrated under standing sedation, chemical restraint is achieved using a combination of detomidine (0.01 mg/kg, IV) and butorphanol (0.01 mg/kg, IV). A twitch may also be applied to facilitate restraint. Lidocaine (up to 20–30 mL/testicle in mature stallions) is always injected intratesticularly followed by subcutaneous injection (approximately 5–10 mL) along the planned incision sites on each side of the median raphe.

In 1 study,[1] 31 horses were castrated while standing, of which 5 (16%) developed complications, compared with 28 of 293 (9.6%) castrated under general anesthesia; however, the odds of developing a complication did not differ between these 2 categories. These findings are similar to those in a previous study[12] in which horses castrated while standing had a complication rate of 22%, compared with a complication rate of 6% for those in which castration was performed under general anesthesia with primary closure of the scrotal incisions. In addition, a recent study[6] of open standing castration in thoroughbred racehorses in Hong Kong found that 60% (150 out of 250 horses) had some type of complication postoperatively, with scrotal swelling, funiculitis, and seroma formation being the most commonly encountered. The most obvious advantage of castration in standing sedated horses is that it minimizes the inherent risks associated with general anesthesia and recovery. It also costs less and often requires fewer personnel to perform safely. However, the consistently higher complication rate observed in different studies deserves mention.

The 3 surgical techniques are open, closed, and semiclosed, with variations in the technique used depending on clinician preference.[1,5,6,8] The open technique requires less dissection than the closed technique and is more commonly used when performed standing castrations.[6] Other retrospective studies[1,7] have reported a higher complication rate associated with the semiclosed technique compared with the open and closed techniques. However, to date, no controlled study has been performed to investigate the superiority of either technique. Potential reasons for an increased complication rate associated with the semiclosed technique include increased tissue handling, increased contamination, or longer duration of surgery, compared with the closed or open techniques.

Scrotal incisions are generally allowed to heal by second intention and left unsutured. Primary closure may also be performed; however, this is not typically performed in the field and is more commonly performed in a hospital setting under aseptic conditions.[12]

The most commonly used emasculators include the Reimer and Serra emasculators.[1,7] These two emasculators differ in jaw profile. With the Serra emasculator, hemostasis is achieved by compression, stretching, and tearing of tissues, and the spermatic cord is simultaneously crushed and transected by a single closing movement of the jaws. With the Reimer emasculator, hemostasis results from the compression of tissues, and resection is performed by the operator at a later stage using a separate handle on the device (**Fig. 1**). One survey[7] reported a higher rate of hemorrhage associated with the use of the Reimer emasculator compared with the Serra emasculator among respondents. However, a more recent an ex vivo study[13] showed the Reimer emasculator resisted significantly higher pressure compared with the Serra emasculator using the open technique of castration, although no difference was noted using the closed technique. One author's (S.S.) preference is to use the Reimer emasculator on younger horses with small spermatic cords and the Serra emasculator on more mature horses with larger cords. The second author (I.K.) uses the Reimer emasculator exclusively, irrespective of size. One additional technique used by the authors where a larger spermatic cord is encountered in a mature horse when performing a closed castration is to separate the cremaster muscle from the cord using blunt dissection either with a hemostat or using a finger. The cremaster muscle is emasculated separately for approximately 30 seconds, which helps to reduce the bulk of the spermatic cord to be emasculated.

In recent years the popularity of the HECI (**Fig. 2**) in clinical practice has increased, with multiple studies[4,14] being published regarding the incidence and type of complications associated with its use. One study, of in 252 horses, found an overall complication rate of 10.7%, most of which were mild and resolved with treatment. This rate is very similar to a previous retrospective study[1] using traditional emasculators in which an overall complication rate of 10.2% (33 of 324) was reported. Similar to previous studies, the most common complications encountered by Hinton and colleagues[4] included seroma formation and mild swelling. Interestingly, no horses included in that study[4] were found to have hemorrhage reported as a complication, compared

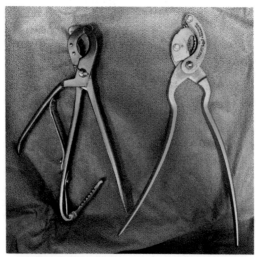

Fig. 1. Reimer and Serra emasculator. The Reimer emasculator (*left*) crushes the cord, and a blade operated by a separate handle severs the cord distally. The Serra emasculator (*right*) crushes and cuts the cord at the same time.

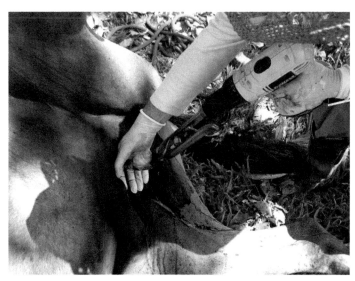

Fig. 2. Use of the HECI for a routine closed castration. Note placement of the emasculator portion just distal to the testicle where it is clamped. With slight tension on the drill and with the instrument held parallel to the cord, the testis is rotated slowly for about 5 turns. The speed of the rotations is gradually increased while keeping slight tension on the cord. After approximately 20 to 25 rotations, the cord separates about 8 to 10 cm proximal to the instrument.

with previous reports using traditional emasculators where postoperative hemorrhage rates ranged from 1.8% to 2.4%.[1,7,15] An additional study[14] has investigated the use of the HECI in horses undergoing closed castration using standing sedation; however, that study reported a postoperative complication rate of 23%.

The importance of properly maintained surgical instrumentation, regardless of which emasculator is used, should be emphasized. Cleaning following use in the field and regular maintenance, including disassembly, thorough cleaning, and resterilization, can help improve longevity and functionality, thus helping prevent complications postoperatively.

Some veterinarians recommend the use of ligatures around the vasculature of the spermatic cord in order to reduce the incidence of postoperative hemorrhage; however, it has also been suggested[7] that placement of a suture could predispose to the development of a scirrhous cord or infection, likely because of the presence of foreign material. In 1 study,[1] only 17 (5.2%) cases of a total of 324 had ligatures placed as part of the castration procedure. The overall rate of hemorrhage as a complication in this study was 6 out of 324 (1.8%), indicating that the use of ligatures may not be necessary to prevent postoperative hemorrhage. Another study[15] did not find that placement of ligatures significantly reduced the incidence of postoperative hemorrhage (2.3%), compared with a reported rate of 2.44% without ligatures.[7] If the clinician choses to use a ligature, it should be placed in a transfixing manner just proximal to the placement of the emasculators on the spermatic cord. An absorbable suture such as polyglactin 910 (Vicryl) is typically used and preferred to polydioxanone (PDS) because of its greater initial breaking strength, excellent handling properties, and most importantly the more rapid resorption time (56–70 days vs 180 days, respectively).[16]

However, the authors do recommend the use of ligatures in all donkeys and mules undergoing castration. This procedure should be performed as a preventive measure against any possible hemorrhage, because blood vessels of the spermatic cord have been reported to be larger in donkeys and mules compared with horses.[17]

COMPLICATIONS AND MANAGEMENT
Postoperative Swelling and Seroma Formation

Postoperative swelling affecting the preputial and scrotal regions (**Fig. 3**) is the most common complication following castration and can be seen up to 4 to 5 days after surgery has been performed. In previous studies, the incidence of swelling and seroma formation was 4.9%,[1] 8.7%,[4] and 8.7%.[5] Excessive swelling may be attributed to inadequate drainage, inadequate exercise following surgery, excessive tissue trauma at the time of surgery, or infection. Older horses have also been reported to be more prone to development of excessive edema following castration, compared with younger horses.[4,18] Following castration, exercise, cold-water hosing of the area, and administration of NSAIDs can help to minimize swelling.[4] Excessive postoperative swelling can be painful and may result in an unwillingness to exercise, causing premature closure of the surgical wound, further exacerbating the problem. Adequate postoperative exercise consisting of hand walking or trotting for 20 minutes twice daily for 10 to 14 days can help prevent premature closure of the surgical wound and seroma formation. Treatment generally involves administration of NSAIDs to reduce swelling and increase the tolerance of the animal to exercise and moving around. Where seroma formation has occurred, it is beneficial to digitally reopen the scrotal wounds to facilitate drainage in an aseptic manner. Therapy with systemic antimicrobials should be administered if discharge is observed, and prophylactically in cases of seroma formation to prevent the development of an infection. Typically, at the author's institution, treatment with oral antimicrobials such as trimethoprim sulfadiazine[a] (24 mg/kg orally twice daily) or minocycline (4 mg/kg orally twice daily) is recommended for 10 to 14 days.

Infection

Local infections of the scrotum and/or spermatic cord occur less commonly than seroma formation.[1,5,7,8] Infection may not be evident until many days after the surgery was performed, with 1 study[5] having documented signs associated with infection being reported an average of 10 days postoperatively. The use of ligatures has been implicated as a cause for postoperative infection, potentially acting as a nidus[7]; however, there are conflicting reports in the literature, with no clear consensus on whether or not ligatures contribute to an increased rate of infection. Infection may also follow formation of a seroma, allowing the development of a septic seroma or scrotal abscess.

Clinical signs of infection may include fever, swelling, lameness or stiffness of gait, and drainage from the incisions. Many horses with seromas have similar clinical signs to those mentioned for infection. Treatment involves opening of the scrotal incisions to facilitate drainage, similar to that performed for a seroma. Exercise to help prevent premature closure of the incisions and promote drainage should also be started. Administration of broad-spectrum systemic antibiotics should be instituted. Ideally a sample taken from deep within the scrotal incisions should be submitted for culture and sensitivity to help direct antimicrobial therapy. Infections that do not resolve

---

[a] Equisul-SDT® Aurora Pharmaceutical, Northfield, MN 55057.

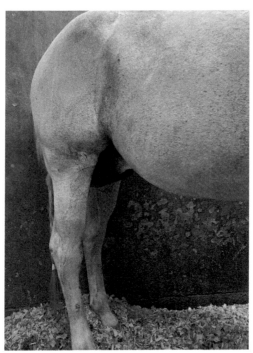

Fig. 3. Marked scrotal swelling in a 4-year-old horse 5 days after castration. The scrotal incisions were reopened in an aseptic fashion to facilitate drainage, and treatment with broad-spectrum antimicrobials was initiated.

with initial medical therapy should be referred to a surgical facility because surgical resection of infected tissue (typically the spermatic cord) may be warranted to resolve the issue completely.[19]

Scirrhous cord, which may also be referred to as funiculitis, refers to the chronic infection of the spermatic cord stump where the scrotal incisions heal but the stump continues to be infected or abscess, eventually forming a draining tract. It may develop as an extension of a scrotal infection or from a contaminated emasculator or ligature. Thorough aseptic palpation and examination of the scrotal and inguinal area can be diagnostic in identifying abnormal tissue; however, ultrasonography can be extremely useful to evaluate for abscesses in the inguinal area and to visualize abnormalities of the spermatic cord that may require surgical resection (**Fig. 4**). In cases where an early diagnosis of scirrhous cord is made, the animal may respond successfully following drainage and long-term (ie, 4–6 weeks) antimicrobial therapy (based on culture and sensitivity testing). However, surgical resection of the infected spermatic cord stump is often required for complete resolution (**Fig. 5**). Surgical excision can be challenging in chronic cases because of the enlargement of the spermatic cord, which can stretch the external inguinal ring, as well as the presence of extensive fibrous adhesions that form in the scrotum. The condition has been historically associated with *Staphylococcus* spp. However, a recent study[19] from 2018 showed growth of *Streptococcus equi* subspecies *zooepidemicus*, *Staphylococcus aureus*, *Actinomyces* spp, and *Bacteroides* spp. from horses that underwent surgical resection of infected tissue. Culture and sensitivity testing of any resected tissue should be performed to ascertain appropriate antimicrobial therapy postoperatively. Prognosis seems to be good with

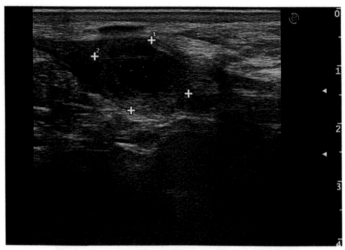

Fig. 4. Transverse ultrasonography image of a persistently infected right spermatic cord remnant measuring 18.0 mm × 12.8 mm, obtained from the inguinal region of a 5-year-old Andalusian gelding 8 months after castration. Treatment required 2 surgical revisions and long-term antimicrobial therapy. Image acquired using a 13-MHz linear transducer at a depth of 4 cm. (*Courtesy of* Betsy Vaughan DVM, DACVSMR, California.)

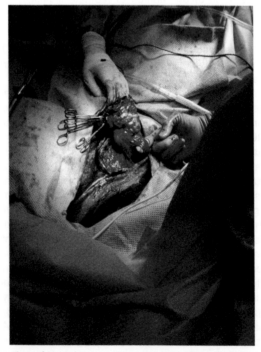

Fig. 5. Surgical resection of a scirrhous cord in a 10-year-old gelding that developed a draining tract at the castration site years after the castration was performed.

appropriate treatment, with complete resolution of clinical signs and return to previous use being documented in 14 of 16 horses that underwent surgical resection and for which long-term follow up was available in 1 study.[19]

In addition, 1 report[20] describing intra-abdominal abscess formation in 61 horses included 3 horses that had abscesses in the inguinal region extending into the abdominal cavity, all of which had undergone castration 21 to 150 days before examination. Although abdominal abscesses are considered a rare complication following castration, it is important to realize that simple infections, if not recognized in an expedited fashion and treated appropriately, may progress to a much more arduous complication.

HEMORRHAGE

Some hemorrhage is normal following castration in the immediate postoperative period when the horse stands following general anesthesia or immediately after the emasculators have been removed. When bleeding occurs in the form of a steady drip or stream (>1 drop/s) for an excessive period of time (>15 minutes), active intervention for hemostasis should be made. The most common source of significant bleeding postoperatively is the testicular artery, but it can also occur from the testicular vein or subcutaneous vessels. Initial therapy should be designed to identify and eliminate the source of hemorrhage. The stump of the spermatic cord can be identified and the individual bleeding vessel isolated and ligated, or, if enough of the cord can be exteriorized, the entire cord can be emasculated again. However, this is usually not possible in a standing animal and necessitates general anesthesia. If the source of the bleeding cannot be identified, the scrotal incision can be packed with sterile laparotomy sponges, which can be left in place for 24 to 48 hours by suturing the scrotal incisions closed. It is important to remember to leave long tails on the scrotal sutures to facilitate easier removal once the packing is to be removed. These horses should be placed on broad-spectrum systemic antibiotics as a precautionary measure to reduce the incidence of infection. They should be maintained on stall rest to allow the clot to stabilize and should not be exercised as per the usual postcastration recommendations.

Adjunctive medical therapies that have been reported to help curtail hemorrhage in horses include use of antifibrinolytic drugs.[21,22] The most commonly used is epsilon-aminocaproic acid, a lysine analogue that works to inhibit plasminogen activator, and stimulate release of a2-antiplasmin from endothelial cells.[23] Typically the authors administer 30 to 40 mg/kg diluted in 1 L of saline IV over 30 minutes, which can be repeated up to 4 times daily; however, usually 1 or 2 doses are sufficient. A dose for continuous-rate infusion is 10 to 15 mg/kg/h; however, this is not practical in a field setting. An alternative to aminocaproic acid is tranexamic acid, also an antifibrinolytic lysine analogue, with a dose in the literature ranging from 5 to 25 mg/kg IV every 8 to 12 hours.[23]

Other reported hemostatic agents include conjugated estrogens[22] (0.05–0.1 mg/kg IV, every 12–24 hours) and 10% formalin (10 mL of 4% formaldehyde solution [ie, 10% formalin] diluted in 1 L of saline IV)[24] (**Table 1**).

Immediate referral should be considered where substantial blood loss has occurred or signs of hypovolemic shock are evident. It is important to remember that the packed cell volume (PCV) may remain normal for up to 12 hours following acute hemorrhage because of the time required for fluid redistribution and the effects of splenic contraction. Serial monitoring of PCV, total solids (TS), and lactate as the horse is rehydrated gives an indication of the extent of blood loss. Loss of a large volume of blood, combined with tachycardia, tachypnea, pale mucous membranes, lethargy, increasing peripheral lactate level (>4 mmol/L), and decreasing TS (<4 g/dL) may lead to the

Table 1
Hemostatic agents that have been reported to help curtail hemorrhage in horses

Drug	Tradename	Dose	Frequency
Epsilon-aminocaproic acid	Aminocaproic Acid Injection USP[a] 250 mg/mL	30–40 mg/kg IV 10–15 mg/kg/h	q6–8 h CRI
Tranexamic acid	Tranexamic Acid Injection[b] 100 mg/mL	5–25 mg/kg IV slowly	q8–12 h
Conjugated estrogens	Premarin[c]	0.05–0.1 mg/kg IV	q12–24 h
10% formalin	—	10–30 mL of 10% formalin in 1 L isotonic fluids	q12–24 h

Abbreviations: CRI, continuous rate infusion; q, every; USP, United States Pharmacopeia.
[a] Hospira, Inc, Lake Forest, IL 60045.
[b] Athenex, Schaumburg, IL 60173.
[c] Wyeth Pharmaceuticals LLC, a subsidiary of Pfizer Inc, Philadelphia, PA, 19101.

decision to transfuse. A blood transfusion is likely to be needed during an acute bleeding episode when the PCV decreases to less than 20%.[25]

The authors have observed horses that have bled into the peritoneal cavity postcastration, resulting in a significant hemoabdomen. This condition can be visualized using ultrasonography to observe the swirling nature of the blood within the peritoneal cavity or the resultant clot formation. These horses are treated as described earlier, with the decision to transfuse based on the hemodynamic stability of the horse; namely, monitoring for clinical evidence of hemorrhagic or hypovolemic shock and changes in laboratory findings (PCV, TS, and lactate). It is important to remember that up to 75% of red blood cells lost into a body cavity (ie, hemoperitoneum) are autotransfused back into circulation within 24 to 72 hours.[25]

EVENTRATION

Eventration, although not a common postcastration complication, occurs when a portion of intestine prolapses through the inguinal canal and out of the scrotal incision. It typically occurs within 4 to 6 hours after castration but it has been reported up to 12 days following surgery.[26] Eventration has been hypothesized to result following increased abdominal pressure (such as straining because of abdominal pain), presence of a large inguinal ring, or potentially during a rough recovery from general anesthesia.[24] Investigators in recent studies reported eventration in 0.4%,[4] 0.8%,[5] and 0.1%[8] of castrations, indicating that the incidence is very low in a general equine population, with seemingly no significant difference in incidence if traditional emasculators or the HECI is used. In another study,[1] eventration occurred in only 1 of 324 (0.3%) horses. In that study, the incidence of eventration was low, despite the lack of use of ligatures as part of the routine procedure in most horses. This finding suggests that further investigation may be needed to determine whether ligatures provide an advantage when castrating horses of breeds other than those reported to be at an increased risk of eventration. One study[15] found that common vaginal (parietal) tunic ligation significantly reduced the incidence of omental herniation and eventration, with only 1 of 131 (0.8%) evaluated horses developing eventration. That study focused on the castration of young draft horses, a breed type reported to be at increased risk of eventration after castration.

If postcastration eventration does occur, prompt emergency care is essential for a successful outcome.[27] Initial therapy should be designed to protect the prolapsed intestine from further damage and contamination and prepare the horse for transport to a referral center. The protruding portion of bowel should be cleaned of all gross contamination with sterile saline and then replaced into the scrotum, which is sutured closed with a nonabsorbable suture or closed with several towel clamps. This procedure is more easily accomplished with the horse under general anesthesia. If this is not possible, either because of the amount of bowel that is prolapsed or because of an inability to reanesthetize the horse, then a moist towel or drape should be made into a sling and used to support the bowel during transport. Treatment with broad-spectrum injectable antibiotics should be instituted along with an antiinflammatory and tetanus prophylaxis. Once at a surgical facility, exploration by both an inguinal and ventral midline approach is warranted, because a better determination of the health of the entire small intestine can be made by fully examining the entire intestinal tract and inguinal rings. Survival rates following surgical treatment of intestinal evisceration range from 36% to 87%, with the lowest survival rates associated with an inguinal-only surgical approach, increased length of prolapsed bowel, and the need to perform a resection and anastomosis.[28,29]

Protrusion of omental tissue through the inguinal rings (**Fig. 6**) can also occur following castration. A thorough examination in a well-sedated horse should be performed to assess the type of tissue protruding because occasionally subcutaneous tissue may be found protruding through the scrotal incision. It is common to find just a small amount of vaginal tunic or connective tissue protruding, which can either be removed using scissors or left to dry without further intervention and close

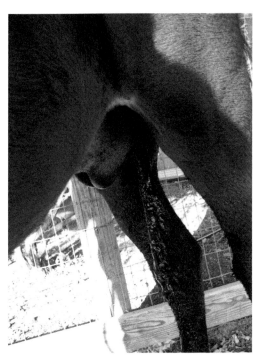

Fig. 6. Omental prolapse in a 6-month-old horse 2 days after being castrated under general anesthesia. The tissue was cleaned thoroughly, and emasculation of the omentum close to the skin incision was performed standing. The horse was placed on broad-spectrum oral antimicrobials for 10 days and recovered without further incident.

monitoring. In most cases of minor omental prolapse, emasculation of the protruding omental tissue can be performed. The animal should be confined to a stall to prevent more tissue prolapsing, and systemic antimicrobial therapy should be instituted to prevent an ascending infection or peritonitis. Where severe herniation of omentum has occurred, surgery under general anesthesia may be necessary to facilitate ligation and transection of the tissue.

Peritonitis

Although cited as a complication of castration, septic peritonitis is a rare complication that has been infrequently reported in the literature. The vaginal tunic derived from the peritoneum continues through the inguinal canal to line the interior of the scrotum. It is composed of 2 layers, the visceral tunic, which attaches firmly to the tunica albuginea around the testis, and the parietal tunic, which is continuous with the parietal peritoneum of the abdomen. As a result of this communication, many horses show a non-septic inflammation or peritonitis, characterized by increased cell counts greater than 10,000 cells/μL for up to 5 days following castration.[30] However, this is usually self-limiting and not particularly clinically significant.

In contrast, bacterial or septic peritonitis is a rare complication that has not been reported in larger retrospective case studies in the recent past, but is limited to case reports involving small numbers of horses.[31,32] Bacterial peritonitis is diagnosed where an increased nucleated cell count with the presence of an increased number of neutrophils (>90%), usually degenerative, is noted on cytologic evaluation of peritoneal fluid following abdominocentesis. The presence of bacteria on cytologic evaluation or a positive culture of the fluid can help confirm the diagnosis. Clinical signs may include fever, depression, inappetence, or mild signs of colic. Treatment should involve administration of systemic antimicrobials based on culture and sensitivity of the peritoneal fluid, antiinflammatories, intravenous fluid therapy, and peritoneal lavage through the use of an indwelling abdominal drain if indicated.

Hydrocoele Formation

A hydrocele is a painless accumulation of fluid within the vaginal cavity in stallions; however, it may also be seen in geldings up to months or years following castration (**Fig. 7**). Hydrocoeles occur infrequently after castration but are reportedly more common in mules.[24] They are reported to form after an open castration is performed, because the parietal tunic is not removed using this technique. The swelling that develops may resemble a scrotal testicle or hernia, and on aspiration a clear, amber-colored fluid is usually obtained. On palpation, the swelling may be reduced by squeezing the fluid proximally toward the inguinal canal and into the abdominal cavity. Drainage of the fluid may only temporarily relieve the condition, and these are considered cosmetic defects. Treatment involves the surgical resection and removal of the parietal tunic under general anesthesia with the equid in dorsal recumbency. However, surgical removal is rarely necessary.

Penile Damage

Penile damage during castration is almost exclusively iatrogenic and usually occurs when a novice surgeon mistakes the penile shaft for a testicle. Although penile trauma is frequently listed as a complication of castration, it is very infrequently reported in the literature.[33] If the penis is transected, the horse should be referred immediately to a surgical facility for surgical repair or phallectomy. A thorough knowledge of the anatomy and the procedure to be performed should prevent this complication.

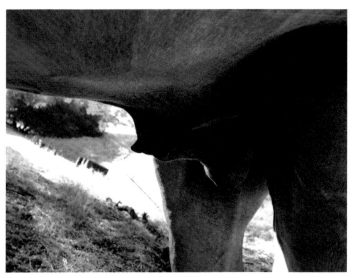

Fig. 7. Hydrocele in a 12-year-old castrated mule. Note the swelling in the scrotal area resembling a residual testicle. On palpation, the swelling was noted to be fluidlike and was easily reduced by squeezing the fluid proximally toward the inguinal canal.

Continued Stallionlike Behavior

Serum concentrations of testosterone and estrogen rapidly decline within 6 hours after castration; however, castration is not always successful in eliminating habitual stallionlike behavior. Historically, causes such as retention of epididymal tissue, adrenal cortex production of testosterone, and heterotopic testicular tissue have been implicated in cases of continued stallionlike behavior, but most commonly the persistent behavior is habitual or represents normal social interaction among horses.[24] In cases where the continued stallionlike behavior is excessive or there is little information pertaining to the castration, hormonal testing is indicated to establish whether there is residual testicular tissue present. Hormonal assays that may be useful to determine whether the horse had undergone a unilateral castration include baseline testosterone concentrations, baseline estrone sulfate concentrations, and testosterone concentrations following human chorionic gonadotropin stimulation.[34] More recently, antimullerian hormone (AMH) has been found to be a sensitive indicator of hemicastrated unilateral cryptorchid horses[35,36] (**Table 2**). Although concentrations of testosterone and estrogen in serum decrease rapidly in serum and stabilize within about 6 hours, clinicians should note that AMH has a longer half-

Table 2			
Hormonal assays to distinguish between geldings and horses with extrascrotal testicular tissue i.e. cryptorchid			
	Mature Stallion	**Gelding**	**Cryptorchid**
Testosterone	800–2000 pg/mL	<50 pg/mL	100–500 pg/mL
AMH	—	<0.15 ng/mL	>0.15 mg/mL
Estrone Sulfate	140–200 ng/mL	<0.1 ng/mL	35–60 ng/mL

Reference laboratory values provided by the Clinical Endocrinology Laboratory at the University of California, Davis (www.vetmed.ucdavis.edu/labs/endo-lab).

life (1.5–2 days) and therefore concentrations take 10 to 14 days to reach baseline after castration.[35]

In general, males should be isolated from mares for 2 days following castration under routine circumstances. After 2 days, ejaculates are highly unlikely to contain sufficient numbers of spermatozoa to cause pregnancy.[37]

DISCLOSURE

The authors have no relationship with a commercial company that has a direct financial interest in subject matter or materials discussed in this article or with a company making a competing product.

REFERENCES

1. Kilcoyne IK, Watson JL, Kass PH, et al. Incidence, management, and outcome of complications of castration in equids: 324 cases (1998–2008). J Am Vet Med Assoc 2013;242:820–5.
2. Schumacher J. Complications of castration. Equine Vet Educ 1996;8:254–9.
3. Searle D, Dart AJ, Dart CM, et al. Equine castration: review of anatomy, approaches, techniques and complications in normal, cryptorchid and monorchid horses. Aust Vet J 1999;77:428–34.
4. Hinton S, Schroeder O, Aceto HW, et al. Prevalence of complications associated with use of the Henderson equine castrating instrument. Equine Vet J 2019;51:163–6.
5. Hodgson C, Pinchbeck G. A prospective multicentre survey of complications associated with equine castration to facilitate clinical audit. Equine Vet J 2019;51:435–9.
6. Rosanowski SM, MacEoin F, Graham R, et al. Open standing castration in Thoroughbred racehorses in Hong Kong: Prevalence and severity of complications 30 days post-castration. Equine Vet J 2018;50:327–32.
7. Moll HD, Pelzer KD, Pleasant RS, et al. A survey of equine castration complications. J Equine Vet Sci 1995;15:522–6.
8. Owens CD, Hughes KJ, Hilbert BJ, et al. Survey of equine castration techniques, preferences and outcomes among Australian veterinarians. Aust Vet J 2018;96:39–45.
9. Busk P, Jacobsen S, Martinussen T. Administration of perioperative penicillin reduces postoperative serum amyloid A response in horses being castrated standing. Vet Surg 2010;39:638–43.
10. Matthews N, van Loon J. Anesthesia, sedation, and pain management of donkeys and mules. Vet Clin North Am Equine Pract 2019;35:515–27.
11. Crandall A, Hopster K, Grove A, et al. Intratesticular mepivacaine versus lidocaine in anaesthetised horses undergoing Henderson castration. Equine Vet J 2020;00:1–6.
12. Mason BJ, Newton JR, Payne RJ, et al. Costs and complications of equine castration: a UK practice-based study comparing 'standing nonsutured' and 'recumbent sutured' techniques. Equine Vet J 2005;37:468–72.
13. Comino F, Giusto G, Caramello V, et al. Do different characteristics of two emasculators make a difference in equine castration? Equine Vet J 2018;50:141–4.
14. Racine J, Vidondo B, Ramseyer A, et al. Complications associated with closed castration using the Henderson equine castration instrument in 300 standing equids. Vet Surg 2019;48:21–8.

15. Carmalt JL, Shoemaker RW, Wilson DG. Evaluation of common vaginal tunic ligation during field castration in draught colts. Equine Vet J 2008;40:597–8.
16. Kummerle JM. Suture materials and patterns. In: Auer JA, Stick JA, editors. Equine surgery. 4th edition. St Louis (MO): Elsevier Saunders; 2012. p. 182–9.
17. Sprayson T, Thielmann A. Clinical approach to castration in the donkey. Practice 2007;29:526–31.
18. May KK, Moll HD. Recognition and management of equine castration complications. Compend Contin Educ Pract Vet 2002;24:150–62.
19. Claffey EF, Brust K, Hackett RP, et al. Surgical management of postcastration spermatic cord stump infection in horses: A retrospective study of 23 cases. Vet Surg 2018;47:1016–20.
20. Arnold CE, Chaffin MK. Abdominal abscesses in adult horses: 61 cases (1993-2008). J Am Vet Med Assoc 2012;241:1659–65.
21. Dechant JE, Nieto JE, Le Jeune SS. Hemoperitoneum in horses: 67 cases (1989-2004). J Am Vet Med Assoc 2006;229:253–8.
22. Arnold CE, Payne M, Thompson JA, et al. Periparturient hemorrhage in mares: 73 cases (1998-2005). J Am Vet Med Assoc 2008;232:1345–51.
23. Fletcher DJ, Brainard BM, Epstein K, et al. Therapeutic plasma concentrations of epsilon aminocaproic acid and tranexamic acid in horses. J Vet Intern Med 2013;27:1589–95.
24. Schumacher J. Testis. In: Auer JA, Stick JA, editors. Equine surgery. 4th edition. St Louis (MO): Elsevier Saunders; 2012. p. 804–36.
25. Mudge MC. Hemostasis, surgical bleeding and transfusion. In: Auer JA, Stick JA, editors. Equine surgery. 4th edition. St Louis (MO): Elsevier Saunders; 2012. p. 35–46.
26. Boussauw B, Wilderjans H. Inguinal herniation 12 days after a unilateral castration with primary wound closure. Equine Vet Educ 1996;8:248–50.
27. Getman LM. Post castration evisceration. Equine Vet Educ 2013;25:563–4.
28. Thomas HL, Zaruby JF, Smith CL, et al. Postcastration eventration in 18 horses: the prognostic indicators for long-term survival (1985-1995). Can Vet J 1998;39:764–8.
29. Shoemaker R, Bailey J, Janzen E, et al. Routine castration in 568 draught colts: incidence of evisceration and omental herniation. Equine Vet J 2004;36:336–40.
30. Schumacher J, Schumacher J, Spano JS, et al. Effects of castration on peritoneal fluid in the horse. J Vet Intern Med 1988;2:22–5.
31. Shearer TR, Smith AD, Freeman DE, et al. Anaerobic peritonitis caused by Clostridium septicum as a complication of routine castration in a 2-year-old Warmblood horse. Equine Vet Educ 2017;29:310–3.
32. Schumacher J, Scrutchfield WL, Martin MT. Peritonitis following castration in 3 horses. Equine Vet Sci 1987;7:220–1.
33. Beavers KN, Mitchell C. Uncommon castration complication: penile amputation and sheath ablation following an iatrogenic phallectomy. Equine Vet Educ 2018;30:415–8.
34. Marshall JF, Moorman VJ, Moll HD. Comparison of the diagnosis and management of unilaterally castrated and cryptorchid horses at a referral hospital: 60 cases (2002-2006). J Am Vet Med Assoc 2007;231:931–4.
35. Claes A, Ball BA, Almeida J, et al. Serum anti-Mullerian hormone concentrations in stallions: Developmental changes, seasonal variation, and differences between intact stallions, cryptorchid stallions, and geldings. Theriogenology 2013;79:1229–35.
36. Murase H, Saito S, Amaya T, et al. Anti-Mullerian hormone as an indicator of hemi-castrated unilateral cryptorchid horses. J Equine Sci 2015;26:15–20.
37. Shideler RK, Squires EL, Voss JL. Equine castration - disappearance of spermatozoa. Equine Pract 1981;3:31–2, 43,36.

Orthopedic Infections— Clinical Applications of Intravenous Regional Limb Perfusion in the Field

Isabelle Kilcoyne, MVB*, Jorge E. Nieto, MVZ, PhD

KEYWORDS

• Equine • Surgery • Orthopedic • Infection • Antibiotics

KEY POINTS

- Intravenous regional limb perfusion is a safe and efficacious modality to deliver high concentrations of antimicrobials to the distal limb of horses.
- It is an easy procedure to perform in the field and has a wide range of applications.
- It can significantly improve clinical outcomes in horses with traumatic injuries to the distal limb in conjunction with systemic antimicrobial therapy.

HISTORY

Regional limb perfusion of medications was first described by August Karl Bier in 1908 and was initially used to describe the technique of exsanguinating the upper extremity and injecting local anesthetic to facilitate surgical procedures in human medicine.[1] Although the Bier block is a commonly used technique in food animal surgery, where anesthesia of the foot may be required for debridement of a foot abscess or potential digit amputation, it was not until 1990 that Dietz and Kehnscherper[2] first described regional intravenous perfusion of antimicrobials in horses.

CLINICAL APPLICATIONS

Traumatic wounds involving the limbs of horses are very common in equine practice and deep punctures or lacerations can potentially threaten the life and athletic career of the horse, particularly when penetration of a synovial structure is involved.[3–5] Poor soft tissue coverage of the distal extremity of horses means wounds and lacerations of the distal limb frequently affect underlying synovial structures, in addition to soft tissue

Department of Surgical and Radiological Sciences, UC Davis School of Veterinary Medicine, One Shields Avenue, Davis, CA 95616, USA
* Corresponding author.
E-mail address: ikilcoyne@ucdavis.edu

Vet Clin Equine 37 (2021) 275–291
https://doi.org/10.1016/j.cveq.2021.04.003
0749-0739/21/© 2021 Elsevier Inc. All rights reserved.

structures such as tendons or ligaments, and bone (**Fig. 1**). These wounds are commonly contaminated with bacteria that typically originate either from the resident microbes of the skin or from microbes that are encountered in the horses' environment.[6] Furthermore, significant infection in postoperative orthopedic cases, such as arthroscopy or fracture repair, or following intra-articular medication can pose a serious complication for the clinician resulting in increased morbidity and necessitating euthanasia in severe cases.

The pathogenic bacteria in equine wounds and infected surgical sites have been categorized in multiple studies spanning the last 30 years. An early study[5] by Schneider and colleagues (1992) looked at 192 horses with septic arthritis/tenosynovitis. As part of that study, they presented the culture results of 156 horses and found that *Staphylococcus* spp. and Enterobacteriaceae species were the most common organisms encountered. More recent studies[7,8] have demonstrated similar findings with *Staphylococcus* spp. more commonly encountered in cases of infection that develop after intra-articular injection or after orthopedic surgery, and Enterobacteriaceae tending to be more common after traumatic wounds. Other bacteria commonly encountered can include *Streptococcus* spp., *Enterococcus* spp., *Pseudomonas* spp., *Proteus* spp., *Actinobacillus* spp., and in the case of puncture wounds, anaerobes.

A thorough examination of the wound/injury, including diagnostics such as radiographs, ultrasound, and synoviocentesis in cases where synovial involvement or

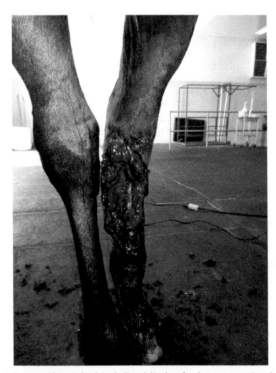

Fig. 1. Extensive injury to the right hind distal limb of a horse sustained after its limb was caught in a fence after kicking out. The horse underwent extensive cleaning and debridement of the wound, bandaging, systemic antimicrobial therapy, and multiple daily intravenous regional limb perfusions. Once a healthy bed of granulation tissue was apparent, skin grafts were recommended to aid epithelialization.

underlying tendon/bone involvement is suspected, is paramount to aid in prompt and aggressive treatment for a better outcome. Radiographs should be performed to rule out fracture, boney lesions or the presence of a radiopaque foreign body. Although radiographs may not be very sensitive for determining involvement of a synovial structure, the presence of gas opacities within the synovial structure should alert the clinician to possible contamination (**Fig. 2**). In cases where involvement of the underlying bone can be ascertained based on clinical assessment, the clinician should remember that radiographic evidence of osteomyelitis or potential sequestrum formation will not be radiographically apparent for at least 10 to 14 days. Contrast radiography, such as fistulograms or the intrasynovial injection of radiographic contrast solution, can also be useful to determine communication of a wound or puncture with a synovial structure.[9,10]

Ultrasound examination can also be useful to determine if a wound or tract communicates with an underlying synovial structure, in addition to assessing for potential injury to the surrounding soft tissue structures. Ultrasonographic findings that may indicate synovial infection most commonly include moderate to severe thickening of the synovial membrane, increased echogenicity of the synovial fluid, and/or the presence of focal hyperechogenic areas within the synovial structure.[11] Ultrasound can also be very useful to rule out the presence of nonradiopaque foreign bodies such as plant awns, wood, and so forth.

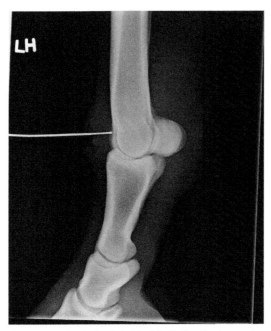

Fig. 2. Lateromedial radiograph of the left hind fetlock of a horse that presented with a wound over the dorsomedial aspect of the joint. Note the insertion of a metallic probe through the dorsal wound tract, which appears to contact the metatarsal condyles. Note also the presence of multiple gas opacities present at the plantar aspect of the distal metatarsal diaphysis, just distal to the splint bones, which are thought to be located within the proximal limit of the plantar recess of the metatarsophalangeal joint.

A definitive diagnosis of synovial sepsis is made based on synoviocentesis. Synovial fluid collection should be aseptically and performed at a site remote from the injury/wound to prevent the possible introduction of microorganisms during synoviocentesis. Following the collection of synovial fluid, the needle can remain within the synovial structure to allow distension of the structure with sterile saline to assess direct communication of the wound with the synovial structure. Similarly, when infection is suspected after surgery (ie, arthroscopy) or intra-articular medication, synoviocentesis remains the primary method of diagnosis. A routine synovial fluid analysis includes evaluation of gross appearance (color, turbidity, viscosity), TP (total protein) concentration, TNCC (total nucleated cell count), and fluid cytology. **Table 1** outlines the normal parameters of synovial fluid constituents and those associated with septic synovitis. Synovial fluid is generally considered to be septic when it has a TP greater than 4.0 g/dL, a TNCC greater than 30,000 cells/µL, and a cellularity greater than 80% neutrophils.[10,12] Biochemical values that may also be evaluated include lactate, pH, and glucose concentration of the synovial fluid compared to serum;[13] however, cytology remains the gold standard.

With regard to puncture wounds of the equine hoof, penetration of the foot, particularly in the frog region (frog and collateral sulci), can lead to serious complications where damage to vital underlying structures such as the distal phalanx, deep digital flexor tendon, navicular bursa, and/or the distal interphalangeal joint (DIPJ) can occur (**Fig. 3**).[14] Radiographs, ideally with the penetrating foreign body in place, are imperative to delineate the depth and direction of the foreign body (usually a nail). If the object has been removed already the use of a sterile probe inserted through the tract can be useful in determining the depth and direction. If synovial structure involvement is suspected, a contrast study can be performed by injecting a radiopaque contrast agent into the synovial structure using aseptic technique and determining if there is communication with the tract. However, the gold standard for determining the involvement of a synovial structure is to obtain a sample via synoviocentesis as outlined earlier. The most common synovial structure to be involved is the navicular bursa because of its more ventral location. Computed tomography and magnetic resonance imaging can also be very useful to determine if damage or injury to underlying soft tissue structures such as the deep digital flexor tendon or impar ligament has occurred or if there has been osseous damage to the distal phalanx not yet detectable on radiographs, particularly in cases where the penetrating object has been removed and the tract is not readily apparent.

In the case of postoperative infection, clinical signs such as increased lameness/discomfort, fever or swelling associated with the surgical site, and/or the presence of a draining tract can help alert the clinician that a possible infection is present. Although serial radiographs can be helpful to demonstrate osteomyelitis of the associated bone, particularly following fracture repair and implant use, ultrasound can also be useful in the earlier stages of infection to identify periosteal reaction or fluid overlying the bony surface. Where a draining tract is present the importance of obtaining a sample for bacterial culture and sensitivity to help dictate antimicrobial therapy cannot be overemphasized.

Depending on the etiology, different treatment modalities may be pursued including wound debridement, or tract debridement in the case of penetrating injuries to the hoof, arthroscopic lavage of a contaminated synovial structure, or curettage of infected bone. Initiation of broad-spectrum antimicrobial coverage is instituted, which should ideally be based on bacterial culture and sensitivity.

Intravenous regional limb perfusion (IVRLP) cannot replace any one of these steps or treatments. For example, arthroscopic lavage of an infected synovial structure will

Table 1
Cytologic and biochemical values of normal and septic synovial fluid in adult horses

Synovial Fluid Variable	Normal Synovial Fluid	Septic Synovial Fluid
Appearance	Transparent, pale yellow, viscous	Cloudy, turbid, nonviscous, may be serosanguinous
TNCC (cells/μL)	<500	>30,000
Neutrophils (%)	<10%	>80–90%
TP (g/dL)	<2	>4
Lactate (mmol/L)	0.42–3.9	>4.9
Serum synovial-glucose difference (mg/dL)	<39.6	>39.6
PH	7.30–7.53	<6.9

Abbreviations: TNCC, total nucleated cell count; TP, total protein.

always be the gold standard treatment for such cases. It is, however, a very valuable adjunctive treatment that has been shown to improve outcomes when used in conjunction with the various treatments outlined earlier. To try to eliminate the pathogenic bacteria, antimicrobial agents must reach adequate concentrations at the site of injury. As there is a relatively poor blood supply to the distal limb of the horse, systemic administration of antimicrobials may not reach adequate synovial concentrations at the site of injury.[15] The technique of IVRLP is based on isolating a portion of the distal extremity from the systemic circulation by applying a tourniquet and then injecting the antimicrobial into the local vasculature. During IVRLP, high concentrations and pressure gradients between the intravascular and extravascular compartments are obtained, which allows diffusion of the selected antimicrobial into the surrounding tissues including soft tissues, synovial structures, and bone. The high local concentration is proposed to create a depot phenomenon that reduces the return of the antimicrobial to the systemic circulation once the tourniquet is removed.[16,17] Obvious advantages include higher antimicrobial concentrations at the site of injury, with lower systemic levels resulting in fewer adverse side-effects.

INTRAVENOUS REGIONAL LIMB PERFUSION TECHNIQUE
Antimicrobial Choice

The goal of any antimicrobial therapy is to achieve antimicrobial concentrations above the minimum inhibitory concentration (MIC) in infected tissue with the least amount of systemic or local adverse effects possible. Aminoglycosides, such as amikacin and gentamicin, are concentration-dependent drugs, therefore a higher peak maximum concentration (C_{MAX}):MIC ratio is associated with a greater bactericidal effect.[18] Human studies evaluating systemic aminoglycosides for the treatment of Gram-negative sepsis have shown that the peak systemic aminoglycoside C_{MAX}:MIC ratio should be at least between 8:1 and 10:1 to maximize the effect of these drugs.[19,20] High concentrations are essential when treating infections caused by less susceptible pathogens with higher MIC of the antibiotic;[21] therefore, the goal of treatment should be optimization of peak concentrations by use of the highest possible nontoxic dose.[20,22] As mentioned, for aminoglycosides to be effective, C_{MAX} should be 8 to 10 times higher than the MIC to be efficacious. For example, if dealing with a susceptible pathogen, that is, has an MIC of 4 μg/mL, ideally you should be targeting concentrations in the region of 40 μg/mL in the vicinity of the injury. For more resistant

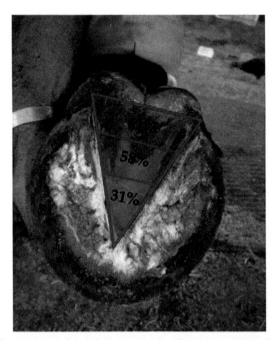

Fig. 3. Picture of the solar surface of the equine hoof with a red triangle outlining the region representing the frog and collateral sulci. According to a study looking at 63 horses with penetration of the frog region by Kilcoyne and colleagues[14] penetration in the cranial aspect of this area resulted in contamination of a synovial structure in 31% of cases, penetration in the middle area resulted in contamination of a synovial structure in 58% of cases and penetration in the most caudal aspect of this area resulted in synovial structure contamination in 63% of cases.

pathogens, that is, has an MIC of 16 μg/mL, therapeutic concentrations of $\geq$160 μg/mL would be required. Although this level of high concentrations of antimicrobials in the synovial cavities of the distal limb is typically impossible to achieve safely by systemic administration of antimicrobials, it has been shown throughout the literature that these levels are quite attainable using IVRLP. These high antimicrobial concentrations (>10 times MIC) not only lead to an increased therapeutic effect but can also help to prevent the emergence of a population of resistant bacteria.[22]

Ideally, the choice of antimicrobial should be based on culture and sensitivity results, either from the wound or synovial fluid in the case of synovial sepsis. However, a positive culture of synovial fluid is not always achievable, with a yield of a positive culture usually in the range of 32.5% to 49%.[23,24] In addition, culture results take up to 48 hours to get back so treatment is usually instituted before obtaining these results.

Amikacin is the most commonly used antimicrobial for IVRLP. As it is an aminoglycoside and a concentration-dependent drug in nature, this favors once-a-day administration, which is more practical in a clinical setting. In addition, because of its spectrum of action, which includes gram-negative aerobes (ie, Enterobacteriaceae) and some *Staphylococcus* species, it is an excellent choice for wounds and orthopedic conditions of the distal limb. Various doses of amikacin have been reported in the literature (250 mg-3g).[7,18,25,26] Typically, at the author's clinic, 2g is the routine dose of amikacin used in an adult (average 500 kg horse) when performing IVRLP. Based on experimental studies,[7,27] it has been shown that synovial concentrations of amikacin drop below the MIC within 24 hrs of performing IVRLP, therefore, daily treatments are usually necessary.

Although it would appear that using time-dependent antimicrobials is less suited to IVRLP compared with the concentration-dependent counterparts, depending on the type of bacteria cultured the more appropriate antimicrobial spectrum may be warranted. For example, when a culture of certain gram-positive isolates such as beta-hemolytic streptococci is obtained. Ceftiofur, a third-generation cephalosporin, is typically thought of as a time-dependent antimicrobial. However, it has been demonstrated in the literature that use of a high dose (2g)[28,29] for IVRLP resulted in concentrations above the MIC in the radiocarpal joint and subcutaneous tissue for greater than 24 hrs, suggesting that daily administration of ceftiofur via IVRLP may be of use in some instances.

Other antimicrobials used for IVRLP reported in the literature (**Table 2**) include enrofloxacin,[26] erythromycin,[30,31] chloramphenicol,[32] vancomycin,[33] imipenem,[34] and meropenem;[35] however, their use clinically would not be common. Given the emergence of new resistant bacterial strains in human and veterinary medicine, the judicious use of certain antimicrobials, particularly vancomycin and carbapenems, should be reserved for infections where results of bacterial culture and susceptibility testing have determined that no other antimicrobial alternatives exist. These drugs have been considered last resort drugs in human medicine and their use in veterinary medicine should be limited as much as possible.

Conflicting evidence exists in the literature as to the use of antimicrobial combinations. Although it would seem intuitive to use a combination of antimicrobials to increase the overall spectrum of action, some evidence exists that drug interactions may render some antimicrobials inactive. A study by Zantingh and colleagues[36] reported the combination of amikacin and ticarcillin-clavulanate in IVRLP resulted in a reduction of amikacin concentration and efficacy of the drug. In addition, a study by Nieto and colleagues[37] showed that, although a combination of sodium penicillin and amikacin reached therapeutic concentrations in the metacarpophalangeal joint after IVRLP, the concentration of penicillin remained above the MIC for only 6 hours. Conversely, a recent study[38] using a combination of sodium penicillin and amikacin resulted in appropriate concentrations of both drugs in the middle carpal joint for at least 24 hrs. At this time, insufficient evidence exists in the literature to support the use of antimicrobial combinations and at this time, the authors recommend using a single antimicrobial.

TYPE OF TOURNIQUET

The efficacy of IVRLP is greatly dependent on the function of the tourniquet, and it has been shown that it is essential to use a wide rubber tourniquet ($\geq$10 cm) or a pneumatic tourniquet.[22,39,40] Although the significant advantage of the pneumatic tourniquet is the ability to standardize tourniquet pressure, it is not practical to use in a field setting, and so a wide rubber or Esmarch tourniquet is more clinically applicable.

The authors typically use a 12 cm Esmarch tourniquet and apply it to the proximal limb, when using the cephalic or saphenous vein, with at least 10 loops around the limb while holding firm pressure. Typically rolled gauze is placed under the tourniquet in the divot where the cephalic vein courses or directly overlying the saphenous vein in the hind limb to produce consistent pressure over the vein and improve tourniquet efficacy (**Fig. 4**).

Table 2
Less commonly used antimicrobials for intravenous regional limb perfusion

Drug	Dose	Spectrum	Cidal/ Static	Reference	Comments
Ceftiofur	2g	Gram + and − aerobes	Cidal	Cox et al,[28] 2016, Pille et al,[29] 2005	After IVRLP synovial fluid ceftiofur concentrations remain above MIC for common pathogens (1 μg/mL) for >24 h
Chloramphenicol	2g	Gram + and − aerobes and anaerobes	Static	Kelmer et al,[32] 2015	T$_{1/2}$ only 3 h — may necessitate twice daily administration
Enrofloxacin	1.5 mg/kg	Gram − aerobes and Staphylococcus spp.	Cidal	Parra-Sanchez et al,[26] 2006	May cause irritation/ vasculitis at the injection site. Associated with developmental cartilage abnormalities in young horses
Gentamicin	500 mg -1g	Gram − aerobes	Cidal	Hyde et al,[46] 2013, Werner et al,[48] 2003	Usually, the next choice if amikacin not available. Limited action against Staphylococcus spp.
Vancomycin	300 mg	Gram + bacteria Clostridial spp. Resistant Staphylococcus and Enterococcus spp.	Cidal	Rubio-Martinez et al,[33] 2005	Limited Gram - activity. Active against Staphylococcus spp.

Note these antimicrobials are typically only used based on bacterial culture and sensitivity results.
Abbreviations: IVRLP, intravenous regional limb perfusion; MIC, minimum inhibitory concentration; T$_{1/2}$, half-life.

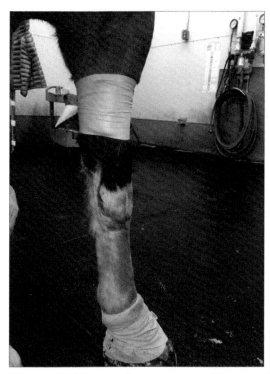

Fig. 4. Placement of a wide rubber Esmarch tourniquet at the proximal antebrachium to facilitate IVRLP at the cephalic vein just below the level of the chestnut. Note that 4 × 4″ gauze pads have been placed under the tourniquet in the grove of the cephalic vein to facilitate adequate compression of the vein.

Another factor to consider is movement during IVRLP, which is considered to be detrimental because it causes leakage of the perfusate and lowers the antimicrobial concentrations in the targeted region due to disruption of the tourniquet. Good sedation practices are paramount to help reduce motion and increase the functionality of the tourniquet. Although general anesthesia has been described in the literature, one study[41] showed higher synovial concentrations of antimicrobials using standing sedation compared with general anesthesia. In addition, placing a horse under general anesthesia to perform daily IVRLP is not practical. Other strategies to reduce movement in addition to good sedation include perineural anesthesia and instillation of local anesthetic as part of the perfusate. A recent study,[42] which looked at the systemic and local effects of lidocaine or mepivacaine when used for IVRLP in standing sedated horses, showed that IVRLP with lidocaine or mepivacaine provided adequate antinociception to the distal limb similar to perineural anesthesia. It is the author's preference to add local anesthetic (lidocaine 2%) to the perfusate rather than performing a regional nerve block, as it has been our clinical experience that this works sufficiently, with reduced time required for the peripheral nerve block to be performed. As previously stated, the appropriate use of sedatives and timing of sedation protocols cannot be overemphasized to optimize the effect of the sedation and reduce movement. The authors typically administer detomidine (0.01 mg/kg IV) and butorphanol (0.01 mg/kg IV) 5 minutes before the application of the tourniquet. Top-up doses are administered as needed if movement or discomfort is noted.

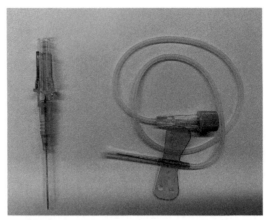

Fig. 5. Two different catheters to facilitate IVRLP. A 23 G butterfly catheter or 22G 2.5 cm catheter can be used to facilitate injection of the perfusate.

Regarding the duration required for tourniquet application, most studies have used application times of 25 to 30 minutes.[22,39,40,43,44] A more recent study[25] looking at the time to peak synovial amikacin concentration in the DIPJ or coffin joint has shown that despite maintenance of the tourniquet, the median peak concentration did not increase past 15 minutes, indicating that application of the tourniquet for 15 minutes should be sufficient to achieve peak concentrations of antibiotics within the DIPJ of the distal limb while performing IVRLP. Use of a shorter tourniquet application time allows the clinician to be more efficient but also reduced the length of time the horse must be sedated. At the author's institution, the tourniquet is typically left in place for 20 minutes.

VESSEL TO PERFUSE

Multiple perfusions, typically 24 hours apart, are usually used to help treat infection in the distal limb. There are no concrete guidelines as to how many are necessary and the decision is usually based on clinician preference and how the horse is responding clinically, that is, degree of lameness, improvement in cytologic parameters of synovial fluid, appearance of the wound, and so forth. Most studies looking at IVRLP have used the cephalic or saphenous vein, which has been shown to be as efficient and effective as using the digital palmar/plantar vessels with similar synovial concentrations achieved in the more distal synovial structures.[16] Both the cephalic and saphenous veins are more accessible and as a result of their larger diameter, they are easier to catheterize than smaller vessels like the palmar/plantar digital vessels, resulting in fewer complications such as thrombosis. Either a 23G butterfly catheter[a] or 22G 2.5 cm catheter[b] can be used to facilitate injection (**Fig. 5**). The author's preference is to use a 22G 2.5 cm over the needle catheter for the cephalic and saphenous vein, as they tend to be more stable in the vessel once placed and less like to result in extravasation. Once inserted in the vessel, a preloaded extension set is connected

[a] Surflo Winged Infusion Set. Terumo Corporation, Tokyo 151-0072, Japan.

[b] BD Instyte, Becton Dickinson Infusion Therapy Systems Inc., Sandy, UT, USA

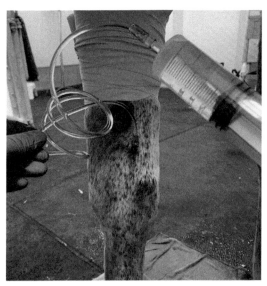

Fig. 6. Instilling the perfusate over 2 minutes following placement of a 22G 2.5 cm catheter in the cephalic vein of a horse that presented for a wound over the dorsal pastern that communicated with the distal interphalangeal joint.

and the perfusate is instilled over 2 minutes (**Fig. 6**). Once all the perfusate has been administered, the catheter is removed and pressure is applied to the site of injection using gauze and tape to prevent hematoma formation. Some irritation at the injection site or hematoma formation can occur, particularly if the movement of the limb occurs during perfusion. Application of 1% diclofenac liposomal cream[44] to the site of injection has been shown to decrease inflammation and may help prolong the period that vessel can be used for IVRLP where multiple treatments are necessary.

For IVRLP of the palmar/plantar digital vessels, the tourniquet is typically placed at the mid to distal third of the metacarpus/tarsus (**Fig. 7**). At the author's institution, a butterfly catheter is the preferred method to instill the perfusate at this level, as it is easier to place in the smaller palmar/plantar digital vessels. Typically, a lower perfusate volume is used when using this method.

Although repeated perfusions are to be performed, or potentially in the case of a poor temperament horse that will not tolerate repeated insertions, an indwelling catheter can be placed at the level of the cephalic or saphenous vein (**Fig. 8**). The authors typically use a 16G, 20 cm over-the-wire polyurethane catheter[c] for this purpose. One study[45] showed that use of an indwelling catheter in the cephalic or saphenous vein provided prolonged venous access and facilitated successive perfusions with minimal complications associated with its use.

VOLUME OF PERFUSATE

The main theory is that the volume of perfusate should be high enough to increase the intravascular pressure, which results in sufficient drug diffusion to the surrounding

---

[c] Arrow International, Inc., 2400 Bernville Road, Reading, PA 19605, USA.

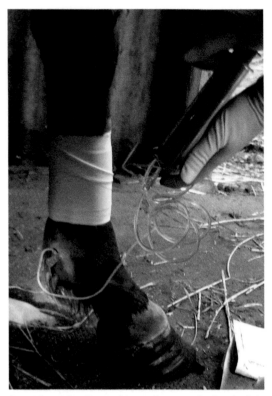

Fig. 7. Placement of a wide rubber Esmarch tourniquet at the level of the mid to distal third of the metacarpus, while performing an IVRLP of the lateral palmar digital vessel, in a horse that presented for a laceration of the coronary band and proximal hoof wall. A 23 G butterfly catheter has been placed in the lateral palmar digital vessel to facilitate the perfusion.

tissues.[27] Different volumes have been reported by different studies and vary greatly from 10 mL to 100 mL.[46,47] A study by Hyde and colleagues[46] found no difference in synovial antimicrobial concentration after using three different volumes (10 mL, 30 mL, or 60 mL) of perfusate during IVRLP. A more recent study[47] found the use of the higher perfusate volume (60–100 mL) resulted in a significantly higher antimicrobial concentration in the synovial fluid compared with lower perfusate volumes (30 mL). These findings highlight the possible importance of venous distention during IVRLP on the antimicrobial concentration in the distal limb, and emphasize the advantage of using a high volume of perfusate (60–100 mL). However, with conflicting evidence in the literature, the optimal volume to use is not clear.

Typically, at the author's clinic, the total volume of perfusate used for regional limb perfusion performed at the level of the cephalic/saphenous vein is 60 mL, consisting of 20 mL 2% lidocaine, 2g amikacin, and ~35 mL sterile saline. A lower total volume of 35 mL perfusate is used if the perfusion is performed using the palmar/plantar digital vessels (**Box 1**).

To help improve the peak concentrations in the synovial structures of the distal limb, it is important to administer the perfusate over 2 minutes at least. Based on the authors' experience, this helps reduce the hydrostatic pressure within the vessel

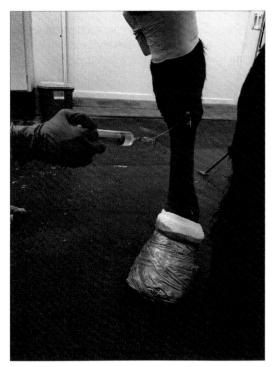

Fig. 8. Performing an IVRLP using an indwelling catheter (16G, 20 cm over-the-wire polyure-thane catheter)[c] placed in the distal saphenous vein in a horse that sustained a penetrating injury to the hoof that communicated with the navicular bursa.

Box 1
General procedure for performing an IVRLP

1. Preparation of the vessel to be injected — the hair is clipped and the area aseptically prepped.

2. The perfusate is prepared. In a 60 mL syringe, 2g amikacin is combined with 20 mL 2% lidocaine or mepivacaine diluted to 60 mL using sterile saline. The extension set is connected and primed. If a butterfly catheter is used, the extension set is not necessary.

3. The horse is sedated. Typically, detomidine (0.01 mg/kg) and butorphanol (0.01 mg/kg) IV is used.

4. After 5 minutes, the tourniquet is placed (wide rubber Esmarch tourniquet ≥10 cm) proximally to the proposed injection site. Gauze is placed below the tourniquet overlying the vessel to be perfused to facilitate complete compression of the vessel.

5. A 23 G butterfly catheter or 22 G 2.5 cm over the needle catheter is placed in the vessel and once blood is observed dripping from the hub, the extension set or syringe is connected.

6. The perfusate is instilled over 2 minutes.

7. A 4 × 4″ gauze pad and white tape is used to apply pressure to the injection site immediately on catheter removal from the vessel.

8. The tourniquet is left in place for 20 minutes.

immediately adjacent to the tourniquet while administering the perfusion, which may result in leakage into the systemic circulation. In addition, placement of the catheter a few cm distal to the tourniquet and not directly below the tourniquet (see **Fig. 6**) can also help reduce the hydrostatic pressure in this region.

SUMMARY

IVRLP is a relatively straightforward procedure, which can be performed easily in a field setting. A multitude of evidence exists in the literature that a higher local concentration of antimicrobial is achievable with IVRLP compared with systemic administration. However, there is also evidence that the concentrations reached can be variable and may not consistently reach therapeutic levels, which can most likely be attributed to tourniquet failure or increased movement during the procedure.[7,25,47,41] Therefore, it is recommended to combine IVRLP with systemic antimicrobial therapy to reduce the risk of treatment failure. Direct intra-articular administration is another alternative therapy to consider, which has been demonstrated to reach therapeutic synovial levels in addition to producing concentrations in adjacent bone similar to those achieved with IVRLP.[48] At the author's clinic, horses with septic synovial structures will typically undergo daily IVRLP following arthroscopic lavage and debridement. Approximately every third day, synoviocentesis is performed instead of IVRLP to facilitate direct intra-articular treatment of the joint and additionally to sample the fluid for cytologic analysis (TNCC and % neutrophils) to assess response to treatment.

As previously stated, there is no clear consensus as to how many IVRLP to perform in each clinical case and this is usually made based on the clinical response to treatment. Clinical parameters such as degree of lameness and the clinical appearance of the wound are important indicators. In the case of a septic synovial structure, cytologic analysis of the synovial fluid, including TNCC and the percentage of neutrophils, is the gold standard in determining response to treatment. Other diagnostics such as the use of ultrasound or radiographs in the case of bone infection can also be useful to assess the progression of the disease process.

In conclusion, although clear advances have been made in the development and use of this procedure, the clinician should also be aware of its limitations. When used appropriately, in conjunction with standard therapeutics such as systemic antibiotics and surgical debridement, IVRLP can help expedite the resolution of infection in the distal limb of horses. Further research is necessary and ongoing to help standardize protocols for its use and refine this useful treatment modality.

CLINICS CARE POINTS

- The typical dose for an average 500 kg horse using the cephalic/saphenous vein would be 2g amikacin diluted to 60 mL using 20 mL 2% lidocaine and sterile saline.
- Tourniquet application for 20 minutes is likely sufficient in most cases.
- Use of a wide rubber tourniquet (≥10 cm) is essential.

DISCLOSURE

The authors have no relationship with a commercial company that has a direct financial interest in subject matter or materials discussed in the article or with a company making a competing product.

REFERENCES

1. Bier A. A new method for anaesthesia in the extremities. Ann Surg 1908;48:780.
2. Dietz O, Kehnscherper G. Intravenose stauugsantibiose bei pyogenen infektionen der distalen gliedmassenabschnitte des pferdes. Der Praktische Tierarzt 1990;8:30.
3. Gibson KT, McIlwraith CW, Turner AS, et al. Open joint injuries in horses: 58 cases (1980-1986). J Am Vet Med Assoc 1989;194:398–404.
4. Milner PI, Bardell DA, Warner L, et al. Factors associated with survival to hospital discharge following endoscopic treatment for synovial sepsis in 214 horses. Equine Vet J 2014;46:701–5.
5. Schneider RK, Bramlage LR, Moore RM, et al. A retrospective study of 192 horses affected with septic arthritis/tenosynovitis. Equine Vet J 1992;24:436–42.
6. Frees KE. Equine practice on wound management: wound cleansing and hygiene. Vet Clin North Am Equine Pract 2018;34:473–84.
7. Harvey A, Kilcoyne I, Byrne BA, et al. Effect of dose on intra-articular amikacin sulfate concentrations following intravenous regional limb perfusion in horses. Vet Surg 2016;45:1077–82.
8. Ahern BJ, Richardson DW, Boston RC, et al. Orthopedic infections in equine long bone fractures and arthrodeses treated by internal fixation: 192 cases (1990-2006). Vet Surg 2010;39:588–93.
9. Morton AJ. Diagnosis and treatment of septic arthritis. Vet Clin North Am Equine Pract 2005;21:627–49.
10. Ludwig EK, van Harreveld PD. Equine wounds over synovial structures. Vet Clin North Am Equine Pract 2018;34:575–90.
11. Beccati F, Gialletti R, Passamonti F, et al. Ultrasonographic findings in 38 horses with septic arthritis/tenosynovitis. Vet Radiol Ultrasound 2015;56:68–76.
12. Steel CM. Equine synovial fluid analysis. Vet Clin North Am Equine Pract 2008;24:437–54.
13. Dechant JE, Symm WA, Nieto JE. Comparison of pH, lactate, and glucose analysis of equine synovial fluid using a portable clinical analyzer with a bench-top blood gas analyzer. Vet Surg 2011;40:811–6.
14. Kilcoyne I, Dechant JE, Kass PH, et al. Penetrating injuries to the frog and collateral sulci - a retrospective study of 63 cases (1998-2008). J Am Vet Med Assoc 2011;239(8):1104–9.
15. Whithair KJ, Bowersock TL, Blevins WE, et al. Regional limb perfusion for antibiotic treatment of experimentally induced septic arthritis. Vet Surg 1992;21:367–73.
16. Kelmer G, Bell GC, Martin-Jimenez T, et al. Evaluation of regional limb perfusion with amikacin using the saphenous, cephalic, and palmar digital veins in standing horses. J Vet Pharmacol Ther 2013;36:236–40.
17. Biasutti SA, Cox E, Jeffcott LB, et al. A review of regional limb perfusion for distal limb infections in the horse. Equine Vet Educ 2020;33(5):263–77.
18. Murphey ED, Santschi EM, Papich MG. Regional intravenous perfusion of the distal limb of horses with amikacin sulfate. J Vet Pharmacol Ther 1999;22:68–71.

19. Lacy MK, Nicolau DP, Nightingale CH, et al. The pharmacodynamics of aminoglycosides. Clin Infect Dis 1998;27:23–7.

20. Moore RD, Lietman PS, Smith CR. Clinical response to aminoglycoside therapy: importance of the ratio of peak concentration to minimal inhibitory concentration. J Infect Dis 1987;155:93–9.

21. Caron JP, Bolin CA, Hauptman JG, et al. Minimum inhibitory concentration and postantibiotic effect of amikacin for equine isolates of methicillin-resistant Staphylococcus aureus in vitro. Vet Surg 2009;38:664–9.

22. Kelmer G. Regional limb perfusion in horses. Vet Rec 2016;178:581–4.

23. Taylor AH, Mair TS, Smith LJ, et al. Bacterial culture of septic synovial structures of horses: does a positive bacterial culture influence prognosis? Equine Vet J 2010;42:213–8.

24. Miagkoff L, Archambault M, Bonilla AG. Antimicrobial susceptibility patterns of bacterial isolates cultured from synovial fluid samples from horses with suspected septic synovitis: 108 cases (2008-2017). J Am Vet Med Assoc 2020; 256:800–7.

25. Kilcoyne I, Nieto JE, Knych HK, et al. Time required to achieve maximum concentration of amikacin in synovial fluid of the distal interphalangeal joint after intravenous regional limb perfusion in horses. Am J Vet Res 2018;79:282–6.

26. Parra-Sanchez A, Lugo J, Boothe DM, et al. Pharmacokinetics and pharmacodynamics of enrofloxacin and a low dose of amikacin administered via regional intravenous limb perfusion in standing horses. Am J Vet Res 2006;67:1687–95.

27. Godfrey JL, Hardy J, Cohen ND. Effects of regional limb perfusion volume on concentrations of amikacin sulfate in synovial and interstitial fluid samples from anesthetized horses. Am J Vet Res 2016;77:582–8.

28. Cox KS, Nelson BB, Wittenburg L, et al. Plasma, subcutaneous tissue and bone concentrations of ceftiofur sodium after regional limb perfusion in horses. Equine Vet J 2016;49(3):341–4.

29. Pille F, De Baere S, Ceelen L, et al. Synovial fluid and plasma concentrations of ceftiofur after regional intravenous perfusion in the horse. Vet Surg 2005;34: 610–7.

30. Kelmer G, Hayes ME. Regional limb perfusion with erythromycin for treatment of septic physitis and arthritis caused by Rhodococcus equi. Vet Rec 2009;165: 291–2.

31. Kelmer G, Martin-Jimenez T, Saxton AM, et al. Evaluation of regional limb perfusion with erythromycin using the saphenous, cephalic, or palmar digital veins in standing horses. J Vet Pharmacol Ther 2013;36:434–40.

32. Kelmer G, Tatz AJ, Famini S, et al. Evaluation of regional limb perfusion with chloramphenicol using the saphenous or cephalic vein in standing horses. J Vet Pharmacol Ther 2015;38:35–40.

33. Rubio-Martinez LM, Lopez-Sanroman J, Cruz AM, et al. Evaluation of safety and pharmacokinetics of vancomycin after intravenous regional limb perfusion in horses. Am J Vet Res 2005;66:2107–13.

34. Kelmer G, Tatz AJ, Kdoshim E, et al. Evaluation of the pharmacokinetics of imipenem following regional limb perfusion using the saphenous and the cephalic veins in standing horses. Res Vet Sci 2017;114:64–8.

35. Fontenot RL, Langston VC, Zimmerman JA, et al. Meropenem synovial fluid concentrations after intravenous regional limb perfusion in standing horses. Vet Surg 2018;47:852–60.

36. Zantingh AJ, Schwark WS, Fubini SL, et al. Accumulation of amikacin in synovial fluid after regional limb perfusion of amikacin sulfate alone and in combination with ticarcillin/clavulanate in horses. Vet Surg 2014;43:282–8.

37. Nieto JE, Trela J, Stanley SD, et al. Pharmacokinetics of a combination of amikacin sulfate and penicillin G sodium for intravenous regional limb perfusion in adult horses. Can J Vet Res 2016;80:230–5.

38. Dahan R, Oreff GL, Tatz AJ, et al. Pharmacokinetics of regional limb perfusion using a combination of amikacin and penicillin in standing horses. Can Vet J 2019; 60:294–9.

39. Alkabes SB, Adams SB, Moore GE, et al. Comparison of two tourniquets and determination of amikacin sulfate concentrations after metacarpophalangeal joint lavage performed simultaneously with intravenous regional limb perfusion in horses. Am J Vet Res 2011;72:613–9.

40. Levine DG, Epstein KL, Ahern BJ, et al. Efficacy of three tourniquet types for intravenous antimicrobial regional limb perfusion in standing horses. Vet Surg 2010; 39:1021–4.

41. Aristizabal FA, Nieto JE, Guedes AG, et al. Comparison of two tourniquet application times for regional intravenous limb perfusions with amikacin in sedated or anesthetized horses. Vet J 2016;208:50–4.

42. Mendez-Angulo JL, Granados MM, Modesto R, et al. Systemic and local effects of lidocaine or mepivacaine when used for intravenous regional anaesthesia of the distal limb in standing sedated horses. Equine Vet J 2020;52(5):743–51.

43. Mahne AT, Rioja E, Marais HJ, et al. Clinical and pharmacokinetic effects of regional or general anaesthesia on intravenous regional limb perfusion with amikacin in horses. Equine Vet J 2014;46:375–9.

44. Levine DG, Epstein KL, Neelis DA, et al. Effect of topical application of 1% diclofenac sodium liposomal cream on inflammation in healthy horses undergoing intravenous regional limb perfusion with amikacin sulfate. Am J Vet Res 2009; 70:1323–5.

45. Kelmer G, Tatz A, Bdolah-Abram T. Indwelling cephalic or saphenous vein catheter use for regional limb perfusion in 44 horses with synovial injury involving the distal aspect of the limb. Vet Surg 2012;41:938–43.

46. Hyde RM, Lynch TM, Clark CK, et al. The influence of perfusate volume on antimicrobial concentration in synovial fluid following intravenous regional limb perfusion in the standing horse. Can Vet J 2013;54:363–7.

47. Oreff GL, Dahan R, Tatz AJ, et al. The Effect of Perfusate Volume on Amikacin Concentration in the Metacarpophalangeal Joint Following Cephalic Regional Limb Perfusion in Standing Horses. Vet Surg 2016;45:625–30.

48. Werner LA, Hardy J, Bertone AL. Bone gentamicin concentration after intra-articular injection or regional intravenous perfusion in the horse. Vet Surg 2003; 32:559–65.

Fracture Stabilization and Management in the Field

Jessica M. Morgan, PhD, DVM[a,b,*], Larry D. Galuppo, DVM[b,c]

KEYWORDS

- Horse • Equine • Splint • Ambulatory • Emergency

KEY POINTS

- Fracture treatment begins with assessment and identification of concurrent systemic compromise.
- An appropriate splint will improve patient comfort, counteract forces on the fracture site, and provide an opportunity for limited weight bearing.
- Splints applied inappropriately can increase soft tissue damage by creating a lever arm at the fracture site.
- Successful splinting is achievable and will improve the success of future fracture repair.

INTRODUCTION

Fractures are inherently distressing for horses and their human caretakers. The general equine practitioner plays a critical role in managing communication, providing initial assessment, and stabilizing these cases. Successful management of these emergencies improves situational safety for humans and horses, protects equine welfare, and is instrumental for the success of fracture repair. Inappropriate first aid and stabilization can result in excessive cutaneous, muscular, and neurovascular trauma. Soft tissue injury that occurs during initial assessment and transport will limit any potential for future fracture repair. Focusing on the treatment goals for emergency fracture stabilization (**Box 1**, **Fig. 1**) in the field is the first step in successful equine fracture repair.

STOCKING THE TRUCK

Although fractures are not the most common emergency in equine practice, they do happen. Being prepared can have a major influence on patient survival. Having the necessary emergency supplies organized and easily obtainable will greatly increase the success of treatment for all orthopedic emergencies. The list of supplies is not

[a] Department of Medicine and Epidemiology, UC Davis School of Veterinary Medicine, Davis, CA, USA; [b] The William R. Pritchard Veterinary Medical Teaching Hospital, University of California, Davis, One Garrod Drive, Davis, CA 95616, USA; [c] Department of Surgical and Radiological Sciences, UC Davis School of Veterinary Medicine, Davis, CA, USA
* Corresponding author. The William R. Pritchard Veterinary Medical Teaching Hospital, University of California, Davis, One Garrod Drive, Davis, CA 95616
E-mail address: jmmorgan@ucdavis.edu

Vet Clin Equine 37 (2021) 293–309
https://doi.org/10.1016/j.cveq.2021.04.004
0749-0739/21/© 2021 Elsevier Inc. All rights reserved.

Box 1
Treatment goals for fracture management in the field

- Stabilize the patient and control hemorrhage
- Relieve pain and anxiety
- Control wound infection
- Prevent additional tissue damage

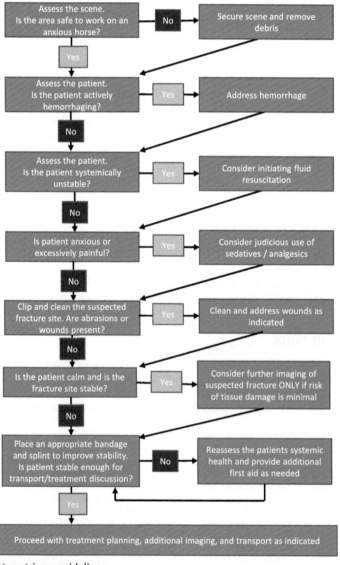

Fig. 1. Fracture triage guidelines.

extensive and most are available in a well-stocked ambulatory vehicle (**Box 2**, **Fig. 2**). The main equipment should include bandage and casting material, splints, fluids for intravenous administration, sedatives and tranquilizers, antibiotics, antiseptics, and tetanus prophylaxis.

INITIAL ASSESSMENT

A horse with a fracture can be difficult to assess at initial presentation due to high levels of anxiety in both the owner and the horse. Successful management of these cases requires the practitioner to assess the situation including potential safety hazards in the environment, access to the patient, and the available personnel. Clear communication regarding handling, restraint, and debris removal will improve safety for all parties involved. Once the situation has been assessed, the initial patient evaluation should focus on determining if the horse is systemically stable and if there is evidence of an unstable fracture causing distress and potential for additional injury.

EMERGENCY FIRST AID

After initial assessment, the most critical concerns should be addressed first (see **Fig. 1**). Every case is unique but in general active hemorrhage should be addressed first followed by addressing pain and anxiety, wound care, and fracture stabilization. Hypovolemic shock can also develop after a traumatic incident due to blood loss or a combination of prolonged stress, sweat loss, and lack of access to water. Potential hypovolemic shock should be addressed in fracture patients at presentation and reassessed regularly throughout treatment to ensure the patient is stable before referral for fracture management.

Trauma leading to fracture can also be associated with internal and/or external hemorrhage. Any active hemorrhage at initial evaluation should be controlled by ligating the offending vessel or vessels. If this cannot be accomplished due to inaccessibility of the vessel, packing the wound and applying a pressure wrap is often a viable alternative. Blood loss may be difficult to assess in cases with internal hemorrhage or hemorrhage that has resolved. Evidence of external hemorrhage in the form of pooled blood can provide a useful indication in some cases, however estimation of total blood loss can be challenging. Internal hemorrhage is often difficult to identify in initial stages but should be considered in cases of thoracic, abdominal, or pelvic trauma as well as

---

Box 2
Supplies for fracture management in the field

- Sedation (xylazine hydrochloride, butorphanol tartrate, detomidine hydrochloride)
- Antiseptic scrub and cleaning supplies
- Clippers with a surgical length blade
- Light weight splints in a variety of lengths for common fractures (distal limb and full limb options)
- Intravenous fluids and delivery methods for treatment of shock and dehydration
- Bandage material (combine bandage, roll cotton, gauze bandages, elastic tape, ace bandage)
- Casting material
- Antibiotics (penicillin, gentamicin, oral antibiotic selection)

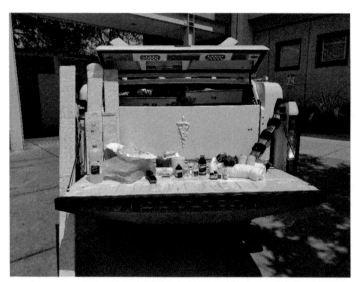

Fig. 2. Ambulatory truck supplies for fracture stabilization including sedation (xylazine hydrochloride, butorphanol tartrate, detomidine hydrochloride), wound cleaning supplies, fluid resuscitation supplies, bandage material and splints, and antimicrobials.

fractures of the humerus or femur. Signs of hypovolemic shock associated with moderate to severe blood loss include tachycardia, tachypnea, prolonged capillary refill times, alterations in pulse pressure, and cool extremities. Hematologic parameters such as pack cell volume and total protein are useful but may be within normal limits if there has not been sufficient time (8–12 hours) for fluid redistribution. In cases in which hemorrhage is ongoing, administration of hemostatic agents such as aminocaproic acid (30–40 mg/kg slowly intravenously [IV]) can help promote clot formation.

IV fluid therapy should be initiated in cases in which hypovolemic shock is identified. In a 500-kg adult horse an initial bolus of 2 L of hypertonic saline followed by 5 to 10 L of isotonic crystalloids or 5 to 10 L of isotonic crystalloids alone and reassessment in 20 to 30 minutes is a reasonable place to start. Fluid boluses can be repeated 2 to 3 times as needed in dehydrated adult horses. Foals have a larger volume of distribution and often require larger boluses relative to size, but are also more susceptible to fluid overload. As a general guideline, an initial bolus of 10 to 20 mL/kg over 30 to 60 minutes followed by reassessment is appropriate for most foals suffering from hypovolemia.[1]

After the initial evaluation and first aid are provided, the practitioner should attempt to relieve the horse's pain and anxiety. The goal is to obtain a patient that is more comfortable, cooperative, and not ataxic to facilitate stabilization of the fracture. Evidence of excessive anxiety, shock, or other signs of systemic disease should be considered when developing a plan for sedation and tranquilization. Judicious administration of sedatives (0.2–0.5 mg/kg xylazine, IV or 0.01–0.02 mg/kg detomidine, IV for adults, and 0.05–0.2 mg/kg diazepam IV for young foals), and analgesics (0.01–0.02 mg/kg butorphanol, IV or 0.05–0.1 mg/kg morphine, IV for adults and 0.01–0.05 mg/kg butorphanol, IV for foals) can alleviate pain and anxiety, and will increase patient cooperation for wound care and limb stabilization. Physical restraint techniques and an experienced handler can also be incorporated to reduce the need for sedation. Excessive sedation can lead to increased ataxia and further trauma to muscle, skin, neurovascular structures, and the fractured bone ends reducing the likelihood of successful repair. It is important to note that the amount of sedative and analgesic administered will vary depending on many factors. For example, if the patient is suffering from extreme hypovolemic shock, these drugs may be contraindicated until the patient is stabilized systemically. Use the preceding recommendations as a guideline, understanding that the exact amount of each agent administered can be variable. In addition, stabilization of the fracture will reduce the pain and anxiety associated with an unstable limb, thereby reducing the need for ongoing sedation.

FRACTURE ASSESSMENT

Once the horse is appropriately sedated, the area of the suspected fracture should be thoroughly evaluated (see **Fig. 1**). Careful palpation should allow the evaluator to identify the involved bone(s) as well as the location along the shaft of the bone. Knowledge of the location of the fracture is important to aid in developing a plan for splint application as well as generating a prognosis. Further evaluation should focus specifically at the fracture site. It is important to assess the amount of soft tissue trauma and determine if the fracture is open or closed. If a wound is not immediately evident, cleaning and clipping the area will prepare the area for bandaging and reveal small wounds that might otherwise be overlooked. If a wound is identified the wound should be addressed before bandaging. In the case of a closed fracture, a light bandage should be placed on the clean dried limb to prevent contamination or further trauma to the region. Although radiographic assessment of the fracture is essential for an accurate diagnosis and prognostication, it is often in the patient's best interest to proceed with wound care and fracture stabilization before taking radiographs. Applying an appropriate bandage, splint, bandage cast or combination thereof to stabilize the limb will minimize the risk of further trauma to the bone, soft tissue, or neurovascular structures while obtaining radiographs. Patients with stabilized fractures are less anxious and more cooperative, which improves the chances of safely and successfully obtaining radiographs. However, there are specific instances when it may be preferable to obtain radiographs before splinting. In horses that are stable and cooperative radiographs before splinting should be considered if the available splinting material is radiodense (eg, metallic) or if a detailed fracture configuration is needed to verify a grave prognosis. A detailed assessment of the fracture and an accurate description of the location, fracture type, presence of comminution, degree of contamination, and associated soft tissue damage are essential to accurately prognosticate and advise the owner.

WOUND CARE

After making the patient tractable with the appropriate sedation and analgesic combination, wound care should be instituted. The goal of wound care is to decrease bacterial contamination and the amount of wound lavage and debridement will depend both on the degree of contamination and the patient's degree of comfort and stability. Ideally wounds would be clipped, cleaned, and debrided to remove any necrotic tissue or debris. Excessive bacterial contamination of the soft tissues surrounding the fracture site greatly increases the risk of developing osteomyelitis during fracture healing. Therefore, reducing bacterial contamination early in the course of therapy, especially for open fractures, is extremely important for patient survival. If surgical site infection and osteomyelitis develop the chances of patient survival decrease significantly.[2] In addition to directly addressing the wound, broad-spectrum antimicrobial therapy should be instituted at the time of initial evaluation in cases with suspect or confirmed open fracture. Details of principals of antimicrobial selection for orthopedic conditions are discussed in Kilcoyne and Nieto's article, "Orthopedic Infections - Clinical

Applications of Intravenous Regional Limb Perfusion in the Field," included in this issue. Tetanus prophylaxis should also be instituted in cases with an open fracture.

STABILIZING THE FRACTURE

Stabilizing the fractured limb is the primary goal of emergency first aid procedures. Stabilization will prevent further tissue damage and relieve patient anxiety, ultimately increasing the overall chance for survival. The key to stabilizing a limb fracture is to apply an appropriate splinting device. If applied correctly the splint will prevent additional skin and muscle trauma, limit neurovascular disruption, and limit eburnation (smoothing) of the fractured bone ends. The splint also provides a strut for the horse to bear a moderate amount of weight. The ability to support some weight on the fractured limb and increasing stability at the fracture site will substantially reduce the patients stress and anxiety. Correct application of all splinting devices is imperative. An incorrectly applied splint or cast can cause more harm than good. The general practitioner faced with an unfamiliar fracture is obligated to be become knowledgeable in appropriate splinting methods described here and in several practical articles in the existing literature to effectively manage the fracture patient.[3,4] The referral center to which the horse is being sent can also be an extremely useful resource. A lack of splinting knowledge is not an appropriate reason for not stabilizing a fractured limb. Ultimately, appropriate stabilization is critical to optimize chances for patient survival.

SPLINT SELECTION

The ideal splint neutralizes damaging forces, is not cumbersome, is easy to apply in the standing horse, and is made of accessible material. Some common materials that work well and are accessible include PVC, wood, conduit, rebar, drainage pipe, and casting material. Although many farms have these materials available, having a good set of various sized splints already on the truck and immediately at hand will improve the speed and reliability of fracture stabilization. Splinting is also more successful when working with familiar lightweight materials rather than makeshift items of inappropriate length. The authors would recommend stocking a basic set of splints for the most common fractures in ambulatory vehicles to facilitate fracture stabilization. In addition, there are several commercially available splints for distal limb fractures that are designed to optimize limb alignment and ease of application in the fractious patient.

The splinting technique for any given case depends on fracture location, and knowledge of how the surrounding muscles and tendons influence the fractured limb when there is loss of an intact bony column (**Fig. 3**). To simplify the splinting procedure, the limbs can be divided into several distinct areas in which some generalized splinting recommendations are available. These can be generally grouped into 4 areas in the forelimb including distal forelimb fractures, mid-forelimb fractures, forearm fractures, and proximal forelimb fractures, as described by Bramlage.[5] The hindlimb can be subdivided into similar areas including distal hindlimb fractures, mid-hindlimb fractures, crus fractures, and proximal hindlimb fractures. Having an understanding of the dominant forces on the limb in each these broad categories will provide the foundation for applying appropriate splinting devices.

DISTAL FORELIMB FRACTURES

Distal limb fractures include phalangeal fractures, sesamoid fractures, and condylar fractures of the distal metacarpus. Loss of a bony strut or the suspensory apparatus in the case of biaxial sesamoid fractures leads to collapse of the limb and compression

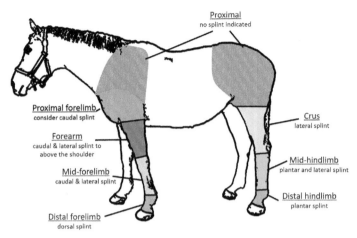

Fig. 3. General regions to guide splint placement.

of the palmar soft tissue structures. The goal of splinting is to align the bony column, and protect the palmar soft tissues in the fetlock and pastern. This can be accomplished by applying a splint on the dorsal aspect of the limb (**Fig. 4**). The splint should incorporate the entire foot and should extend to the proximal aspect of the metacarpus. Due to the relative frequency of fractures in these locations there are several commercially available splints designed for these injuries. Most widely used of these is the Kimzey Leg Saver Splint.[a] This splint provides a dorsal splint secured with reusable straps and lifts the heel to align the bony column (**Fig. 5**). This splint is easy to

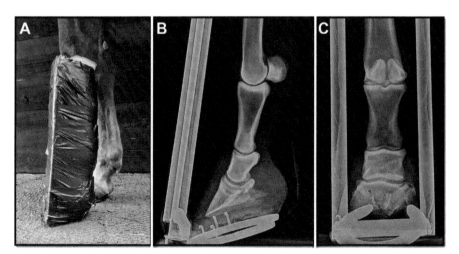

Fig. 4. Dorsal splint application to align the boney column. (*A*) Splint of metal and cast material placed on dorsal aspect of limb with the toe incorporated in the bandage to prevent dorsal migration of the splint. (*B*) Lateral projection of the bony column with dorsal splint in place. (*C*) Dorsal palmar projection of the bony column with dorsal splint in place.

[a] Kimzey Welding, Woodland, California.

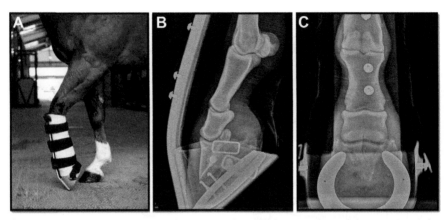

Fig. 5. Kimzey Leg Saver splint application to align the boney column (*A*). Lateral and dorsomedial projections of the distal limb illustrating alignment of the bony column and the ability to assess integrity of the proximal and middle phalanx with the splint in place (*B, C*).

apply under emergency conditions and is very effective for stabilizing the injuries listed above. One weakness of the Kimzey splint compared with other splint configurations is the lack of medial lateral support as the Velcro straps may loosen with load. Increased support can be achieved with this splint by bolstering the straps with duct tape.

MID-FORELIMB FRACTURES

Mid-forelimb fractures include fractures of the diaphysis or proximal epiphysis of the third metacarpal bone, carpal bone fractures and distal radial fractures. Carpal luxations, although not true fractures, represent a similar mechanical situation and can be grouped with carpal fractures for the purpose of splinting. When horses attempt to bear weight on complete mid-forelimb fractures the distal portion of the limb can deviate in 4 directions: cranial, caudal, lateral, or medial. The multiple planes of motion involved and limited soft tissue coverage overlying these areas make the fracture site vulnerable to trauma and increases the risk of bone fragments penetrating the skin (**Fig. 6**). This is especially true for metacarpal bone fractures.

The main goal of splinting is to realign the bony column, and prevent deviation of the distal limb. The main forces that will cause damage at the fracture site in these locations are bending forces in the craniocaudal, and lateromedial directions, and axial compression. If the bony column is aligned, the limb will have increased resistance to axial compression, which will allow the horse to bear some degree of weight on the fractured limb. Stabilization of mid-forelimb instability is best accomplished by applying 2 splints placed at right angles. A caudal splint placed from the ground to the most proximal aspect of the olecranon will prevent deviation of the limb in the craniocaudal direction. A lateral splint, placed from the ground to the elbow, will prevent limb deviation in the mediolateral direction (**Fig. 7**). In cases with transverse fracture, alignment of the boney column to achieve bone-on-bone contact of the proximal and distal segments of the fracture greatly enhances stability and patient comfort.

FOREARM FRACTURES

Radial fractures consisting of complete fractures from the proximal metaphasis to the distal diaphysis make up the forearm fracture category. Due to the ulna's role in triceps

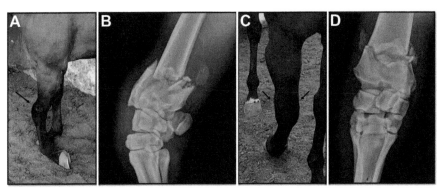

Fig. 6. This is an example of a mid-forelimb fracture and a candidate for a caudal and lateral splint. This comminuted distal radial fracture has trauma to the skin and soft tissues medially and laterally at the fracture site (*black arrow, A, C*). The distal fragment is displaced proximally and cranially. There is evidence of luxation at the antebrachial carpal joint (*B, D*).

function, ulnar fractures are more mechanically similar to fractures of the humerus and scapula than radial fractures and will be discussed in the proximal limb section. The main forces that should be addressed in unstable radial fractures are craniocaudal bending, lateromedial bending, and axial compression. This is best observed when

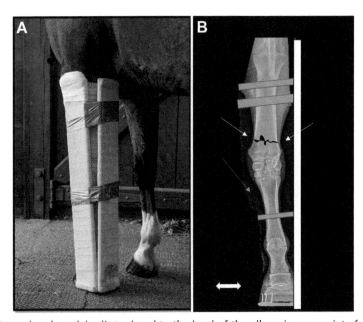

Fig. 7. Lateral and caudal splints placed to the level of the elbow is appropriate for a mid-forelimb fracture (*A*). These splints should be further secured with a large amount of duct tape to prevent rotation about the limb. The lateral splint (*B*) secured to the bandage (*blue arrow*) with nonelastic tape prevents medial lateral movement (*wide white arrow*) at the fracture site and reduces the risk of sharp bone ends (*thin white arrow*) traumatizing the surrounding soft tissues. The caudal splint reduces the risk of cranial caudal displacement in a similar fashion.

horses attempt to bear weight, and the distal portion of the limb can deviate cranially, caudally, laterally and/or medially. The musculature of the forearm helps protect the soft tissues and skin during cranial, caudal and medial deviation of the distal limb. However, when the limb deviates laterally the lack of musculature on the medial aspect of the radius can lead to more serious soft tissue trauma as this is the location of the main neurovascular supply to the distal limb including the median artery, vein, and nerve. If the distal portion of the limb deviates laterally, sharp bone ends can lacerate the medial skin and neurovascular structures. Compromise of the skin leads to open fracture prone to infection and significant trauma to the neurovascular supply compromises future viability and function of the distal limb. These complications often ultimately result in humane destruction of the horse.

The goal of splinting in this region is to realign the bony column, and prevent deviation of the distal limb with a particular focus of preventing lateral deviation. Alignment of the bony column will improve resistance to axial compression, and will allow the horse to bear some degree of weight on the fractured limb. As in the mid-forelimb, stability is best accomplished by applying 2 splints placed at right angles (**Fig. 8**). A caudal splint identical to that used for mid-forelimb fractures, placed from the ground to the most proximal aspect of the olecranon, will prevent deviation of the limb in the craniocaudal direction. However, the lateral splint recommended for mid-forelimb fractures which extends to the level of the elbow is inappropriate for radial fractures. For radial fractures, the lateral splint should extend from the ground to above the shoulder to prevent limb deviation in the mediolateral direction. If the lateral splint is not placed above the shoulder, it will act as a lever arm and increase soft tissue trauma at the fracture site. The lateral splint, placed above the shoulder, effectively prevents

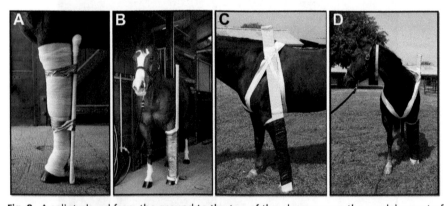

Fig. 8. A splint placed from the ground to the top of the olecranon on the caudal aspect of the limb fixes the carpus and achieves stability for horses with a loss of triceps function associated with radial nerve damage or olecranon fractures (*A*). This splint type can also be used in cases with humeral or distal scapular fractures as fixing the carpus can reestablish limb alignment, which can increase overall comfort. However, be aware, depending on fracture type that a caudal splint may increase risk of neurovascular trauma at the fracture site. Splinting scapular or humeral fractures should be assessed on a case by case basis. A long lateral splint extending above the shoulder is appropriate for radial fractures and reduces the risk of the fracture ends traumatizing the vulnerable medial soft tissues (*B*). The upper portion of the splint should be secured to the trunk with a Figure 8 pattern to stabilize the upper portion of the splint as illustrated (*C, D*). A Caudal splint applied together with a long lateral splint is appropriate for radial fractures involving the metaphyseal or distal diaphysis regions (*A, B*). A caudal splint can increase stability but should be assessed on a case by case basis in radial fractures.

lateral deviation of the distal limb. Attaching the proximal portion of the splint to the shoulders should be accomplished with elastic bandage material in a figure-of-8 pattern as in **Fig. 8**C.

PROXIMAL FORELIMB FRACTURES

Proximal forelimb fractures include fractures of the ulna, humerus, or distal scapula. Similar splinting principals also apply to radial nerve paralysis. All of these conditions result in a loss of triceps function. Without triceps function, horses cannot straighten the limb and fix their carpus and therefore cannot bear any weight. Horses become extremely stressed and anxious, which is exacerbated by transportation where horses must balance on 3 legs during the entire trailer ride.

The main goal of splinting for proximal forelimb fractures is to mimic the triceps apparatus by fixing the carpus. Aligning the bony column is best achieved by applying one splint, extending from the ground to the elbow, on the caudal aspect of the limb (see **Fig. 8**A). Reestablishment of triceps function by placing a caudal splint is extremely effective in cases of olecranon fracture or radial nerve paralysis as it allows full weight bearing through an intact boney column. This translates to less stress and anxiety, as well as protecting the contralateral limb from excessive weight bearing and will make the patient a better candidate for fracture treatment.

In cases with complete humoral or scapular fractures, applying a caudal splint to reestablish triceps function may allow some weight-bearing, but has the potential to increase neurovascular and muscle trauma at the fracture site. This is especially a concern for the radial and suprascapular nerves in fractures of the humerus and scapula respectively. Depending on fracture configuration, placing a caudal splint may allow the surrounding musculature to provide sufficient support to allow the horse to bear some weight, which may improve patient comfort. In adult horses, it is worth applying a caudal splint to evaluate patient comfort. If improved, then the horse can be managed with the splint. If the horse is not improved or more uncomfortable then the patient is best managed without a caudal splint. For foals, splinting humeral and or scapular fractures is not recommended.

DISTAL HINDLIMB FRACTURES

Distal hindlimb fractures include phalangeal fractures, sesamoid fractures, and condylar fractures of the distal metatarsus. Similar splinting strategies will apply to horses with disruption of the soft tissue structures the suspensory apparatus in the absence of a fracture. Once there is loss of a bony strut or suspensory apparatus, the limb will collapse and compress the plantar soft tissue structures. The goals of splinting are to align the bony column, and protect the plantar soft tissues in the fetlock and pastern form excessive compression, as in the forelimb. In the hindlimb, this can best be accomplished by applying a splint on the plantar aspect of the limb (**Fig. 9**A, B). The splint should incorporate the entire foot and should extend to the proximal aspect of the cannon bone. The Kimzey Leg Saver, designed for stabilizing distal limb fractures, can be easily applied and is very effective for stabilizing injuries in the distal hindlimb (**Fig. 9**C, D). It is important that any splint applied maintain the bony column in alignment with the toe pointed distally (see **Fig. 9**B, C).

MID-HINDLIMB FRACTURES

Mid-hindlimb fractures include fractures of the diaphysis or proximal epiphysis of the third metatarsal bone and tarsal bone fractures. Tarsal luxations, although not true

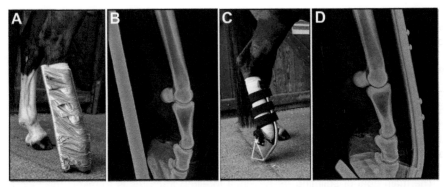

Fig. 9. Plantar splint applied to the distal hindlimb is appropriate for distal limb fractures (A). An effective plantar splint will align the boney column as illustrated in this lateral radiographic projection (B). This is accomplished by incorporating the hoof and extending the splint to the proximal metatarsus. Alternatively, distal hindlimb fractures can also be stabilized with commercial splints such as the Kimzey leg saver splint pictured here applied to a hindlimb over a modified Robert Jones bandage (C, D).

fractures, will follow similar splinting principals to tarsal bone fractures. The main forces that will cause damage at the fracture site in unstable third metatarsal bone fractures are dorsoplantar and lateromedial bending forces, and axial compression. When horses attempt to bear weight on mid-hindlimb fractures the distal portion of the limb can deviate in 4 directions; dorsal, plantar, lateral or medial. There is limited soft tissue coverage overlying the metatarsus, which makes the fracture site vulnerable to trauma. In addition to bending and axial compression forces, tarsal fractures and luxations are also subject to collapsing forces from the reciprocal apparatus. Each time the limb is flexed or extended the fracture or luxation will collapse in a dorsoplantar direction.

The main goal of splinting third metatarsal bone fractures is to realign the bony column, and prevent deviation of the distal limb. In complete tarsal bone fractures or tarsal luxations, the reciprocal apparatus also requires stabilization. As with midforelimb fractures, splinting is best accomplished by applying 2 splints placed at right angles. In the hindlimb a caudal splint placed from the ground to the most proximal aspect of the calcaneus will prevent deviation of the limb in the dorsoplantar direction (**Figs. 10**B and **11**). The calcaneus provides enough bone proximal to the fracture to allow rigid splinting of proximal third metatarsal and tarsal bone fractures. A lateral splint, placed from the ground to the calcaneus, will prevent limb deviation in the mediolateral direction for third metatarsal fractures (**Fig. 10**A), but will not give enough support for tarsal bone fractures or tarsal luxations. A lateral splint bent in the shape of the hindlimb can be used to extend the splinting device more proximally for fractures or luxations involving the tarsal bones (**Fig. 10**C). This will increase rotational and mediolateral stability for third metatarsal bone fractures, and will counteract the collapsing forces of the reciprocal apparatus in tarsal bone fractures and tarsal luxations.

CRUS FRACTURES

Tibial fractures make up the crus fracture category. The main damaging forces for complete tibial fractures are fracture collapse and mediolateral bending. When the bony strut of the tibia is lost, the reciprocal apparatus causes collapse of the fracture

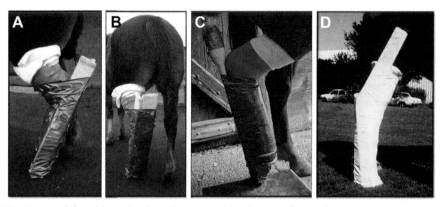

Fig. 10. Caudal and lateral splints that extend to the top of the calcaneus are appropriate for mid-shaft and proximal metatarsal fractures (*A, B, C*). Fractures that involve the tarsal bones will require extension of the lateral splint. This can also be accomplished with pliable materials bent to follow the shape of the hind limb as pictured in panel (*D*).

as the horse attempts to use the leg. The sharp bone ends repeatedly traumatize skin, muscle, and surrounding neurovascular structures every time the limb is flexed or extended. Eburnation of the bone ends also occurs readily. As with radius fractures there is minimal soft tissue covering over the medial aspect of the tibia. The cranial, lateral and caudal musculature of the gaskin region helps protect the fracture site and skin during cranial, caudal and medial deviation of the distal limb. However if the distal limb deviates laterally, sharp bone ends can lacerate the medial skin and neurovascular structures. This increases the risk of an open fracture and subsequent infection. Trauma to the neurovascular supply to the distal limb can compromise the chances of repair and lead to humane destruction of the horse.

The goal of splinting is to realign the bony column, prevent fracture collapse, and lateral deviation of the distal limb. If the bony column is aligned and the reciprocal apparatus stabilized, the splinted limb will have increased resistance to axial

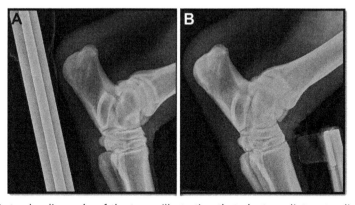

Fig. 11. Lateral radiographs of the tarsus illustrating that plantar splints extending to the top of the calcaneus provide additional support through the tarsus for proximal metatarsal and distal tarsal bone injuries (*A*). In contrast, the dorsal support of the Kimzey splint is only appropriate for fractures of the distal metatarsal condyles or distal limb because the splint ends at the proximal metatarsus (*B*).

compression, torsion, and medial lateral bending. Because of the shape of the hindlimb, this is best accomplished by applying one lateral splint extending from the ground to the hip. In this location, the lateral splint helps prevent fracture collapse and lateral deviation of the distal limb, and will increase resistance to torsion and axial compression. If the lateral splint is not secured and extended to the level of the hip, it will act as a lever arm, increasing soft tissue trauma at the fracture site. It is very important to affix the proximal aspect of the splint to the hind quarters with strong elastic tape to enhance the function of the splint (**Fig. 12**).

PROXIMAL HINDLIMB FRACTURES

Proximal hindlimb fractures include femoral and pelvic fractures. These fractures cannot be stabilized with external splinting devices, therefore splinting fractures located proximal to the stifle is contraindicated. Applying any splinting device below the fracture will act as lever arm, increasing trauma directly at the fracture site.

FRACTURES OF THE SKULL AND AXIAL SKELETON

Fractures of the skull and axial skeleton present unique challenges compared with fractures of the limbs. These fractures are not generally amendable to stabilization with external devices and are often contaminated. They are also often associated with marked hemorrhage due to the highly vascular nature of these regions. Once hemorrhage is addressed, the horse should be evaluated for any evidence of neurologic deficits secondary to trauma to the brain, spinal cord, or cranial nerves. In horses with suspected brain trauma mannitol, diuretics, dimethyl sulfoxide, and corticosteroids can be used to manage brain edema in the acute phase.[4,6] Horses with fractures of affecting the cranial vault or the axial skeleton may present with paraplegia or quadriplegia. In these cases transport to a referral facility must be performed recumbent and is often associated with a grave prognosis.[5]

Conversely, suspected orbital fractures can be readily assessed with palpation of the orbital rim under sedation. Follow-up imaging, including radiography and in

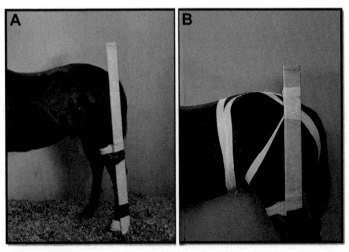

Fig. 12. Proximal hindlimbs splints (*A*) should be secured to the pelvisor shoulder with a figure 8 using nonelastic tape (*B*). Fixation of the proximal aspect of the splint effectively stabilizes the limb, which reduces the risk for additional soft tissue and boney trauma at the fracture site.

some cases advanced imaging is recommended to fully characterize the extent of these fractures before pursuing repair.[7] Orbital fractures have a good prognosis particularly if the globe, nasolacrimal duct, or sinus cavity are not involved. Epistaxis is often reported in these cases and sinus involvement should be ruled out due to an increased risk of complications. If sinus involvement is apparent these horses usually responds well to sinus trephination and lavage.[7]

Mandibular and maxillary fractures are common. Although assessment with an open mouth is critical, the practitioner must be careful not to exacerbate the fracture with a full mouth speculum.[8] Use of a gag on the unaffected side can be effective in cases in which the fracture appears unilateral. Thorough evaluation of the involved structures such as the cranium, eye, sinus, oral cavity, cranial nerves, and central nervous system will aid in prognostication and direct ultimate treatment. Rostral maxillary and mandibular fractures are often amenable to fixation using wires which can be performed in the field or at a referral center. In cases where the clinician is suspicious a fracture may extend more caudal in the mandible or maxilla, referral for further imaging including radiographs and possible computed tomography is indicated as these fractures may necessitate a more involved surgical fixation.[8] In general, in the absence of central nervous system involvement skull fractures carry a good prognosis even when open due to the vascularity of the region.

PROGNOSIS AND DECISION MAKING

Once the fracture has been stabilized the equine practitioner can focus on discussing the decision to pursue treatment. Owners are often emotional and faced with an unexpected series of decisions, thus the practitioner plays a vital role in communicating with the owner and consulting with equine surgeons who have expertise in fracture management. When determining if a patient is a candidate for treatment, factors such as overall patient health and condition, patient size, financial constraints, and the fracture itself should be considered.

The fracture location, configuration, degree of comminution, degree of contamination, and regional soft tissue damage influence prognosis. In general, a small horse (200–350 kg) with a closed, simple fracture of the distal limb, that is in good physical condition, and has an excellent temperament, has the best overall chance for survival. Large horses, with highly comminuted open fractures of the proximal limb have poor to grave prognoses for survival. Horses that have lost blood supply to the limb are not candidates for fracture repair. The prognosis for a specific fracture is best determined by consulting with regional surgical specialists that would be receiving the referral. Reaching out to a regional referral facility early in the process of treating these cases will aid in setting appropriate client expectations and optimizing patient care.

Discussing expectations and financial limitations with the owner before referral plays a vital role in ensuring patient welfare is protected and the horses are not transported for long distances with unrealistic treatment goals. Although there are many factors to consider for each patient, finances are a major influencing factor. The cost for internal fixation and fracture repair varies widely based on the local economics and the fracture itself. However, costs often range from $10,000 to $15,000 and in cases with complications can easily exceed $20,000 without guarantees of survival. Keeping this in mind if there is any doubt about the fracture's prognosis or the owner's wishes referral to a facility equipped to provide additional diagnostics and with surgical and anesthetic support can aid in the decision process. Ultimately, referral for additional information gathering can provide a valuable service to owners and the larger equine community.

Box 3
checklist for fracture management in the field

- Hemodynamic stabilization (fluid support if needed)
- Wound care and assessment
- Fracture stabilization
- Fracture assessment
- Consultation with local specialists if considering referral
- Tetanus prophylaxis
- Antimicrobial coverage as appropriate for fracture type
- Appropriate trailer for transportation if indicated with ramp or small step

---

TRANSPORTATION

Transportation is extremely stressful for horses with an unstable limb. Even with an appropriate splinting device, they must still balance most of their weight on 3 legs. Anything that can be done to improve transportation of the fracture patient will increase the chances for a successful outcome. If available, horses should be transported in a specialized trailer containing a sling. The sling allows the patient to rest intermittently if desired and will prevent the horse from falling down. However, in most cases a specialized trailer cannot be obtained. Therefore, a large trailer that has movable partitions, is low to the ground or has a ramp is the best choice. Horses require a lot of room to load and unload, but need a firm wall to lean on during transportation.[5] Loading seems to be less traumatic than unloading, but under both circumstances, horse will require assistance.

Having a step trailer that is low to the ground or a trailer with a ramp will greatly facilitate loading and unloading the fracture patient. With both forelimb and hindlimb fractures, horses should be loaded forward. During transportation, horses with forelimb fractures should be positioned facing backward in the trailer. It is much easier for them to support their weight if there is need to make a sudden stop. For similar reasons, horses with hindlimb fractures should be transported facing forward. When unloading, horses with forelimb fractures should be unloaded backward, and horses with hindlimb fractures should be unloaded forward. A large trailer with movable partitions will facilitate changing a horse from facing forward to backward throughout the transportation process.

SUMMARY

Fracture stabilization in the field is a critical part of fracture management and treatment. Successful fracture repair begins with assessment of the fracture and the horses overall health in the field. Timely treatment of wounds, assessment of hydration status, and fracture stabilization are critical. Application of an appropriate splint will minimizes damaging forces and avoid creating a lever arm at the fracture site that risks causing additional tissue damage. Stabilizing the patient by addressing the fracture and systemic health allows time for the owner and clinicians to assess the fracture and make informed treatment decisions. These steps are summarized for in a checklist for fracture management in the field (**Box 3**). A stable patient will improve the health of the patient during transport and increase the opportunities for successful fracture repair.

CLINICS CARE POINTS

- Fracture stabilization in the field is critical to potential future repair
- Addressing systemic condition of the patient will ultimately improve outcomes
- Splints are invaluable but are contraindicated in some proximal limb fracture due to the potential to cause additional injury
- Radiographs obtained after splinting are often sufficient for initial assessment and referral

DISCLOSURE

The authors have no conflicts of interest to report.

REFERENCES

1. Magdesian KG. Replacement fluids therapy in horses. In: Langdon C, Magdesian KG, editors. Equine fluid therapy. Ames, Iowa: John Wiley & Sons, Inc; 2015. p. 161–74. https://doi.org/10.1002/9781118928189.ch12.
2. Curtiss AL, Stefanovski D, Richardson DW. Surgical site infection associated with equine orthopedic internal fixation: 155 cases (2008–2016). Vet Surg 2019;48(5): 685–93.
3. Davison EJ, Orsini JA. Musculoskeletal system. In: Orsini JA, Divers TJ, editors. Equine emergencies treatments and procedures. 4th ediition. St Louis, MO: Elsevier Inc.; 2014. p. 155–70. https://doi.org/10.1016/B978-1-4557-0892-5.00021-0.
4. Mudge MC, Bramlage LR. Field fracture management. Vet Clin North Am Equine Pract 2007;23(1):117–33. Available at: http://www.sciencedirect.com/science/article/pii/S0749073906000897.
5. Bramlage LR. First aid and transportation of equine fracture patients. In: Equine fracture repair. Wiley Online Books; 2019. p. 83–90. https://doi.org/10.1002/9781119108757.ch6.
6. Tremaine H. Management of skull fractures in the horse. In Pract 2004;26(4):214 LP–22 LP. Available at: http://inpractice.bmj.com/content/26/4/214.abstract.
7. Gerding JC, Clode A, Gilger BC, et al. Equine orbital fractures: A review of 18 cases (2006-2013). Vet Ophthalmol 2014;17(SUPPL. 1):97–106.
8. Ramzan PHL. Management of rostral mandibular fractures in the young horse. Equine Vet Educ 2008;20(2):107–12.

Respiratory Distress in the Adult and Foal

Ashley G. Boyle, DVM, DACVIM*

KEYWORDS

- Upper respiratory • Lower respiratory • Trachea • Nasopharynx • Lung • Pulmonary
- Obstruction

KEY POINTS

- It is important to identify the anatomic source of the respiratory distress (upper vs lower respiratory tract [noise/no noise] vs nonrespiratory).
- Establish or maintain an airway if necessary using a nasogastric tube or via tracheostomy.
- Ultrasound, endoscopy, and tracheostomy tubes are useful tools to have on the truck.
- Try to avoid the use of sedation in these animals owing to respiratory compromise.

 Video content accompanies this article at http://www.vetequine.theclinics.com.

INTRODUCTION

Respiratory distress in the horse and foal is an emergency. Managing equine respiratory distress in the field starts with appropriate assessment of the patient to determine whether the breathing obstruction stems from the upper or lower respiratory tract or is nonrespiratory in origin. The veterinarian must assess the severity of the situation, take action to attempt to relieve the distress mechanically or medically, and determine the need to triage the animal for hospitalization if possible. Establishing an airway in upper respiratory distress is a lifesaving procedure and should be followed by maintaining adequate breathing and circulation. Diagnosing the cause of respiratory distress is necessary to direct treatment appropriately.

DEFINITIONS AND PATHOPHYSIOLOGY

Respiratory distress is an excessive degree of effort to breathe based on an assessment of respiratory rate, rhythm, and character. It often suggests that breathing is

Department of Clinical Studies New Bolton Center, University of Pennsylvania School of Veterinary Medicine, 382 West Street Road, Kennett Square, PA 19348, USA
* Corresponding author.
E-mail address: boylea@vet.upenn.edu

Vet Clin Equine 37 (2021) 311–325
https://doi.org/10.1016/j.cveq.2021.04.005
0749-0739/21/© 2021 Elsevier Inc. All rights reserved.

labored.[1] The term dyspnea is sometimes used interchangeably with respiratory distress, but is more accurately used in human medicine owing to it being a subjective feeling of difficult breathing or shortness of breath.[1] Respiratory distress is caused by hypoxia (PaO_2 lower than 80 mm Hg), which is most commonly due to a lack of proper movement of oxygen-containing air into and out of the lungs, but can also be due to the inability of the blood to carry oxygen or the inability of the tissues to process the oxygen.[1]

CLINICAL SIGNS

Horse and foals that are in respiratory distress will have abnormal respiratory rates, rhythm, and character to their breathing or various combinations of these signs.[1] Tachypnea is a common finding in animals with respiratory distress. The normal respiratory rate at rest for the horse is 8 to 16 breaths per minute and can be slightly faster in the foal depending on its age. Increased ambient temperature can raise the respiratory rate of the horse as the horse attempts to cool itself. In the normal horse, breathing should be regular and not be labored. Horses in respiratory distress often have increased abdominal effort and flared nostrils. Severe respiratory distress may result in retractions. Horses may have a concurrent cough, have nasal discharge, and usually have exercise intolerance. Special attention should be paid to the presence or absence of upper respiratory noise (stridor on inspiration [most common] or stertor on expiration). Auscultation of the trachea can help identify more subtle noises originating from the upper respiratory tract.

The animal's stance should be noted. Horses with abducted elbows or reluctance to walk may have a pleural component to their disease. Animals may have an inspiratory or expiratory grunt (see Video 1). The grunt is an attempt to maintain an adequate lung volume (usually on expiration) against a partially closed glottis.[2] Expiratory grunts have been considered the cardinal sign of lobar pneumonia in humans and provides physiologic advantages to the compromised patient. It was the mainstay for the development of positive-pressure breathing therapy. It is thought to physiologically help prevent lung edema by preventing the release of serum from the lung capillaries by positive pressure on pulmonary circulation.[3]

PHYSICAL EXAMINATION FINDINGS

Examination of the mucous membranes should be the first thing performed in physical examination. The veterinarian must assess mucous membrane color, capillary refill time, and the presence of petechia and ecchymoses. Cyanotic mucous membrane is a sign of central cyanosis and does not occur until PaO_2 is lower than 40 mm Hg, indicating a dire situation unless corrected immediately. It represents inadequate oxygenation of arterial blood or the presence of abnormal hemoglobin.[4] In addition to respiratory rate, heart rate and temperature should be obtained. Note the character, regularity, and pattern of breathing as well as the symmetry and synchronicity of the chest excursions.

Determine the amount of airflow from each nostril. Percussion of the sinuses may reveal a change in density and facial asymmetry, revealing a mass effect resulting in upper respiratory distress. Palpation of the submandibular and retropharyngeal regions may reveal enlarged lymph nodes, resulting in secondary airway obstruction. Auscult the trachea to assess for tracheal rattles and upper respiratory stridor. The normal lung field should extend from the shoulder musculature cranially to the seventeenth intercostal space at the level of the tuber coxae caudodorsally, with a curve returning cranioventrally to the level of the olecranon. The epaxial muscles border dorsally. Auscultation may reveal adventitial lung sounds that consist of crackles and wheezes. Crackles are short sounds caused by sudden pressure equalization when part of the airway opens during breathing, which are most commonly heard with pneumonia, interstitial fibrosis, chronic obstructive lung disease, congestive heart failure, and atelectasis. Wheezes result from the vibration of the airway walls at the end of the expiration or beginning of the inspiration.[5] Pleural friction rubs indicate pleural disease. Percussion can be used to determine a fluid line within the pleural space. Cardiac sounds may radiate owing to a consolidated lung field. Chronic respiratory distress may result in hypertrophy of the ventral abdominal muscles, resulting in a heave line. Cardiac auscultation should also be carefully examined for murmurs, dysrhythmias, and muffling of heart sounds in case respiratory distress is cardiac in origin.

PROCEDURES, EQUIPMENT, AND DIAGNOSTICS

The first and foremost issue to determine is whether the animal is in enough distress that emergency, lifesaving procedures need to occur before any other diagnostics. In the case of an upper respiratory obstruction, airway patency needs to be established. If severe nasal swelling has occurred, owners can pass cut pieces of the garden hose up the ventral meatus while they wait for the veterinarian's arrival. These can remain intact for as long as necessary while the veterinarian examines the animal. Another noninvasive technique to establish an airway is to pass a small nasogastric tube partially into the trachea if it will pass through the glottis. It then can be secured in place with medical tape. Emergency tracheotomy can also be performed to establish an airway via vertical incision through the skin and ventral neck muscles and horizontal incision between the tracheal rings (**Box 1**) (**Fig. 1**).

In addition to one's physical examination, additional diagnostics can be performed to determine the location and severity of the disease causing the respiratory distress. If upper respiratory noise is present, then upper airway endoscopy examination and radiography can be performed. Other reasons to perform an upper respiratory endoscopy examination include concurrent nasal discharge, epistaxis, coughing, dysphagia, and sometimes exercise intolerance. Ultrasonography is a particularly useful imaging modality to examine the lungs in the field. Owing to the limit of the

---

Box 1
Steps for performing a tracheotomy/temporary tracheostomy in the field

- Palpate the trachea on the ventral midline of the neck in the region between the upper and middle third of the neck in the horse.

- Clip the surgical area, and perform a sterile scrub.

- Place a local anesthetic (5–10 mL of 2% lidocaine) subcutaneously and into the paired sternothyrohyoideus muscles over the trachea.

- Using sterile technique, a 10-cm incision is made through the skin, subcutaneous tissue, and cutaneous colli muscle. The paired sternothyrohyoideus muscle bellies are bluntly divided along the ventral midline for a distance of about 8 cm and held in a retracted position using a self-retaining retractor.

- An incision is then made in the annular ligament between two adjacent cartilage rings such that the incision is parallel to the orientation of the cartilage rings and perpendicular to the skin incision. The incision between the rings is lengthened to allow placement of a tracheal cannula. The incision should not exceed one-half the circumference of the trachea.

- The tracheal tube is inserted through the incision (see **Fig. 1**).

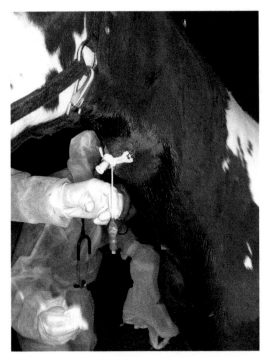

Fig. 1. Weanling with the tracheostomy tube in place that was experiencing severe upper respiratory stridor owing to retropharyngeal lymph node enlargement secondary to strangles.

radiographic plate size and x-ray penetration of mobile units, field thoracic radiography is typically only useful in the neonate or animals of similar size and stature. Ideally, a 2.5 to 5 mHz curvilinear probe that can penetrate to a depth of 30 cm works best for the thorax, but a rectal probe will also work. A linear probe will give you more definition but less depth.[6] Point-of-care ultrasound is now readily available, making ultrasound more affordable to put in every equine veterinary truck. The convenience of these handheld units that can be displayed on a mobile device makes them ideal for examining acute pathologies during time-sensitive emergencies.[7]

Additional equipment that can be helpful in the field includes a portable, handheld blood analyzer in which an arterial blood gas test could be performed (**Box 2**). Accessible arteries for blood collection include the facial artery or the brachial or greater metatarsal artery of a foal. A portable, battery-operated suction device can be useful to relieve pneumothorax.

Diagnostics that can assist in assessing the patient's systemic status and determining clinical management include a complete blood count, the clinical chemistry profile, and inflammatory proteins such as fibrinogen and serum amyloid A. Other diagnostics to consider are submissions for viral and bacterial testing.

UPPER RESPIRATORY CONDITIONS THAT CAUSE RESPIRATORY DISTRESS (WITH NOISE)

Many upper respiratory conditions can cause respiratory distress of the horse and foal. These conditions affect the nasal passages, nasopharynx, larynx, or trachea. Because horses are obligate nasal breathers, a bilateral nasal obstruction will prevent

---

Box 2
Equipment for respiratory emergencies in the field

Essential
  Narrow-diameter nasogastric tube
  Tracheostomy tube
  1-m Endoscope
  Ultrasound

Helpful
  Two 12-inch pieces of cut garden hose
  Portable suction device
  Handheld blood gas analyzer
  Portable oxygen tank for nasal insufflation (should be anchored in the vehicle during motion)

---

breathing. Nasal and laryngeal swelling secondary to edema can be life-threatening as in the case of anaphylaxis or snake envenomation. Rarely, horses have inhaled foreign bodies that become lodged in the trachea or a main stem bronchus, or potentially severe trauma to the nasal cavity may preclude smooth air flow. Establishing an airway in the case of respiratory distress with noise is essential. The following conditions are upper respiratory conditions that are causes of respiratory distress in the equid.

Strangles

Enlargement of the retropharyngeal lymph nodes from infection with *Streptococcus equi* subsp. *equi*, especially when swelling develops axially into the pharyngeal space, can result in significant narrowing of the nasopharynx and result in asphyxiation. These horses will often stand with an extended head and neck, and palpation of the retropharyngeal region will be turgid and sensitive to the touch (**Fig. 2**). When swelling is severe, these horses need emergency tracheostomies. Axial swelling into the pharynx and guttural pouch makes lymph nodes inaccessible for safe drainage via lancing. A tracheostomy can be performed as a preventative measure while the animal is concurrently treated with penicillin and nonsteroidal anti-inflammatories to resolve swelling.[8]

Nasopharyngeal Cicatrix

This condition is caused by inflammation that results in the scarring of the pharynx, guttural pouch openings, epiglottis, and/or arytenoid cartilages, which results in narrowing of the nasopharyngeal region. It is most commonly seen in older horses that are on pasture in the eastern and southern states bordering the Gulf of Mexico. Horses can present acutely, with less than 50% of the airway patent. These horses may have nasal discharge and exercise intolerance, but they typically do not cough. On endoscopy, the nasopharyngeal region will be hyperemic. Emergency tracheostomy may be required if the animal is in respiratory distress. Referral for diode laser treatment to break down the scarring in the nasopharyngeal region may improve airway patency, but some horses do require a permanent tracheostomy.[9]

Epiglottic Cyst/Subepiglottic Granuloma

A rare cause of respiratory distress is conditions affecting the epiglottis such as epiglottic cysts and granulomas. Depending on the size of the lesion, partial or full obstruction of the rima glottis can occur, resulting in upper respiratory noise, exercise

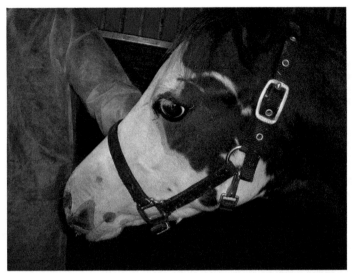

Fig. 2. Weanling with severe axial swelling of retropharyngeal lymph nodes secondary to infection with *Streptococcus equi* subsp. *equi* resulting in head and neck extension at rest.

intolerance, coughing, nasal discharge, and respiratory distress. Referral for surgical correction is required for these conditions.[10]

Arytenoid Chondropathy

Although arytenoid chondropathy typically presents with progressive upper respiratory noise and/or coughing, if ignored, the horse could present with acute respiratory distress, requiring an emergency tracheostomy. Arytenoid chondropathy is an upper airway condition in which the arytenoid cartilage mucosa is inflamed secondary to a bacterial or viral infection via hematogenous spread. It most commonly presents as a performance-limiting condition in thoroughbred racehorses. A recent Australian study highlighted the importance of common respiratory bacteria as causative agents of opportunistic infections in this disease as well as the importance of appropriate broad-spectrum antimicrobial usage and the possibility of involvement of multidrug-resistant bacteria.[11]

Snake Envenomation

Rattlesnake envenomation is a common cause of severe nasal swelling and resultant respiratory distress in horses in endemic areas. Horses are often bit on the nose, resulting in swelling and edema. Maintaining an airway for these horses is essential, and often, the horses are seen by the primary veterinarian before the nasal swelling is at its worst. Passage of a cut garden hose or nasogastric tube up the ventral nasal meatus can help prevent full obstruction in these horses until swelling is brought under control with steroidal or nonsteroidal anti-inflammatories, broad-spectrum antibiotics, and antivenom if available and financially feasible. A tetanus toxoid should also be administered if vaccination status is not up to date. Alternatively, in cases with severe swelling, a temporary tracheotomy may be necessary (see **Box 1**). These horses often need concurrent management of tissue necrosis, possible coagulopathies, and hemolytic anemia. Cardiac abnormalities are common in affected animals, so serial monitoring of cardiac troponin 1 and electrocardiogram (ECG) recordings is recommended.[12,13]

Tracheal Collapse

Noncongenital tracheal collapse in miniature horses and ponies occurs as the result of degeneration of the hyaline cartilage rings, weakening of the dorsal trachealis muscle, and elongation of dorsal tracheal ligament.[14,15] Donkeys may be predisposed to tracheal ring deformities.[16] Most commonly, this condition affects the extrathoracic trachea, presenting as an inspiratory stridor, but can present as expiratory noise if the intrathoracic trachea is affected.[17] Mild cases can be managed by keeping the animal calm and cool as well as managing any concurrent respiratory conditions such as lower air inflammatory disease. Animals that are hyperventilating will benefit from nasal insufflation oxygen therapy, decreasing the amount of collapse. More severe cases may require surgical stenting, but this has had varying success owing to the involvement of the dorsal tracheal ligaments and the intrathoracic component to this condition.[14]

Hyperkalemic Periodic Paralysis Pharyngeal Dysfunction

Hyperkalemic periodic paralysis (HYPP) is caused by the inherited defect in skeletal muscle sodium channels and can present in the adult as an acute attack with paralysis of the upper respiratory muscles. These animals may present with dysphagia and respiratory distress. This is most commonly seen in horses that are homozygous for HYPP, resulting in pharyngeal collapse, pharyngeal edema, and laryngeal paralysis.[18,19] Homozygous and heterozygous foals have presented with severe pharyngeal dysfunction at birth, resulting in respiratory distress and dysphagia. In both the adult and the neonate, an emergency tracheostomy may be needed to prevent asphyxia. As the foal matures, pharyngeal function may improve with time. Acute distress cases should also be managed by stabilizing the muscle membrane with slow administration of 23% calcium gluconate diluted in 0.9% NaCl (0.2–0.4 mL/kg) and reducing extracellular potassium levels with intravenously (IV) 5% dextrose solution alone (4–6 mL/kg) or in combination with 8.4% sodium bicarbonate (0.5–1.0 mEq/kg or 0.5–1.0 mL/kg).[18]

Atresia Choanae

A rare neonatal upper respiratory cause of distress is atresia choanae that is a respiratory emergency with a long-term guarded prognosis. It is a congenital malformation resulting in a membranous obstruction, preventing communication between the nasal cavity and the pharynx. If the condition is bilateral, the condition can be fatal unless an emergency tracheostomy is performed at birth because horses are obligate nasal breathers. The foal will require referral for repeated transendoscopic laser fenestration and bougienage procedures to prevent recurrent stenosis as the animal grows.[20]

Esophageal Obstruction

Although not respiratory in origin, esophageal obstruction can be a cause of respiratory distress with concurrent noise. Usually caused by a food bolus lodged in the proximal two-thirds of the esophagus, physical obstruction of the neighboring trachea or larynx may occur. In addition, horses are often quite stressed owing to the inability to swallow. As this condition is not primarily respiratory in origin, sedation is indicated to relax the horse's disposition and the esophagus. In acute, but mild, cases, esophageal relaxation with alpha-2 agonists may be sufficient to result in dislodgement and swallowing of the food bolus. Most cases require additional passage of a nasogastric tube to dislodge the bolus. In more severe cases with a dehydrated bolus, copious lavage via the nasogastric tube is required with or without systemic rehydration via intravenous fluids. Oxytocin (0.11–0.22 IU/kg IV) or buscopan (0.3 mg/kg IV or intramuscularly [IM]) can be used to relax the distal third of the esophagus that contains smooth muscle.[21] Nonsteroidal anti-inflammatories are used to control inflammation at the site of the bolus, and systemic broad-spectrum antibiotics are useful to prevent secondary aspiration pneumonia in cases that were obstructed for a prolonged period or required aggressive lavage.[22]

RESPIRATORY DISTRESS CAUSED BY LOWER RESPIRATORY CONDITIONS

A variety of lower respiratory conditions affecting the lung can cause respiratory distress. Many of the conditions require intensive monitoring and may require referral. Emergency triage should still focus on establishing an airway and then restoration of breathing, followed by circulation.[23] The underlying cause for the distress must be determined in order to focus on management.

Pneumonia and Pleuropneumonia

Severe pneumonia and pleuropneumonia, both viral and bacterial in origin, can result in acute respiratory distress. Animals may present with pleurodynia and be unwilling to move, but usually horses present with coughing, nasal discharge, fever, and/or anorexia. Increased bronchovesicular sounds may be evident on auscultation, with crackles and wheezes. The presence of pleural fluid can be identified on auscultation (evident by lack of lung sounds or radiating heart sounds) or by thoracic ultrasound, and thoracocentesis can be performed to relieve the respiratory distress. Aerobic and anaerobic culture and sensitivity of any pleural fluid retrieved should be analyzed in addition to samples obtained by means of a transtracheal wash. Broad-spectrum antibiotics such as penicillin (22,000–44,000 U/kg) and aminoglycosides are often the mainstay of bacterial pneumonia treatment until culture and sensitivity results are available, with metronidazole (15–25 mg/kg PO/PR QID) added when pleural involvement is evident.[24] Extensive supportive care may be required in cases of evidence of toxemia, and hospitalization would be indicated.

Pulmonary Edema

Pulmonary edema is typically secondary to a cardiogenic or noncardiogenic pathologic condition. The underlying pathologic condition results in alterations in forces that change the surface area and pore size of the blood-gas barrier, resulting in accumulation of extravascular fluid in the lung. Accumulation can also result owing to decreased lymphatic drainage.[25] Examples of underlying conditions are upper airway obstruction, fluid overload, anaphylaxis, and smoke inhalation. In order to relieve the pulmonary edema, both the resultant damage to the lung as well as the underlying cause must be treated. Horses present with shallow breathing and dyspnea; crackles and wheezes are heard on auscultation. Venous distension can be present in fluid overload. Fluid from the nose can be clear, yellow, or pink-tinged. Red fluid carries a poor prognosis. These animals often cough continuously and typically need referral for intensive monitoring and treatment with nasal insufflation of oxygen. They may need to be stabilized first with a combination of furosemide (1 mg/kg IV), bronchodilators (albuterol, 1–2 µg/kg q 1 hour via a metered-dose inhaler), steroids or nonsteroidal anti-inflammatories, and diphenhydramine (0.75–1 mg/kg IV). Epinephrine may be needed in case of anaphylaxis (0.02 mg/kg IV).[6]

Acute Respiratory Distress Syndrome

Acute respiratory distress syndrome is defined by severe pulmonary dysfunction as the result of injury to the lung or an exaggerated pulmonary immune response.[26] As the name suggests, this syndrome presents within 72 hours of the known insult such as a viral infection, bacterial infection such as that caused by *Rhodococcus equi*, smoke inhalation, or an extrapulmonary cause such as sepsis. Hypoxemia is present secondary to a dysregulated inflammatory response that results in pulmonary capillary leakage.[26] These animals typically require referral for intensive treatment, including nasal insufflation of oxygen for hypoxemia in combination with steroids and antibiotics.[27]

Pneumothorax

Pneumothorax occurs when air is present in the pleural space and not confined to the lung parenchyma. An open pneumothorax occurs when there is trauma to the thoracic wall and air moves freely in and out of the chest through the opening (see Video 2). The chest wall is intact in a closed pneumothorax in which the air moves in and out of the pleural space from the lung parenchyma secondary to infection such as pleuropneumonia, ruptured bullae, or a laceration from a fractured rib. A tension pneumothorax occurs when a one-way valve develops either in the thoracic wall or in lung parenchyma and air is trapped in the pleural space but cannot be exhaled. In a tension pneumothorax, if the intrathoracic pressure starts to exceed the atmospheric pressure, sudden death can occur owing to cardiopulmonary collapse.[28] These horses will typically present with flared nostrils and an increased respiratory rate. On auscultation, lung sounds will be absent, and there will be increased resonance dorsally on percussion. The lack of movement of the hyperechoic visceral pleural line (lack of the gliding lung sign) on ultrasound is indicative of a pneumothorax[29] (see Videos 3A and 3B). M-mode ultrasound has been described as a useful tool to identify pneumothorax. The normal lung has a seashore appearance, and the pneumothorax has a barcode appearance (also called the stratosphere sign)[29] (**Fig. 3**A and **B**).

Initial treatment should be instituted by providing temporary closure of any chest wound by packing or bandaging to minimize the severity of the pneumothorax (**Figs. 4** and **5**). Kitchen cling wrap works well, but in the field, any bandage that keeps it closed is sufficient. Once the wound is sealed, remove the pleural air by inserting a sterile teat cannula or 14 g catheter using a stylet into the dorsal thorax between the 11th and 15th intercostal space just cranial to the rib. Attach an extension set with a 3-way stopcock and a 60-mL syringe or attach to a portable suction pump. If the wound is acting like a one-way valve causing a tension pneumothorax, a teat cannula into the wound will normalize the pressure.[23] Broad-spectrum systemic antibiotics and triage to a referral hospital may be necessary once stabilized in order to provide effective monitoring.

Hemothorax

Hemothorax can be differentiated from pneumothorax on auscultation and percussion by reduced lung sounds ventrally and percussion of a fluid line. Hemothorax can then be differentiated from pleural effusion via the evidence of anechoic swirling on ultrasonographic examination. A thorough history may also help differentiate hemothorax from pleural effusion. Drainage is not recommended unless the animal is in severe respiratory distress. The blood within the thoracic cavity can inhibit further bleeding if the active site is below the blood fluid line and some of the red blood cells will be reabsorbed. Initial treatment with broad-spectrum systemic antibiotics to prevent infection and possibly hemostatic agents such as aminocaproic acid to curtail hemorrhage can be instituted. Stabilization and monitoring of these patients is intensive, and referral to a hospital setting is prudent.[23]

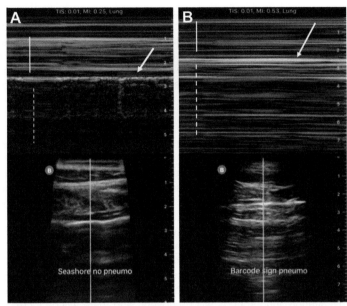

Fig. 3. (*A*) Transverse M-mode ultrasonographic images of the caudodorsal aspect of the thoracic cavity of the normal horse. The solid white line represents the body wall and subcutaneous tissues. The white arrow represents the parietal pleural line. The white dashed line represents the seashore pattern created by the constant movement of the lung parenchyma. (*B*) Transverse M-mode ultrasonographic images of the caudodorsal aspect of the thoracic cavity of a horse with a pneumothorax. The solid white vertical line represents the body wall and subcutaneous tissues. The white arrow is pointing at the hyperechoic region that represents the parietal pleural line. The white dashed line represents the stratosphere or barcode sign indicative of a pneumothorax. (*A*) (*Courtesy of* Dr. Cristobal Navas de Solis, University of Pennsylvania, New Bolton Center.) (*B*) (*Courtesy of* Dr. Cristobal Navas de Solis, University of Pennsylvania, New Bolton Center.)

Equine Asthma

Severe equine asthma can cause a range of clinical distress. More severe episodes often stem from an exacerbation of more mild disease or a lack of control of the condition. Sudden attacks can develop owing to poor air quality and environmental conditions. Horses present with a significant abdominal component to their breathing pattern and exercise intolerance (see Video 4). In severe cases of respiratory distress, the horse may not eat because the horse is using all of its effort to breathe. These horses lose weight quite quickly if not adequately controlled. More mild distress may present with coughing and exercise intolerance, but the horse may still be seen eating. Asthmatic horses in distress usually require a combination of systemic corticosteroids (dexamethasone, 0.04 mg/kg IV or IM) for immediate relief in combination with bronchodilators (albuterol, 1–2 μg/kg q 1–2 hours via a metered-dose inhaler or clenbuterol, 0.8 μg/kg PO). Inhaled corticosteroids (ciclesonide, 2744 μg/kg BID for 5 days and then 4116 μg/kg SID for 5 days or fluticasone, 1–6 μg/kg q 12 hours) can be used instead for acute and longer term management along with the necessary environmental managements such as soaked hay or a complete pelleted diet. It is important to remember to not use only bronchodilators for this will further expose the airways to irritants and not treat the inflammation in the lower airway.[30]

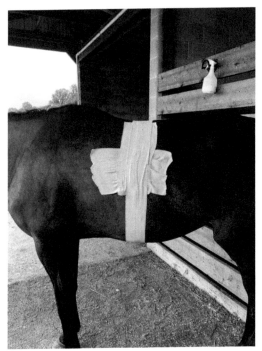

Fig. 4. Thoracic wall wound with pneumothorax bandaged with elasticon.

Rib Fractures in Foals

Rib fractures in foals are more commonly seen in fillies, on the left side, and in foals from multiparous dams. They typically occur just dorsal to the costochondral junction of ribs 3 to 8. Rib fractures are easily overlooked but can cause respiratory distress. Closely examine the chest wall for asymmetry between sides and trauma at the level of the costochondral junction or evidence of crepitus. Ultrasound was found to be more accurate than radiography for identification of rib fractures in an emergency. Additionally, ultrasound permits characterization of concurrent thoracic abnormalities such as pleural fluid accumulation, pulmonary contusion, or pericardial effusion. If a foal is in respiratory distress secondary to a rib fracture, one should consider additional pathology internally such as visceral lung and arterial lacerations.[31] Flail chest develops when two or more adjacent ribs are fractured, resulting in an unstable section of the rib cage and paradoxic movement during respiration. Stabilization in the field consists of analgesia and movement restriction for up to 4 weeks. Other supportive care may include antibiotics and antiulcer medications. Referral may be necessary depending on the degree of compromise, and although surgical intervention is usually not necessary, it should be considered in cases wherein there is potential for intrathoracic injury. Bandaging of a flail chest in contraindicated because it causes inward stabilization of the section and can result in pulmonary injury and more respiratory distress.[23]

Selenium and Vitamin E Deficiency

Nutritional myodegeneration in foals secondary to selenium or vitamin E deficiency in the dam's diet during gestation most commonly presents with a slower onset of

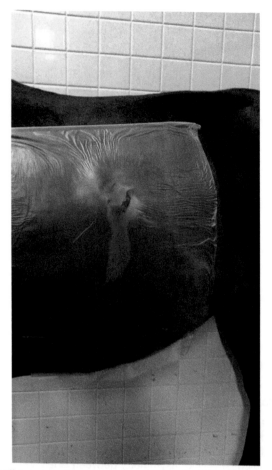

Fig. 5. Thoracic wall wound with pneumothorax closed with sterile brown gauze packing and wrapped with sterile adhesive dressing.

muscle weakness, trembling, or recumbency, but can affect the muscles of the diaphragm and intercostal muscles, resulting in respiratory distress. Foals may present with respiratory distress, which originates from the upper airway, owing to weakened pharyngeal and laryngeal musculature. Diagnosis is based on the geographic location and clinical signs. Blood can be drawn to measure levels of selenium, with levels lower than 10 mg/dL indicative of deficiency. The need for intensive supportive care will depend on the severity of clinical signs along with supplementation of selenium and vitamin E.[32,33]

NONRESPIRATORY CAUSES OF RESPIRATORY DISTRESS

There are many causes of respiratory distress that do not originate from the respiratory tract. A thorough physical examination, history taking, and a complete blood count are important to identify these nonrespiratory causes of distress. Oxygen exchange can be limited by altered hemoglobin (as in red maple toxicity), significant anemia, and acute blood loss. Acute cardiac disease that results in left-sided cardiac overload will lead to respiratory distress with a poor prognosis. This emphasizes the importance of careful cardiac auscultation in these horses. Horses with hyperthermia will also present with respiratory distress because the respiratory tract tries to assist in cooling the body. Hyperthermia can be due to exercise in excessive heat, which is seen in racehorses, endurance horses, and buggy horses. Anhidrosis can also result in tachypnea as the horse's body tries to cool itself through the respiratory tract owing to lack of sweating. Drug-induced hyperthermia is common in foals during high ambient temperatures while on treatment with erythromycin and, less commonly, other macrolides. Animals with hyperthermia need to be moved to a cool environment. These animals can be hosed with cool water with special attention to the large vessels of the body, and then the water removed with a scraper.[34,35] Alpha-2 agonist sedatives cause tachypnea and a drop in body temperature in febrile horses.[36] One of the hallmark signs of the systemic inflammatory response syndrome is either tachypnea or hyperventilation.[37] Finally, pain can result in respiratory distress in the horse.

SUMMARY

When dealing with the equid in respiratory distress, a thorough but efficient physical examination should be performed to determine if the cause is originating from the upper respiratory tract (most commonly with noise), is originating from the lower respiratory tract, or is nonrespiratory in origin. Establishing an airway is paramount, followed by maintaining breathing and circulation, to allow for proper airway exchange and eliminate hypoxia. Endoscopy and ultrasound are helpful imaging modalities when dealing with respiratory distress and can be easily performed in the field. It is also important to try to avoid sedation in animals with respiratory compromise, for this could worsen the condition further.

CLINICS CARE POINTS

- It is important to identify the anatomic source of the respiratory distress (upper vs lower respiratory tract [noise/no noise] vs nonrespiratory).
- Establish or maintain an airway, if necessary, using a nasogastric tube or via tracheostomy.
- Ultrasound, endoscopy, and tracheostomy tubes are useful tools to have on the truck.
- Try to avoid sedation in these animals owing to respiratory compromise.

DISCLOSURE

The author has nothing to disclose.

REFERENCES

1. Lakritz J. Alterations in respiratory function. In: Smith B, Van Metre D, Pusterla N, editors. Large animal internal medicine. Sixth edition. St. Louis: Elsevier; 2019. p. 43–81.
2. Wilkins PA. Lower respiratory problems of the neonate. Vet Clin North Am Equine Pract 2003;19(1):19–33.
3. Barach AL. Physiologic advantages of grunting, groaning, and pursed-lip breathing: adaptive symptoms related to the development of continuous positive pressure breathing. Bull N Y Acad Med 1973;49(8):666–73.
4. Krotje L. Cyanosis: physiology and pathogenesis. Compend Contin Educ Pract Vet 1987;9:271.
5. West J. Pulmonary pathophysiology. Baltimore: Williams and Wilkins; 1982.

6. Lascola K, Wilkins P, Woolums A. Diseases of the respiratory system. In: Smith B, Van Metre D, Pusterla N, editors. Large animal internal medicine. Sixth edition. St. Louis: Elsevier; 2019. p. 515–701.
7. Baribeau Y, Sharkey A, Chaudhary O, et al. Handheld point-of-care ultrasound probes: the new generation of POCUS. J Cardiothorac Vasc Anesth 2020; 34(11):3139–45.
8. Boyle AG, Timoney JF, Newton JR, et al. Streptococcus equi infections in horses: guidelines for treatment, control, and prevention of strangles-revised consensus statement. J Vet Intern Med 2018;32(2):633–47.
9. Chesen AB, Whitfield-Cargile C. Update on diseases and treatment of the pharynx. Vet Clin North Am Equine Pract 2015;31(1):1–11.
10. Aitken MR, Parente EJ. Epiglottic abnormalities in mature nonracehorses: 23 cases (1990–2009). J Am Vet Med Assoc 2011;238(12):1634–8.
11. Johnston GCA, Lumsden JM. Antimicrobial susceptibility of bacterial isolates from 33 thoroughbred horses with arytenoid chondropathy (2005-2019). Vet Surg 2020;49(7):1283–91.
12. Fielding CL, Pusterla N, Magdesian KG, et al. Rattlesnake envenomation in horses: 58 cases (1992-2009). J Am Vet Med Assoc 2011;238(5):631–5.
13. Gilliam LL, Holbrook TC, Ownby CL, et al. Cardiotoxicity, inflammation, and immune response after rattlesnake envenomation in the horse. J Vet Intern Med 2012;26(6):1457–63.
14. Aleman M, Nieto JE, Benak J, et al. Tracheal collapse in American Miniature Horses: 13 cases (1985-2007). J Am Vet Med Assoc 2008;233(8):1302–6.
15. Ida KK, Sauvage A, Gougnard A, et al. Use of nasotracheal intubation during general anesthesia in two ponies with tracheal collapse. Front Vet Sci 2018;5:42.
16. Powell RJ, du Toit N, Burden FA, et al. Morphological study of tracheal shape in donkeys with and without tracheal obstruction. Equine Vet J 2010;42(2):136–41.
17. Dallap Schaer B, Orsini J. Respiratory system. In: Orsini J, editor. Divers T equine emergencies: treatment and procedures. Fourth ed. St. Louis: Elsevier; 2014. p. 450–84.
18. Naylor JM. Hyperkalemic periodic paralysis. Vet Clin North Am Equine Pract 1997;13(1):129–44.
19. Rudolph JA, Spier SJ, Byrns G, et al. Linkage of hyperkalaemic periodic paralysis in quarter horses to the horse adult skeletal muscle sodium channel gene. Anim Genet 1992;23(3):241–50.
20. James FM, Parente EJ, Palmer JE. Management of bilateral choanal atresia in a foal. J Am Vet Med Assoc 2006;229(11):1784–9.
21. Meyer GA, Rashmir-Raven A, Helms RJ, et al. The effect of oxytocin on contractility of the equine oesophagus: a potential treatment for oesophageal obstruction. Equine Vet J 2000;32(2):151–5.
22. Chiavaccini L, Hassel DM. Clinical features and prognostic variables in 109 horses with esophageal obstruction (1992–2009). J Vet Intern Med 2010;24(5):1147–52.
23. Radcliffe RM. Thoracic trauma. In: Orsini J, Divers T, editors. Equine emergencies treatment and procedures. Fourth edition. St. Louis: Elsevier; 2014. p. p728–34.
24. Arroyo MG, Slovis NM, Moore GE, et al. Factors associated with survival in 97 horses with septic pleuropneumonia. J Vet Intern Med 2017;31(3):894–900.
25. Mellins RB, Stalcup SA. Pulmonary edema. In: Kendig EL, Chernick V, editors. Disorders of the respiratory tract in children. Fourth edition. Philadelphia: WB Saunders; 1983. p. 458.

26. ARDS Definition Task Force, Ranieri VM, Rubenfeld GD, Thompson BT, et al. Acute respiratory distress syndrome: the Berlin Definition. JAMA 2012;307(23): 2526–33.

27. Dunkel B, Dolente B, Boston RC. Acute lung injury/acute respiratory distress syndrome in 15 foals. Equine Vet J 2005;37(5):435–40.

28. Peroni J. Thoracic trauma: gasping for air. In: Proceedings, ACVS symposium. 2011. p. 52–4.

29. Partlow J, David F, Hunt LM, et al. Comparison of thoracic ultrasonography and radiography for the detection of induced small volume pneumothorax in the horse. Vet Radiol Ultrasound 2017;58(3):354–60.

30. Couëtil LL, Cardwell JM, Gerber V, et al. Inflammatory airway disease of horses–revised consensus statement. J Vet Intern Med 2016;30(2):503–15.

31. Jean D, Picandet V, Macieira S, et al. Detection of rib trauma in newborn foals in an equine critical care unit: a comparison of ultrasonography, radiography and physical examination. Equine Vet J 2007;39(2):158–63.

32. Dill S, Rebhun W. White muscle disease in foals. Compend Contin Educ Pract Vet 1985;7(11):S627–32.

33. Maylin GA, Rubin DS, Lein DH. Selenium and vitamin E in horses. Cornell Vet 1980;70(3):272–89.

34. Stratton-Phelps M, Wilson WD, Gardner IA. Risk of adverse effects in pneumonic foals treated with erythromycin versus other antibiotics: 143 cases (1986-1996). J Am Vet Med Assoc 2000;217(1):68–73.

35. Brownlow MA, Dart AJ, Jeffcott LB. Exertional heat illness: a review of the syndrome affecting racing Thoroughbreds in hot and humid climates. Aust Vet J 2016;94(7):240–7.

36. Kendall A, Mosley C, Bröjer J. Tachypnea and antipyresis in febrile horses after sedation with alpha-agonists. J Vet Intern Med 2010;24(4):1008–11.

37. Bone RC, Balk RA, Cerra FB, et al. Definitions for sepsis and organ failure and guidelines for the use of innovative therapies in sepsis. The ACCP/SCCM Consensus Conference Committee. American College of Chest Physicians/Society of Critical Care Medicine. Chest 1992;101(6):1644–55.

Approach to Toxicologic Emergencies

Julie E. Dechant, DVM, MS

KEYWORDS

- Toxicant • Decontamination • Antidotes • Activated charcoal

KEY POINTS

- Intoxication should be considered as a differential diagnosis when multiple herd mates are affected, there are unexplained deaths, or there is a collection of unusual clinical signs.
- Management should focus on stabilizing the patient and less emphasis on identifying an antidote or specifically counteracting the toxicant.
- A successful case outcome depends on prompt stabilization, good nursing and supportive care, and use of appropriate decontamination methods for the situation and patient.
- Be mindful of the legal implications of some toxicologic emergencies and the veterinarian's role in documenting, collecting, and securing evidence for a toxicologic event.

INTRODUCTION

Toxicologic emergencies in horses are relatively infrequent, especially when compared with humans or dogs;[1] however, intoxication is an important differential diagnosis to consider when multiple animals are affected, or presented with unusual clinical signs, unexplained deaths, or history of exposure to a potential toxicant. Historical events that have been associated with an increased risk of intoxication include recent introduction of animals to a property, feeding of poor-quality or inadequate feed, use of overgrazed pastures, change in management, change in feeding routine, feeding of a new feed or new batch of feed, administration of medication (especially, compounded medications) or supplements, recent wind storms that fell branches or trees, or recent yard work by gardeners or landscapers.[2] It is important for veterinarians to be familiar with plant-associated or environmental toxicants that have regional distributions and are relevant to their practice area.

Emergency management of an intoxication is simplified when there is exposure to a known toxicant because the treatment and monitoring can be targeted toward that specific toxin. It is much more common that the veterinarian will be presented with a sick animal or group of animals, without specific knowledge that an intoxication has occurred. Even if a toxicologic emergency is highly suspected, the veterinarian

Department of Surgical and Radiological Sciences, School of Veterinary Medicine, University of California, Davis, 2112 Tupper Hall, Davis, CA 95616, USA
E-mail address: jedechant@ucdavis.edu

Vet Clin Equine 37 (2021) 327–337
https://doi.org/10.1016/j.cveq.2021.04.006
0749-0739/21/© 2021 Elsevier Inc. All rights reserved.

should remain mindful of other differential diagnoses. There is a tendency in toxico-logic emergencies to unduly focus on identification of an antidote; however, antidotes are not available for many toxicants or not feasible or affordable for large animals, such as horses. Management should be prioritized at addressing the patient's needs and stabilizing clinical signs.

The intent of this review is to provide a broad overview of the approach to the field management of toxicologic emergencies, including triage, stabilization, collection of diagnostic samples, and decontamination. There will also be a predominant focus on causes of toxicologic emergencies in North America, although some of these tox-icants have relevance or correlates that are not geographically specific.

GENERAL APPROACH

Field management of toxicologic emergencies are challenging because available diagnostic, therapeutic, and personnel resources are limited compared with hospital situations. An important advantage to field assessment is context of the clinical envi-ronment, which means that the field veterinarian is able to recognize and identify pat-terns of locations, signalment, and distribution, as well as other environmental and management observations that may have important implications in the diagnosis of an intoxication.

Knowledge of the toxicant simplifies the approach to patient management because it allows the veterinarian to better anticipate the clinical course and to triage multiple patients. Regardless, a general approach to suspected intoxications, espe-cially those involving herd presentations, includes triage, emergency patient stabili-zation, complete physical evaluation, history taking, collection of diagnostic samples, decontamination and/or antidote administration, and supportive care and monitoring. The exact approach taken for each patient will vary, depending on specific clinical presentation, availability of treatment modalities, financial con-straints, availability of diagnostic tests, and knowledge of the toxicologic etiology. It is important to recognize that clinical signs may vary between individuals exposed to the same toxicant at the same time or different presentations of the same intox-ication. Age, individual sensitivity, dose, duration since exposure, source of expo-sure, and general health and nutritional status of the patient can produce a range of clinical severities and clinical presentations.[3]

If there is no known or witnessed exposure to a toxicant, the initial management of a suspected intoxication includes early consideration of toxicosis as a differential diag-nosis for the clinical presentation (**Box 1**). If multiple animals are exposed or affected, the initial step will be to triage the group of animals to prioritize and direct treatment efforts. Triage in situations involving multiple animals or multiple owners may be complicated by nonmedical issues, emotional factors, and financial considerations. It is important for the veterinarian to quickly assess these situations, identify these is-sues, and determine the best course of action for each scenario. For these compli-cated or multiple animal intoxications, it is equally important to recognize when additional help is needed and to recruit the assistance of colleagues or other veterinary personnel. Another important consideration early in the management of a toxicologic emergency is to prevent or eliminate exposure of other animals to the potential source of the toxicant. If the toxicant and its source are unknown and because ongoing expo-sure may be a possibility, herd mates should be moved from the current housing and provided with new feed and water, if possible. Any medications, supplements, feed, or topical products used on affected animals should not be used until the source of the intoxication is identified and those products are deemed safe. Although a relatively

---

Box 1
Characteristics associated with potential intoxications

- Multiple herd mates affected
- Unexplained deaths
- Collections of unusual clinical signs
- Presence of historical risk factors
  - Introduction of animals to a new property
  - Use of new feed or a new batch of feed
  - Feeding poor-quality or inadequate feed
  - Change in management or feeding routine
  - Recent windstorm that fell branches or trees
  - Yard work by landscapers

Data from Poppenga RH, Puschner B. Toxicology. In: Orsini JA, Divers TJ, editors. Equine Emergencies: Treatment and Procedures, 4th edition. St. Louis: Elsevier; 2014. p. 580-606.

---

uncommon circumstance, if there is a possibility of inhaled or dermal intoxicants, inadvertent exposure of personnel should be considered and prevented.[4]

STABILIZATION

Following initial triage of the situation, the next step is to focus on stabilizing the individual patient. Stabilization is not toxicant specific. The primary goal of emergency stabilization is to support essential organ function in order to provide time for other treatments (decontaminants, antidotes) to have an effect and to provide time for the body to eliminate the toxicant.[5] Vital signs (temperature, heart rate, respiratory rate and effort) and perfusion parameters (mucous membrane color, capillary refill time, pulse quality, extremity temperature) are assessed to direct and prioritize stabilization efforts.[6] Mentation changes can reflect either perfusion abnormalities and shock or the effects of the toxicant on the central nervous system. At least one large gauge intravenous catheter should be placed in severely poisoned patients.[7]

Stabilization is focused on the airway (A), breathing (B), circulation (C), and dysfunction (D) of critical patient care. The airway should be secured in any patient with respiratory obstruction or potential for airway obstruction owing to swelling of tissues, especially considering that horses are obligate nasal breathers.[1] Unconscious animals or animals with neuromuscular weakness may benefit from a secured airway and sternal positioning, if possible, to improve ventilation. The options to support ventilation by providing supplemental oxygen or assisted ventilation for management of hypoxemia or hypoventilation, respectively, are extremely limited and challenging in field situations, and immediate referral to a facility that can provide that level of care should be pursued.

Circulation is supported by administering intravenous fluids to correct hypovolemia and stabilizing cardiac function (rate, rhythm, contractility), as appropriate to the patient. The need for resuscitation and correction of fluid deficits will vary between patients because of differences in toxicant effects, the amount of toxicant exposure, duration since the exposure occurred, and patient variability. Fluid therapy can be further complicated if the toxicant impairs cardiac function. Small-volume fluid resuscitation in the field with hypertonic saline (2–4 mL/kg or 1–2 L/500 kg of horse) and small boluses (10–20 mL/kg or 5–10 L/500 kg of horse) of balanced electrolyte fluids should aid in stabilization of the patient, with the goal of allowing time for transportation to a referral center (**Table 1**).

Table 1
List of emergency drugs and dosages that may be useful in emergency management of toxicologic emergencies in horses

Target of Treatment	Emergency Drug	Dosage
Hypoxemia	Supplemental oxygen	100–150 mL/kg/min or 10–15 L/min if >100–150 kg
Intravenous fluid resuscitation	Hypertonic (7.0%–7.5%) saline	2–4 mL/kg IV administered no faster than 1 mL/kg/min
	Synthetic colloids (eg, hetastarch)	5–10 mL/kg IV
	Isotonic crystalloid fluids	10–20 mL/kg IV bolus, can repeat once for resuscitation
Hemorrhagic blood loss	Whole blood	10–20 mL/kg IV
Cholinergic-associated bradycardia	Atropine	0.005–0.01 mg/kg IV or IM
	Glycopyrrolate	0.002–0.01 mg/kg IV
	Butylscopolammonium bromide	0.3 mg/kg IV or IM
Ventricular arrhythmias	Lidocaine	0.25–0.5 mg/kg as IV bolus up to a total of 2 mg/kg
	Magnesium sulfate	2.2–5.6 mg/kg/min for 10 min up to a total of 25 g/500 kg
Seizure control	Diazepam	0.05–0.44 mg/kg IV
	Midazolam	0.1–0.2 mg/kg IV
	Phenobarbital	5–15 mg/kg IV q 8–12 h
Coagulopathy	Fresh or fresh frozen plasma	5–20 mL/kg IV
Decontamination	Activated charcoal	1–3 g/kg PO, followed by 0.25–0.5 g/kg PO every 1–6 h

Data from Hackett ES, Divers TJ, Orsini JA. Appendix 9: Equine emergency drugs: approximate dosages and adverse drug reactions. In: Orsini JA, Divers TJ, editors. Equine Emergencies: Treatment and Procedures, 4th edition. St. Louis: Elsevier; 2014. p. 835-860.

Organ dysfunction is the final category of critical patient stabilization. Metabolic derangements, such as hypoglycemia, metabolic acidosis, and electrolyte abnormalities, can often be present with intoxications, but these will typically not be identified without supportive laboratory data. The most life-threatening organ dysfunctions that can be identified clinically and would need to be addressed on an emergency basis include central nervous system derangements (seizures, muscle tremors, altered consciousness), body temperature alterations (hyperthermia or hypothermia), and coagulopathies (see **Table 1**).

Body temperature derangements should not be overlooked in the stabilization of toxicologic emergency patients. Of the two body temperature derangements, hyperthermia is the more difficult and life-threatening abnormality to modify. Toxicants that induce seizures or tremors are likely to be associated with hyperthermia; therefore, control of seizures or tremors is important to manage hyperthermia.[5] If body temperature is dangerously high, active cooling of the horse with ice water or alcohol baths and fans may be helpful. Hypothermia may be a problem in stuporous or comatose patients. Animals in cardiovascular shock may have subnormal body temperature, although this usually improves if resuscitation is successful. The disadvantage of hypothermia is the resulting reduction in the metabolic rate, which slows toxicant degradation and elimination.[5] Hypothermia can be managed with blankets, forced air warming systems (eg, 3M Bair Hugger), administration of warmed intravenous fluids, and careful use of heat lamps. Some of these rewarming strategies would be better deferred to hospital management rather than being instituted during field management.

Following initial stabilization, the veterinarian can direct attention to obtaining a thorough history and complete physical examination and developing a diagnostic plan.[6,8] The detailed history and physical examination can help identify comorbidities as well as provide further characterization of abnormalities to aid in the diagnosis of the intoxication.[2] Important historical details that should be investigated include timeline and progression, the number of animals affected or potentially exposed, initial clinical signs, potential feed or environment changes, and details of management, medications, and supplements.[2] Signs of intoxication can be subtle, and recognition of these subtle signs can be the key to a good clinical outcome.[9] The management plan should include diagnostic investigation of both the affected patient and of potentially exposed, nonclinical animals to address or prevent issues before they arise. Ongoing monitoring of the patient and response to stabilization is indicated as the clinical progression evolves or new clinical signs develop.

DIAGNOSTIC SAMPLING

A minimum database consisting of a complete blood count, biochemistry panel, including electrolytes, venous blood gas, and urinalysis is useful in attempting to differentiate toxicologic from nontoxicological etiologies and will identify important metabolic derangements.[4] Coagulation panels may be useful in certain situations. The use of point-of-care analyzers, such as lactate meters or handheld blood gas and laboratory analyzers, can provide valuable patient-side information to guide stabilization during field management of toxicologic emergencies.

It is important for the veterinarian to recognize that there is potential for legal action to be pursued by horse owners following intoxications.[2] This is most likely if the source of the toxicant is feed, supplements, or compounded medications. Veterinarians should carefully document the situation and their observations, including photographs, and collect, secure, and catalog any suspected sources of toxicants, including feed, medications, supplements, and so forth.[2]

A minimum of 10-mL volumes of EDTA-anticoagulated whole-blood and serum samples should be collected and submitted or stored for toxicologic analysis.[2,8] Urine (minimum volume: 20 mL) should be collected and stored, if not submitted immediately. Gastric contents or reflux and feces (a minimum of 100g) are important samples to collect, as is feed and water.[2,8] These samples should be stored in a leakproof container and labeled with patient information and the date of collection. Samples should be kept chilled or frozen (whole blood should be refrigerated, not frozen).[2,8] Bagged or baled feed, medication, or supplements should be secured, cataloged, and stored, in case there is future legal action.[2,8] The collection and submission or storage of appropriate samples can be selected in collaboration with the clinical toxicologist at the diagnostic laboratory.[2,3,8]

DECONTAMINATION

The purpose of decontamination is to prevent continued exposure to the toxicant.[4,6,7] Decontamination may be useful early in the patient's management, but it may not be appropriate or effective for all situations.[7] However, many decontamination strategies are applicable for field situations and can be performed before referral. Patients should be stabilized, and diagnostic samples should be collected before decontamination, if possible. Typical methods of decontamination used in veterinary medicine and applicable to field management of toxicologic emergencies are ocular, dermal, and gastrointestinal approaches.

Ocular decontamination is relevant to a very small minority of toxicant exposures and involves prolonged (a minimum of 20–30 minutes) eye lavage with isotonic saline solution.[10] Dermal exposure in large animals is often related to dosing errors of topically applied insecticide or pesticide products, and they are a relatively uncommon source of intoxication in horses. The most important consideration when doing dermal decontamination is the protection of personnel from inadvertent exposure to the toxicant while handling or bathing the animal.[4] Dermal decontamination is usually accomplished by bathing with liquid dishwashing soap (eg, Dawn) and copious rinsing with warm tap water.[10] Another form of dermal decontamination would be wound debridement in situations of wound botulism or tetanus; however, these are relatively unique situations.

It is estimated that oral ingestion is the route of exposure for approximately 80% of all intoxications in people.[11] This route is expected to be involved at least as commonly, if not higher proportions, in equine intoxications. Gastrointestinal decontamination methods applicable in small animals and people do not uniformly apply to horses owing to anatomic and physiologic differences.

Although not described in the literature, oral rinsing or flushing should be considered in horses that have ingested highly toxic plants, such as oleander. Horses can retain feed in their cheek pouches, which may be significant when a few leaves of a highly toxic plant (eg, oleander) can be fatal. Although this step is unlikely to guarantee successful treatment, it would reduce ongoing exposure to a highly potent toxicant.

Gastric lavage may be used as a substitute to remove ingested toxins from the stomach. It is much less effective in evacuating gastric contents than emesis, but emetics are contraindicated in horses. Gastric lavage uses irrigation to remove ingested contents from the stomach (instilling 10–12 mL/kg through a large-bore nasogastric tube and retrieving the fluid using a siphon).[12] There is a risk that the procedure will increase outflow of contents into the small intestine, where it is more readily absorbed.[4,10] Similarly, the procedure could induce electrolyte changes if large amounts of the lavage fluid are retained. Horses should be well sedated to lower their head and neck to reduce the risk of aspiration of lavage fluids. Use of warm water has been suggested to slow gastric emptying compared with cold water,[12] but this will not eliminate risks of the technique.

Activated charcoal is the most commonly used method for gastrointestinal decontamination in horses, but its use is not without controversy. The American Academy of Clinical Toxicology recommends against the use of activated charcoal in the management of human intoxications because of the risk of complications and the inability to demonstrate a survival benefit.[13–15] Activated charcoal remains a valuable therapeutic strategy in management of equine intoxications owing to its cost-effectiveness, efficacy, and applicability to toxicologic emergencies.[15]

Activated charcoal is a nonspecific absorbent that binds many toxicants and drugs, which then facilitates excretion of the adsorbed substance and reduces the amount of free agent available for absorption. The efficacy depends on the time since the toxicant was ingested, the ability of activated charcoal to adsorb the toxicant, and the potency of the ingested dose.[16] It is ineffective for treatment of ingestion of inorganic toxins, heavy metals, corrosive and caustic acids, petroleum products, and small polar molecules.[4,10,16,17]

Activated charcoal should be considered in the management of an ingested toxicant if administered early after exposure or if the toxicant undergoes enterohepatic circulation. Use of activated charcoal is contraindicated in an unconscious or regurgitating animal or for a toxicant that is, not adsorbed by activated charcoal.[15] If the dose of the toxicant is known, dosing of activated charcoal should be 10 times the toxicant dose by weight.[16,18] In reality, the toxicant dose is generally not known and activated charcoal should be dosed at 1 to 3 g/kg.[16] If the toxicant undergoes enterohepatic circulation, a loading dose of 1 to 2 g/kg should be administered, followed by repeated doses of 0.25 to 0.5 g/kg every 1 to 6 hours.[4] If sorbitol (70%; 3 mL/kg) is used concurrently with activated charcoal, sorbitol should not be administered repeatedly.

Other adsorbents are not recommended as substitutes for activated charcoal. Di-tri-octohedral smectite (250 g–1 kg/500 kg of horse q 24 hours) and kaolin-pectin have been suggested as alternatives, but their ability to adsorb toxicants is far inferior to activated charcoal.[10,19] The concurrent use of cathartics has been suggested to prevent stasis of gastrointestinal contents, regardless of whether activated charcoal is used or not; however, many cathartics can reduce the efficacy of activated charcoal or have the potential to cause additional derangements. Mineral oil is contraindicated in management of intoxications because it will reduce the efficacy of activated charcoal and may enhance absorption of certain toxicants.[20]

ANTIDOTES

Antidotes are therapeutic agents that act directly on a toxicant to decrease toxicity or increase elimination, to competitively inhibit the toxicant at its site of action, or to counteract the clinical effects produced by the toxicant.[10] Antidotes are often perceived as a critical intervention in the management of toxicologic emergencies; however, antidotes are often not available for the toxicant involved or are too costly for large animal patients. With rare exceptions, it is unlikely that an antidote will be available for use in field management of toxicologic emergencies. If an antidote is available and feasible to use, the timing of administration will depend on the toxicant, the antidote, and the situation (**Table 2**).[10]

REFERRAL

For most equine toxicologic emergencies, the primary goals of field management are to triage the situation, recognize intoxication as a differential diagnosis, reduce exposure of unaffected animals, and stabilize the affected animals before referral. Decontamination procedures can and should be initiated in the field, if appropriate, providing that patients are stable for decontamination. The field veterinarian is ideally positioned to collect a variety of samples for diagnostic purposes because the field veterinarian has access to the feed sources, supplements, medications, and the environment, as well as the patient. Referral hospitals should be contacted to discuss concerns and clinical findings, especially if multiple animals will be transferred to their care. The referral hospital can also be a resource for advice on triage, stabilization, selection of diagnostic samples, and decontamination. Clinical toxicologists at local diagnostic laboratories can provide advice on the workup of the case, possible toxicologic diagnoses, collection of samples, and preventative measures.[2]

TOXICITY BASED ON CLINICAL SIGNS

Veterinarians should prioritize treatment and management of their patient and its clinical signs, instead of becoming distracted by attempts to diagnose the toxicant or identify the antidote. Good supportive care and stabilization of physiologic derangements are the cornerstone to a successful outcome. However, there is no doubt

Table 2
Antidotes potentially available for use in equine toxicologic emergencies (Note that some of these antidotes are not readily available or cost-effective for use in horses.)

Potential Antidotes	Toxicant
Atropine (0.1–0.5 mg/kg; 25% of initial dose administered IV with remainder IM or SQ; given to effect)	Organophosphate/carbamate insecticides
Botulinum antitoxin, polyvalent and monovalent	Botulism neurotoxin
CaNa$_2$EDTA (75 mg/kg/d slow IV divided q 12 h; alternatively, 25 mg/kg SQ q 6 h for 5 d)	Lead, zinc
Calcitonin, bisphosphonates (dose not determined)	Cholecalciferol
Crotalid antivenom (dose to clinical signs; 1–5 vials)	Crotalid snake envenomation
Deferoxamine mesylate (10 mg/kg IM or IV slowly)	Iron
Digoxin Fab fragments (in people, 80 mg/1 mg of digoxin ingested; alternatively, 400–800 mg of Fab fragments IV)	Cardiac glycosides
D-penicillamine (copper, 10–15 mg/kg/d PO; lead, 110 mg/kg/d PO for 7–14 d)	Copper, lead
Pralidoxime chloride (2-PAM) (20 mg/kg slow IV, IM, or SQ q 12 h)	Organophosphate insecticides
Sodium nitrite (16 mg/kg IV once)	Cyanide
Sodium thiosulfates (30–40 mg/kg slow IV; may be repeated)	Arsenic, cyanide
Succimer (chelator; 10 mg/kg PO q 8 h for 5 d, then 10 mg/kg PO q 12 h for 14 d)	Lead, arsenic
Vitamin K1 (0.5–2 mg/kg SQ q 6 h for the first 24 h, followed by 1 mg/kg PO q 24 h for 4–6 d [first-generation anticoagulants] or 2.5–5.0 mg/kg PO q 24 h for 14–21 d [second-generation anticoagulants])	Anticoagulant rodenticides
Yohimbine (0.15 mg/kg slow IV; if clinical signs) or atipamezole (0.1 mg/kg slow IV; if clinical signs)	Amitraz

Data from Refs.[1,4,21]

that there are advantages in identifying the presence of a toxicant because it allows for better tailoring of targeted treatment for the patient, and prevention of further exposure of this patient or other animals to the toxicant, as well as alleviating some of the stress for the owner and veterinarian in not having a diagnosis. Human medicine has identified collections of signs and symptoms, termed toxidromes, that are associated with different classes of potential toxicants.[6,22] These toxidromes are well defined in human medicine and help the clinician in directing specific treatments. Toxidromes have not been defined in veterinary medicine, but they can be helpful in identifying the primarily affected organ or distinctive clinical sign attributable to various toxicants (**Table 3**).

SUMMARY

The most important aspect of treating any toxicologic emergency is to focus on treating the patient and the patient's clinical signs rather than focusing on the toxicant itself. It is important to be open to other differential diagnoses when treating these

Table 3
Predominant localizing body system effect or localizing clinical signs associated with toxicants

Localizing Body System or Clinical Sign	Toxicant
Gastrointestinal	Amitraz Tropane alkaloids/atropine toxicosis Blister beetle/cantharidin (also hematuria) Oak (also renal injury) Oleander (also cardiac arrhythmias and renal injury) Organophosphate and carbamate insecticides (also salivation, lacrimation, sweating, muscle tremors, dyspnea) Red clover (salivation) Arsenic and mercury
Neurologic	Avocado (cardiac arrhythmias possible) Botulism Fumonsin mycotoxins Ivermectin/moxidectin Lead Locoweed Marijuana/hemp (also colic) Phosphide salts (also sweating, muscle tremors, pyrexia, hypoglycemia) Ryegrass Selenium Sudan grass (cystitis, +/– cyanide) White snakeroot (also arrhythmias, cardiac failure) Yellow star thistle
Hepatic injury or failure	Aflatoxins Alsike clover (also photosensitization) Blue-green algae (also neurotoxic, sudden death) Iron Kleingrass or fall panicum Pyrrolizidine alkaloids (hepatic encephalopathy)
Cardiac	Cyanide (also erythrocyte changes) Ionophore Oleander/cardiac glycosides (also gastrointestinal and renal) Yew
Renal injury	Cantharidin Oak (also gastrointestinal) Oleander (also gastrointestinal and cardiac)
Erythrocyte changes	Cyanide *Pistacia* leaves Red maple Wild onion
Coagulopathy	Anticoagulant rodenticide poisoning Moldy sweet clover
Pigmenturia	Cantharidin (also gastrointestinal) Ionophores (also cardiotoxin) *Pistacia* leaves Red maple Seasonal atypical pasture myopathy (box elder)

Data from Refs.[1,2,8]

cases, regardless of whether intoxication is highly suspected or not. It is equally important to balance the benefits and risks of decontamination or antidote treatment. A successful case outcome depends on prompt stabilization, good nursing and supportive care, and the use of appropriate decontamination methods for the situation and the patient.

CLINICS CARE POINTS

- Direct treatment on the patient and the clinical signs.
- Do not focus on a specific treatment or intervention to the detriment of the patient's overall wellbeing.
- Completely evaluate the patient and obtain a thorough history.
- Balance risks of decontamination procedures against the benefits.
- Be mindful of potential exposure of yourself or others to the toxicant when handling or decontaminating animals, particularly those with dermal (e.g., topical organophosphates) or inhalational (e.g. phosphide salt ingestion) intoxicant exposures.
- Do not use mineral oil for management of a gastrointestinal toxicant—at a minimum, it is unlikely to provide a benefit and at worst, it will interfere with potentially efficacious treatments or facilitate absorption of toxins.
- Collect and test a variety of sample types, because different samples may be needed to identify the toxicant and establish a diagnosis.
- Perform necropsy examinations on deceased animals when investigating unexplained deaths, especially in a herd situation, so that a variety of samples and tissues can be collected for pathological, microbiological, and toxicological testing.
- Be aware of the legal implications of some intoxication exposures, and be careful to collect, catalog, and secure diagnostic samples and document clinical findings.
- Become familiar with poisonous plants and environmental toxins present in your geographical area.

DISCLOSURE

The author has nothing to disclose.

REFERENCES

1. Poppenga RH. Toxicology. In: Southwood LL, Wilkins PA, editors. Equine emergency and critical care medicine. Boca Raton: CRC Press; 2015. p. 555–620.
2. Poppenga RH, Puschner B. Toxicology. In: Orsini JA, Divers TJ, editors. Equine emergencies: treatment and procedures. 4th edition. St. Louis: Elsevier; 2014. p. 580–606.
3. McGuirk SM, Semrad SD. Toxicologic emergencies in cattle. Vet Clin Food Anim 2005;21:729–49.
4. Poppenga RH. Treatment. In: Plumlee KH, editor. Clinical veterinary toxicology. St. Louis: Elsevier; 2004. p. 13–21.
5. Landolt GA. Management of equine poisoning and envenomation. Vet Clin North Am Equine Pract 2007;23:31–47.
6. Thompson TM, Theobald J, Erickson TB. The general approach to the poisoned patient. Dis A Month 2014;60:509–24.
7. Boyle JS, Bechtel LK, Holstege CP. Management of the critically poisoned patient. Scand J Trauma Resus Emerg Med 2009;17:29.

8. Puschner B, Dechant JE. Common toxins in equine practice. In: Sprayberry KA, Robinson NE, editors. Robinson's current therapy in equine medicine. 7th edition. St Louis: Elsevier; 2015. p. 922–7.

9. Kirk M, Pace S. Pearls, pitfalls, and updates in toxicology. Emerg Med Clin North Am 1997;15:427–49.

10. De Clementi C. Prevention and treatment of poisoning. In: Gupta RC, editor. Veterinary toxicology: basic and clinical principles. 3rd edition. London: Elsevier; 2018. p. 1141–59.

11. Holstege CP, Dobmeier SG, Bechtel LK. Critical care toxicology. Emerg Med Clin North Am 2008;26:715–39.

12. Beasley V. Diagnosis and management of toxicosis. In: Beasley V, editor. Veterinary toxicology. New York: International Veterinary Information Service; 1999. Available at: http://www.ivis.org/advances/Beasley/Cpt1B/chapter_frm.asp?LA=1. Accessed August 31, 2020.

13. Anonymous. Position statement and practice guidelines on the use of multi-dose activated charcoal in the treatment of acute poisoning. American Academy of Clinical Toxicology; European Association of Poison Centres and Clinical Toxicologists. J Toxicol Clin Toxicol 1999;37:731–51.

14. Chyka PA, Seger D, Krenzelok EP, et al. Position paper: single-dose activated charcoal. Clin Toxicol (Phila) 2005;43:61–87.

15. Juurlink DN. Activated charcoal for acute overdose: a reappraisal. Br J Clin Pharmacol 2015;81:482–7.

16. El Bahri L. Pharm profile: activated charcoal. Compend Contin Educ Vet 2008;30: 596–8.

17. Neuvonen PJ, Olkkola KT. Oral activated charcoal in the treatment of intoxications. Role of single and repeated doses. Med Toxicol Adverse Drug Exp 1988; 3:33–58.

18. Peterson ME. Toxicologic decontamination. In: Peterson ME, Talcott PA, editors. Small animal toxicology. 3rd edition. St. Louis: Elsevier; 2013. p. 73–83.

19. Tiwary AK, Poppenga RH, Puschner B. In vitro study of the effectiveness of three commercial adsorbents for binding oleander toxins. Clin Toxicol (Phila) 2009;47: 213–8.

20. Qualls HJ, Holbrook TC, Gilliam LL, et al. Evaluation of efficacy of mineral oil, charcoal, and smectite in a rat model of equine cantharidin toxicosis. J Vet Intern Med 2013;27:1179–84.

21. Hackett ES, Divers TJ, Orsini JA. Appendix 9: Equine emergency drugs: approximate dosages and adverse drug reactions. In: Orsini JA, Divers TJ, editors. Equine emergencies: treatment and procedures. 4th edition. St. Louis: Elsevier; 2014. p. 835–60.

22. Rasimas JJ, Sinclair CM. Assessment and management of toxidromes in the critical care unit. Crit Care Clin 2017;33:521–41.

Managing Reproduction Emergencies in the Field

Part 1: Injuries in Stallions; Injury of the External Portion of the Reproductive Tract and Gestational Conditions in the Mare

Kim A. Sprayberry, DVM[a],*, Kristina G. Lu, VMD[b]

KEYWORDS

- Vaginal • Trauma • Placentitis • Uterine torsion • Penile injury • Testicular injury
- Paraphimosis • Priapism

KEY POINTS

- Injuries or emergent conditions involving the reproductive tract are common in equine practice, and initial care measures can play a substantial role in determining short- and long-term outcomes.
- Interventions for the various injuries of the male external genitalia have in common the goal of mitigating inflammation and edema, preventing secondary problems from dependent positioning, and preserving neurologic function.
- Placentitis does not represent a life risk for the dam but is an emergency condition for the fetus; foals should be considered at risk for sepsis and encephalopathy after birth, and monitored accordingly.
- Hydropsic conditions can be detected and monitored sonographically, and elective controlled reduction of the voluminous fluid is often the intervention of choice.
- Uterine torsion can be challenging to definitively diagnose and manage in the field.

INTRODUCTION

In the gamut of reproduction-related emergency conditions in horses, dystocia in the mare may be the problem most familiar to equine veterinarians and horse owners—the specter of birth-related problems rightfully elicits much preparation and client education from veterinarians to recognize and prepare for parturition-related emergencies— but there are many other conditions affecting the reproductive tract that also represent

Funded by: CSU2020.
[a] Department of Animal Sciences, Cal Poly University San Luis Obispo, Cal Poly University, 1 Grand Avenue, San Luis Obispo, CA 93407, USA; [b] Hagyard Equine Medical Institute, 4250 Iron Works Pike, Lexington, KY 40511, USA
* Corresponding author.
E-mail address: kspraybe@calpoly.edu

significant problems in which timely intervention is imperative. As with emergencies involving any other organ system, minimizing the time to diagnosis and intervention is key to a positive outcome. Therefore, the ability to recognize and intervene in these conditions is an important part of the knowledge base for veterinarians whose practice includes breeding animals. This article will review guidelines for managing selected emergency conditions involving the reproductive tract in stallions, and that involve the external portion of the tract or arise during gestation in mares. The goal is to help prepare the veterinarian to recognize and confidently undertake or at least initiate effective interventions for these problems in the field.

Conditions of the External Portion of the Reproductive Tract of Mares

Injury of the vestibule and vagina

Lacerations of the vagina, transverse fold, and vestibule most commonly occur during breeding and foaling. The vulva and vestibule are also an occasional site of injury from kicking wounds from other mares; the hind foot of the kicking mare can abrade and lacerate the vulva and enter the vestibule and tear the mucosa (**Fig. 1**). Mares found with vulvar injury should be examined to determine whether abrasion or laceration extended into the vestibule.

Blood on the stallion's penis or in a dismount sample after natural-cover breeding may be the initial indicator of reproductive tract trauma[1] and should prompt immediate examination. Blood in a dismount sample may also originate from an episiotomy performed in the mare to facilitate breeding. Breeding injury often takes the form of laceration of the cranial part of the vagina, in the dorsolateral aspect of the wall near the cervix, but may also also result in full-thickness rupture of the wall or laceration of the uterine wall.[1] Methods of examining the vagina and vestibule include manual palpation; visualization of the tract through a disposable or glass speculum as it is gradually withdrawn from the cervix to the vestibule; evaluation with a Caslick speculum, which can allow a broader visual field, especially of the cranial extent of the vagina; and use of an endoscope that is passed manually or through a speculum.

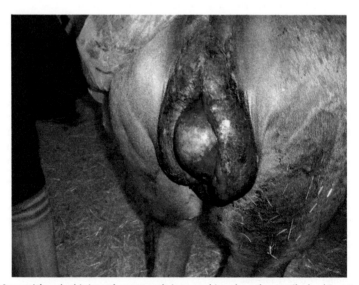

Fig. 1. Mare with vulval injury that extends into and involves the vestibule. (*Courtesy of* Dr. Peter Morresey, *BVSc MVM MACVSc DipACT DipACVIM CVA, Kentucky.*)

If vaginal injury is suspected after a live breeding, initial evaluation can be performed with a speculum or endoscope to confirm a lesion and site. Injuries involving only the mucosa or submucosa often heal spontaneously. Injuries that appear suspicious for deeper penetration may be best evaluated with a scrubbed and disinfected bare hand, lubricated with sterile jelly, and slowly and gently advanced into the vagina for careful digital exploration in the adequately restrained mare. Deep lacerations or full-thickness tears in the cranial aspect of the vagina are likely to open into the peritoneal cavity and warrant immediate emergency care, including administration of antimicro-bials and a nonsteroidal anti-inflammatory drug (NSAID), and preparation or referral for surgery, if possible.[1–3] Diagnostic workup for peritonitis, and monitoring for it over the next several days, with peripheral blood testing, sonographic imaging, or abdomi-nocentesis is also indicated (see section on uterine rupture in the accompanying article in this issue). It should be kept in mind that deep lacerations or near-ruptures that approach but do not actually penetrate the serosal surface can still facilitate transloca-tion of bacteria and induce peritonitis and the same clinical changes as a true perfora-tion. Vaginal lacerations and perforations arising caudal to the peritoneal reflection can be managed with medical treatment and second-intention healing. In one report[4] of cra-nial vaginal lacerations and caudal uterine lacerations repaired with the mare in a Tren-delenburg position, 5 of 8 mares with vaginal laceration recovered, whereas 2 of 4 mares with uterine lacerations were euthanized because of severe, diffuse peritonitis. If the equipment and technical support are available on site for general anesthesia and hoisting the mare's hindquarters into the Trendelenburg position, this surgery can be performed in the field if surgical expertise is available.

Lacerations in the cranial part of the vagina can also arise as a foaling injury, with clinical signs appearing in the postpartum period and ranging from mild, bloody vaginal discharge to peritonitis and intestinal evisceration through the vagina or vulva. Mares with bloody discharge and signs of systemic illness (depression, pyrexia, strong digital pulses) should not have uterine lavage until they have been examined to rule out a vaginal or uterine perforation.

Summary: Suspicion of a vaginal injury should prompt visual evaluation of the tract to locate a lesion, and possibly manual evaluation to determine the site and depth of the injury. Deep lacerations of the uterus or cranial part of the vagina carry a risk of communicating with the peritoneal cavity; these wounds and outright perforation should be sutured and the mare treated with broad-spectrum antimicrobials and anti-inflammatories while being monitored for peritonitis. Caudal lacerations or perfo-rations may be manageable with medical treatment.

Conditions of the External Portion of the Stallion Reproductive Tract

Traumatic injury of the external genitalia
Scrotal and testicular injury. Traumatic injury of the external genitalia in a stallion is considered a reproductive emergency because prompt intervention is required to reduce damage to fertility or breeding ability. Most such injuries arise during breeding from a kick by a mare,[5–7] but stallions can also sustain injury to this area while attempt-ing to jump a fence or by impaling accidents at pasture. Scrotal swelling, asymmetry, or heat, skin abrasion or laceration, and pain upon palpation make the diagnosis visu-ally straightforward. In addition to traumatic orchitis, less-acute causes of testicular inflammation, such as septic orchitis,[8–10] may also be considered emergent in nature once they are noticed in a breeding stallion, because of the need to quickly and effec-tively reduce scrotal inflammation in the interest of preserving fertility.

Direct blows to the scrotal area result in a gamut of severity: blunt trauma may cause testicular contusion and associated edema, may disrupt the parietal layer of the tunica vaginalis and result in hydrocele or hematocele (**Fig. 2**), or may penetrate the tunica albuginea and directly damage testicular parenchyma, including causing testicular rupture.[11,12] The third severity can lead to disruption of the blood-testis barrier and exposure of seminiferous tubule contents to the circulation, causing the downstream complication of immune-mediated orchitis as a threat to future fertility.[5,13]

The immediate goals in managing traumatic scrotal and testicular injury are reducing swelling and attenuating the inflammatory response that will develop in response to the trauma. Administration of a NSAID and local application of a cold pack are important first-aid measures. Nonsteroidal anti-inflammatory medications (flunixin meglumine, 1.1 mg/kg, intravenously [IV] or orally or phenylbutazone, 4.4 mg/kg, IV or orally) pharmaceutically attenuate the prostaglandin release and cytokine cascade that are activated upon traumatic injury and lead to increased blood flow, local vascular leak, and pain in the injured tissue. An NSAID should be continued for as long as clinically dictated by the severity of injury and response to treatment. The edema or hemorrhage in the scrotum may preclude precise determination of injury by means of palpation; diagnostic ultrasonography is very useful in aiding the examiner to determine the nature, location, and extent of injury inside the scrotum, as well as the response to treatment and development of delayed complications such as formation of adhesions.[14–16] Color Doppler ultrasonography can be used to confirm blood flow to an injured testis, or impairment thereof.[16]

Cold application is an effective countermeasure for inflammation. Cold application can be started with hydrotherapy, but use of a sling to hold a cold pack in place and provide prolonged contact between it and the scrotal area is a superior method of reducing local tissue temperatures and inflammation.[11] Depending on the severity of injury, additional treatments should encompass broad-spectrum systemic antimicrobials, furosemide, and topical wound treatments as parts of the treatment regimen. Corticosteroids can be used as an additional source of anti-inflammatory activity and

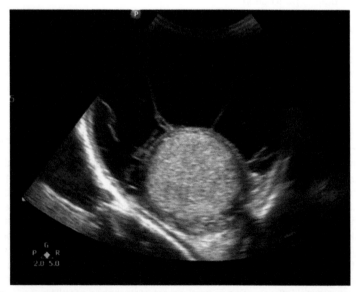

Fig. 2. Transcutaneous sonogram of testicular hydrocele in a stallion following previous traumatic injury in the scrotal area. Notice the strands of fibrin extending from the surface of the testicle to the parietal layer of the tunic.

are warranted in an animal with immune-mediated orchitis, but should be used with care in stallions, particularly individuals with confirmed or phenotypic metabolic syndrome. Intentional sexual stimulation should be avoided in the initial period following the injury; stallion rings or any other device to discourage masturbation should not be used.[17]

The sequelae of ineffective inflammation and temperature control in testicular trauma can include decreased semen quality in the future. Trauma induces edema and swelling that effectually insulate the testicles and impair fertility. Even a transient period of increased temperature can reduce spermatogenesis for 60 days.[6] In one study,[18] serial sperm chromatin structure assays were used to evaluate the effect of scrotal heat stress on spermatozoal DNA content. Scrotal heat was created by applying a plastic-coated wool covering for 48 hours, which resulted in a 2- to 3-degree increase in scrotal temperature. The susceptibility of spermatozoal DNA to denaturation was dependent on the spermatogenic cell stage that the ejaculated sperm were in at the time of the heat stress, with the spermatid, late primary spermatocyte stage, and early primary spermatocyte stages being the most susceptible.

In one case report,[13] fine-needle testicular aspirates were used to follow testicular function following severe trauma of the penis, prepuce, and scrotum in a stallion. Aspirations were performed under sedation with a 22-gauge needle connected to a 10-mL syringe. The first aspirate was obtained 1 month after the injury, and the second aspirate was obtained 1 month later. The first aspirate revealed testicular degeneration, with observation of chiefly primary spermatocytes with a few late-stage spermatids and spermatozoa and an increased Sertoli cell-to-germ cell ratio. Macrophages were also seen in the first sample. The second aspirate revealed a marked decrease in Sertoli cell-to-germ cell ratio and an increase in early and late spermatids, findings consistent with improvement. Giant multinucleated cells were seen in both aspirates, consistent with heat-associated testicular inflammation and degeneration. The stallion of that report was able to breed and settle mares 2 months after the second aspirate.

Penile injuries. Injuries of the penis most often arise during live-cover breeding, in the form of blunt trauma from a kicking mare, sudden movement by the mare during coitus, or laceration from the mare's tail hairs stretched across the vulva. The engorged penis can also be inadvertently bent during semen collection with an artificial vagina (AV) or during mounting of the phantom. Clinical signs of swelling, heat, and pain are usually quickly apparent, but sometimes may not manifest for a period of hours to days after breeding (**Fig. 3**). Hematomas form if there is disruption of the venous plexuses running along the dorsal aspect of the penis and can arise anywhere along the shaft of the penis.

The basic first aid measures are similar to those discussed for scrotal injury and are aimed at reducing swelling: application of cold through cold-water hosing or compression with a covered ice pack and administration of an NSAID medication. These should be initiated as quickly as possible. Other helpful measures are massage of the swollen tissue, applying a length of stockinette to the penis to provide continuous compression support, administration of a diuretic, topical application of a hydrophilic agent (glycerin) or osmotic agent (mannitol, sugar) to reduce edema, topical and systemic antimicrobials if there is a wound, and application of a nonirritating emollient (nitrofurazone, petroleum jelly) to protect the exposed penile epithelium. Penile skin quickly becomes inflamed and excoriated with exposure, and cracking of the epidermis facilitates infection and further inflammation with eventual fibrosis. If the penis can be pushed back through the preputial orifice into the external preputial fold, placement of a purse-string suture at the orifice will retain the penis there

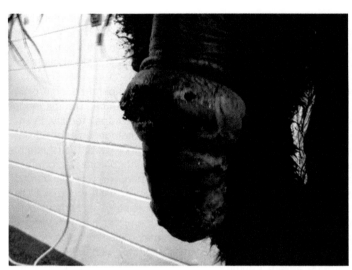

Fig. 3. Penile injury with secondary swelling and paraphimosis in a stallion. (*Courtesy of* Dr. Peter Morresey, *BVSc MVM MACVSc DipACT DipACVIM CVA, Kentucky.*)

temporarily in a physiologic position and the prepuce will help provide counterpressure. If the preputial area is also injured and abraded or edematous, the tissue will be friable and placement of a purse-string suture is not indicated. An alternative to this technique is using a penile repulsion (probang) device to maintain the penis inside the prepuce, using easily obtainable materials.[19] If the horse cannot retract the edematous penis and it cannot be manually repelled into the prepuce, it should be supported against the abdomen with a sling to prevent dependent edema from exacerbating the initial swelling. Continuation of an NSAID, daily hosing, massaging, and light exercise through hand walking will aid resorption of edema. Failure to effectively resolve edema and enable retraction of the penis will result in progressive edema, fatigue of the penile retractor muscle, and stretch injury of the pudendal nerves, which lead to the inability to self-correct and paraphimosis. As with scrotal injuries, ultrasound imaging is helpful in identifying the internal nature and extent of penile injuries[14,20] and for objectively monitoring response to treatment.

Summary: Quick administration of NSAIDs and cold application are the first-line treatments to attenuate swelling and control pain. Manual massage, application of external compression, application of topical emollients to aid in reducing edema and protect the penile epidermis, and prevention of additional edema secondary to dependent positioning are also necessary.

Priapism. Priapism refers to vascular penile engorgement not arising from sexual stimulation. Priapism has been categorized as high flow or low flow, from either excessive arterial inflow through an arteriovenous communication or decreased venous outflow of blood from the cavernosus, respectively. In horses, priapism is nearly always low flow, or veno-occlusive, in etiology.[21] Unmitigated priapism can progress into paraphimosis. In horses, priapism can also occur secondary to administration of a phenothiazine-derivative tranquilizer such as acepromazine, although in the past it was associated with propriopromazine. Priapism has also been reported following general anesthesia, neoplasia, and nematodiasis.[22,23]

Priapism can present as persistent, full, penile erection or as partial erection with persistent protrusion of only part of the penis from the prepuce, with palpable turgidity of the corpus cavernosum.[22] Ultrasonographically, the priapic corpus cavernosum tissue appears hyperechoic.[20]

Acetylcholine antagonists can be used in the short term when priapism is the result of α-adrenergic blockade such as following administration of acepromazine. The use of benztropine mesylate (8 mg/average-sized horse, given slowly IV) has been described.[22,24] Other drugs that may be useful for treatment of priapism include terbutaline and clenbuterol, beta-specific agonists that cause vasodilation and are thought to improve venous outflow from the corpus cavernosum.[22]

Injection of alpha-1-selective agonist phenylephrine (10 mg phenylephrine diluted in saline solution to a concentration of 1 mg/mL) into the corpus cavernosum can be effective for reducing priapism. A single treatment may be efficacious in acute cases. This treatment may only be effective for several hours in chronic cases.[22,23]

Irrigation of the corpus cavernosum with heparinized saline (10 units/mL) to flush out sludged erythrocytes and thrombotic material may be necessary in cases that do not respond to medical treatment. With the horse under anesthesia, heparinized saline is instilled under pressure through a 12- or 14-gauge needle introduced into the corpus cavernosum just proximal to the glans penis, and the saline is drained through a similarly placed needle or stab incision made 10 to 15 cm distal to the ischium until fresh hemorrhage is present in the effluent. Phenylephrine can also be infused following irrigation.[22,23] Failure of fresh blood to appear may indicate permanent vascular damage.[22]

Erection that persists following irrigation suggests that venous outflow remains occluded, whereas arteriolar inflow continues. This situation may warrant a corpus cavernosum penis shunt through the corpus spongiosum penis.[22,25]

Paraphimosis. The term paraphimosis refers to the condition of being unable to retract the penis because it is paralyzed, it has become engorged and enlarged secondary to hanging in an extended position and will not fit through the preputial orifice, or the prepuce has become edematous and swollen to the extent that it cannot accommodate retraction of the penis. The most common cause is traumatic injury to the genital area, with preputial swelling that reduces the preputial opening size. In addition to traumatic injury, neurologic injury or any other condition that leads to prolonged penile protrusion and dependent positioning has the potential to result in paraphimosis. Known causes include severe bodily debilitation, herpesvirus 1 infection, rabies, purpura hemorrhagica, unresolved priapism, inguinal abscess, and systemic hypo-oncotic conditions, among others.[26,27] Administration of tranquilizers of the phenothiazine class, notably acepromazine, has been linked to the development of paraphimosis. This development occurs as a result of α-adrenergic receptor blockade; blockade of α receptors may directly block activity in the motor neurons supplying the retractor penis muscle and may also prevent vasoconstriction of the arterial vasculature delivering blood to the corpus cavernosum, impairing detumescence.[28–30] Whatever the initial insult, once the penis has dangled in a ventral and unretracted state for a brief period of time, venous and lymphatic return are impaired and the organ will grow increasingly edematous. Progressive swelling makes the problem more dire by exacerbating the penile size and heft, decreasing the likelihood that the retractor muscles can return the penis to the prepuce, even if they have normal innervation and function. In long-standing cases, chronic stretching of the internal pudendal nerves can result in permanent paralysis and the need for surgery to amputate a portion of the penis.

Recognition of paraphimosis is visually straightforward (see **Fig. 3**). Measures to reduce edema should immediately be started, whatever the cause. Intervention is the same as described for traumatic injury of the externa genitalia at the beginning of the article. External compression with an Esmarch bandage or other means,[14,17,31] manual massage, application of ice packs, administering anti-inflammatory drugs, topical application of osmotic agents and emollients to protect the penile skin, and preventing progression of swelling by replacing and retaining the penis in the prepuce or holding it up against the body wall with a sling are all helpful. A recent case study[31] described favorable results with the novel use of a 5-L fluid bag compression device to provide external compression to stallions with paraphimosis.

CONDITIONS ARISING DURING GESTATION
Placentitis

Placentitis can be considered a reproductive emergency because prompt intervention may improve the outcome for the mare and foal, especially if the intervention is initiated early in the disease process. In most instances, it can be recognized through physical examination and ultrasonography and appropriately managed on the farm. Placentitis is a common infectious cause of abortion and perinatal foal mortality. Nearly 25% of placentas from aborted, stillborn, or premature foals examined over a 2-year period at one diagnostic laboratory had evidence of placentitis, and nearly one-third of 3514 aborted fetuses, stillborn foals, and foals that died less than 24 hours after birth were associated with placentitis.[32,33]

Cause

Most cases of placentitis are caused by bacteria ascending from the vulva or vagina and breaching the cervical barrier to colonize the caudal pole of the chorioallantois, at the cervical star. Mares may have acquired anatomic conditions of the caudal part of the reproductive tract that permit introduction of bacteria into the tract, such as pneumovagina or vaginovestibular reflux, or may have conditions that impair the integrity of the tract's normal barriers, such as cervical tears, adhesions, or fibrosis.[34]

Placentitis can take one of several clinical manifestations. Chronic, late-gestational placentitis most commonly causes focal disease, with lesions located at the cervical star.[32] However, bacterial placentitis can also manifest acutely, with either focal or diffuse placental lesions. This form of placentitis is the type most associated with fetal bacteremia and most frequently found in the placenta from fetuses aborted before or around midgestation.[32] In contrast, placentitis caused by nocardioform actinomycetes causes no changes at the cervical star, but rather a focal to focally extensive placentitis at the base of the uterine horns or the juncture between the horns and uterine body, with accumulation of mucoid exudate causing a plane of separation between the fetal membranes and endometrium (**Figs. 4** and **5**).

Major causative pathogens in one large study included *Streptococcus zooepidemicus*, *Leptospira* spp, *Escherichia coli*, nocardioform actinomycetes, fungi, *Pseudomonas aeruginosa*, *Streptococcus equisimilis*, *Enterobacter agglomerans*, *Klebsiella pneumoniae*, and α-hemolytic *Streptococcus*.[32] *Leptospira* spp induced diffuse placentitis, regardless of gestational age.[32] Leptospiral abortion in the mare is usually associated with *Leptospira interrogans* serovar Pomona type kennewicki.[35] The most frequent nocardioform actinomycete species associated with equine abortion were *Amycolatopsis* spp and *Crossiella equi*.[36] Fungal organisms generally induced focally extensive placentitis at the cervical star, usually observed in late gestation, with *Aspergillus* spp being the most common organism isolated.[32]

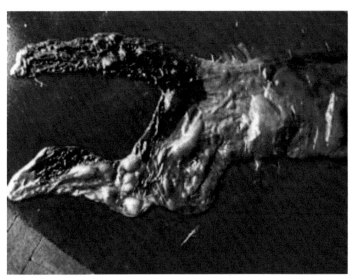

Fig. 4. Placenta from mare with nocardioform placentitis. Notice the diffuse nature of the thickening and tan discoloration in the pregnant horn (bottom) along its length and at its junction with the body.

Pathogenesis

The inflammation caused by infection is an important cause of abortion in ascending placentitis. Colonization of the placental tissues with bacteria causes upregulation of proinflammatory mediators (interleukin [IL]-6 and IL-8) and increased prostaglandin production, immune cell infiltration, and placental thickening at the site of infection. In

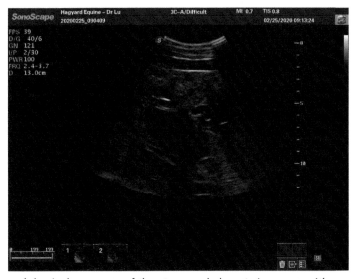

Fig. 5. Transabdominal sonogram of the uterus and placenta in a mare with nocardioform placentitis. The image was obtained in the pregnant horn; an area where hypoechoic exudate is accumulating (*asterisk*) and creating separation between the endometrium and chorioallantois (*arrow*) is seen.

an ascending placentitis model induced by cervical inoculation of S zooepidemicus, inflammation was seen at the cervical star and in the umbilical cord and amnionic fluid.[37] Premature birth was not always associated with fetal bacterial infection, and not all mares with placentitis had clinical signs or placental pathology. High concentrations of allantoic fluid prostaglandin E_2, and prostaglandin $F_{2\alpha}$ were detected within the 48 hours preceding abortion or delivery.[37] Proinflammatory cytokines in the chorioallantois, amnionic fluid, endometrium, cervix, and fetal tissues were higher in the experimentally infected mares, compared with controls.[37–41] The placental infection, although typically not affecting the dam, results in an infectious, proinflammatory gestational environment that can lead to impaired fetal growth, fetal sepsis, and early parturition or abortion.

Clinical Signs

The most common clinical signs of placentitis are premature mammary development or appearance of mammary secretions, vulvar discharge, ligamentous relaxation around the tail head, and abortion. Other differentials for these clinical signs include incorrect breeding date, twin pregnancy, or other noninfectious (eg, umbilical cord torsion, hydrops) and infectious (herpesvirus) causes of impending abortion.

Diagnosis

Transrectal ultrasonography is an important diagnostic tool for detection of ascending or diffuse placentitis, as it allows detailed imaging of the uterus and placenta at the cervical star where most placentitis lesions occur. Any pregnant mare with vulvar discharge should be scanned transrectally, as 90% of placentitis is ascending and can be detected at the cervical star (**Fig. 6**). If no abnormality is seen in that area, the mare should next be evaluated with transabdominal ultrasonography to rule out nocardioform placentitis. For transrectal imaging, a linear rectal transducer is advanced to a point immediately cranial to the cervix and entrained on the ventral arm of the uteroplacenta. The combined thickness of the uterus and placenta (CTUP) is measured at the ventral uterine body and compared with known reference ranges. In a prospective study, from 4 to 8 months of gestation, the mean CTUP in light-horse mares was 4 mm. The upper limit of reference range was 6.7 mm at 10 months, 8.54 mm at 11 months, and 11.77 mm at 12 months. Detachment of the placenta from the endometrium and echogenicity of the allantoic and amniotic fluids can also be evaluated[42] (see **Fig. 6**).

Transabdominal ultrasonography is valuable for assessing fetal and placental health and for detection of nocardioform placentitis. Parameters that can be assessed include fetal presentation, fetal heart rate and rhythm, fetal activity and size, fetal stomach measurements, uteroplacental thickness, fetal fluid depth, and presence of multiple fetuses.[43] An equine biophysical profile score was developed for late gestation (298 days to term) based on fetal heart rate, aortic diameter, fetal activity level, uteroplacental thickness, uteroplacental contact, and maximal allantoic fluid depth. Each parameter is scored from 0 to 2 for a maximal score of 12, with a score of 8 or less being associated with a negative fetal outcome. Negative outcomes can occur regardless of the score.[44]

Not all mares with placentitis have vulvar discharge, but in those that do, culture of the fluid is useful to determine the causative organism and its antimicrobial sensitivity pattern to guide treatment. The sample should be obtained by donning a sterile sleeve and using a guarded swab to sample the fluid from where it exits the external cervical os.

Serial progestin measurement may aid in assessing fetoplacental function in a mare with placentitis. Progestins cross-react with the progesterone antibody used in commercial progesterone assays, although the ranges for normal values can vary between laboratories. Abnormal patterns that may be observed in progestin profiles include a

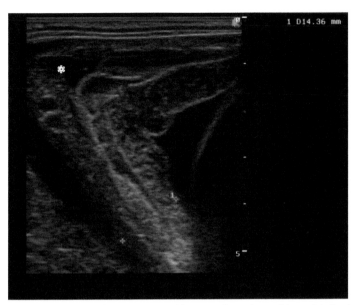

Fig. 6. Transrectal sonogram from a mare with ascending placentitis and infection of the caudal pole of the chorioallantois. The transducer is positioned immediately cranial to the cervix, at the cervical star. Shown are the electronic calipers in use to measure the combined thickness of the uterus and placenta (CTUP). The CTUP is thickened, and separation of the chorioallantois from the uterus at the cervical star can be seen (*asterisk*).

premature rapid decline, a marked increase occurring earlier than the expected increase around 3 weeks before parturition, or a failure to increase prepartum.[34,45–47] A rapid decline usually indicates fetal death or imminent expulsion, a premature increase is seen with placental pathology or fetal stress, and a failure to increase shortly before the expected time of parturition is seen with exposure to ergopeptine alkaloids produced by the endophyte fungus in fescue toxicosis.[34]

Mares with placentitis rarely have changes in complete blood cell count or chemistry profiles unless they have concurrent disease.[34] Serum amyloid A (SAA) is an acute-phase protein secreted in response to inflammatory stimuli that is low or undetectable in healthy horses. Mares with experimentally induced placentitis had a significant increase in SAA within 96 hours after bacterial inoculation. This increase in SAA was prevented by treatment with trimethoprim sulfamethoxazole (30 mg/kg, by mouth, every 12 hours), pentoxifylline (8.5 mg/kg, by mouth, every 12 hours), and altrenogest (0.088 mg/kg, by mouth, every 24 hours) beginning at the onset of clinical signs and ending at the time of abortion or delivery.[48] Anecdotally, SAA has not been reliably observed to increase in clinical cases of chronic placentitis; this may be the result of the short duration of SAA in the early stages of inflammation preceding the appearance of overt clinical signs.

Management

The goals of treatment are to limit bacterial growth and expansion, maintain myometrial quiescence, and reduce the inflammation associated with bacterial infection of the fetal membranes. Thus the primary treatments for placentitis consist of antimicrobials, anti-inflammatory drugs, and altrenogest. Duration of each of these treatments varies by clinician and response to treatment. Periodic reevaluation of the fetus is necessary to ensure that the fetus is still alive.

Several studies have evaluated the penetration of antimicrobials into fetal fluids. Both systemically administered penicillin (penicillin G potassium, 22,000 IU/kg, slowly IV, every 6 hours) and gentamicin (6.6 mg/kg, IV, every 24 hours) reach the allantoic fluid at concentrations similar to and 20% less than systemic concentrations, respectively.[49] Systemically administered trimethoprim sulfamethoxazole (30 mg/kg, by mouth, every 12 hours) and pentoxifylline (8.5 mg/kg, by mouth, every 12 hours) also reached the allantoic fluid at concentrations similar to serum.[50] Enrofloxacin (5 mg/kg, IV, every 24 hours) reached therapeutic concentrations in fetal fluids in 7 normal mares at 260 days gestation treated for 11 days, with no detected fetal lesions. The investigators cautioned that further research is needed to determine if enrofloxacin is toxic at other stages of pregnancy, after a longer duration of treatment, or once foals are delivered and weight-bearing.[51] Doxycycline (10 mg/kg, by mouth, every 12 hours) was found to diffuse through the fetoplacental unit of late pregnant mares with the highest concentration in the allantoic fluid of 73 ng/mL.[52] The minimum inhibitory concentration to inhibit growth of 90% of organisms (MIC_{90}) for intragastric administration of a similar dose of doxycycline was determined to be ≤ 1.0 µg/mL for *S zooepidemicus*.[53] Ceftiofur sodium (4.4 mg/kg, intramuscularly [IM], every 24 hours) and ceftiofur crystalline free acid (6.6 mg/kg, IM, every 96 hours) were found to incompletely transfer across fetal membranes in pony mares.[54,55]

Duration of treatment influenced recovery of bacteria from the postpartum uterus in mares with induced placentitis. Mares with negative postpartum uterine culture results were treated for at least 3 weeks. This fact also suggests the need for postpartum uterine treatment in mares with placentitis.[56]

In a combination treatment experiment in mares inoculated with *S zooepidemicus* to induce ascending placentitis, mares treated with trimethoprim sulfamethoxazole (30 mg/kg, by mouth, every 12 hours), pentoxifylline (8.5 mg/kg, by mouth, every 12 hours), and altrenogest (0.88 mg/kg, by mouth, every 24 hours) carried pregnancies longer and delivered more live foals than untreated, inoculated mares. Treatment was initiated when clinical signs of placentitis were observed, such as ultrasonographic evidence of increased CTUP, placental separation, or a change in fetal fluid character, or the onset of mammary development or vulvar discharge.[56]

A study evaluated the use of antibiotics alone or in combination of immunomodulators to prevent preterm birth or increase neonatal viability in induced placentitis. Mares with induced placentitis were treated with trimethoprim sulfamethoxazole alone (30 mg/kg, by mouth every 12 hours), trimethoprim sulfamethoxazole and tapering dexamethasone doses (40 mg IV every 24 hours for 2 days, followed by 35 mg IV every 24 hours for 2 days, followed by 25 mg IV every 24 hours for 2 days), or trimethoprim sulfamethoxazole and aspirin (50 mg/kg, by mouth, every 12 hours). Pregnancy outcomes were similar between groups suggesting that strategic treatment with antimicrobials can substantially improve pregnancy outcome.[57]

In a study assessing the value of firocoxib (0.3 mg/kg, by mouth, one time loading dose; 0.1 mg/kg, by mouth, every 24 hours) in induced placentitis, some cytokine concentrations were significantly lower in allantoic fluid in treated mares. Prostaglandin concentrations were variable between groups. Results suggested a trend toward suppressive effects of firocoxib treatment on cytokine and prostaglandin concentrations in fetal fluids of mares with induced placentitis.[58]

Progestin treatment has been described for use in women for preterm labor and mares to promote uterine quiescence and is often prescribed for placentitis in mares.[59] However, it may be warranted to discontinue progestin therapy before parturition depending on the case. One study of the effect of altrenogest administration on parturition and neonatal viability in normal mares revealed a prolonged second stage of parturition, lower neonatal respiratory rate, and higher plasma pH during the first 30 minutes of life. Altrenogest did not inhibit parturition.[60]

The addition of long-acting altrenogest (0.088 mg/kg, IM, every 7 days) and estradiol cypionate (10 mg/mare, IM, every 3 days) to trimethoprim sulfamethoxazole (30 mg/kg, IV, every 12 hours) and flunixin meglumine (1.1 mg/kg, IV, every 24 hours) for treatment of induced placentitis has been evaluated. Foal survival at parturition and 7 days after delivery was similar between treatments; however, the few foals deemed high risk after parturition originated in groups treated with both trimethoprim sulfamethoxazole and flunixin meglumine or a combination of sulfamethoxazole, flunixin meglumine, and estradiol cypionate.[61]

Hydrops Allantois and Hydrops Amnion

Hydrops allantois and hydrops amnion are conditions of excessive fetal fluid accumulation, with intrauterine volumes of 120 to 220 L reported.[62] The reference range for allantoic fluid volume near the end of gestation is 8 to 18 L, and the reference range for amnionic fluid volume is 3 to 7 L.[63] Hydrops allantois and hydrops amnion are considered reproductive emergencies in the mare because of their association with prepubic tendon rupture, uterine rupture, and abdominal wall herniation.[64,65] Spontaneous abortion and sudden loss of the excessive fetal fluid can result in hypovolemic shock.[66] Dystocia and retained placenta are common due to the marked uterine distension,[63] with other potential complications including delayed uterine involution and metritis.[67]

Presentation

Hydrops allantois and amnion are uncommon in the mare[62,63] but have been reported across a wide age range, a variety of breeds, and in both nulliparous and multiparous mares.[62,67] In one report, 5 cases of hydrops allantois were identified out of 364 high-risk pregnancies.[67] Mares are typically in or near the last trimester[62,63] of gestation when the condition arises. Hydrops allantois is more common than hydrops amnion, and the clinical patterns of the 2 conditions differ somewhat in that with hydrops amnion, the fluid volume is not as marked as with hydrops allantois[64] and the abdominal distension develops more gradually over a period of weeks to several months during the last half of gestation, whereas with hydrops allantois, fluid volume and abdominal distension are marked and arise more acutely, over 1 to 2 weeks, also during the last part of gestation. Suspicion of a hydropsic condition is made by visual observation of abdominal distension greater than what would be expected for the stage of gestation (**Fig. 7**) or by usually rapidly developing, gross abdominal distension (**Fig. 8**) accompanied by signs of increasing discomfort and distress. Differential diagnoses include twin pregnancy, colic, ascites, abdominal wall herniation, prepubic tendon rupture, hypoproteinemia, and other causes of ventral edema.

Cause

Hydrops allantois is most commonly thought to be caused by a vascular disturbance in the allantois,[63] although other pathogeneses have been suggested, including umbilical cord torsion, hereditary factors, and fetal abnormalities.[62,67,68] Fetal growth retardation has also been observed.[63] In a report of 5 cases of hydrops allantois, placentitis was observed to an extent in all cases, but it was not determined whether the hydropsic condition caused the placentitis, or vice versa.[67] *L interrogans* serogroup Pomona has been associated with hydrops allantois, which may warrant testing of affected mares and fetal tissues, and maintaining a mindfulness of the zoonotic potential during treatment.[69,70]

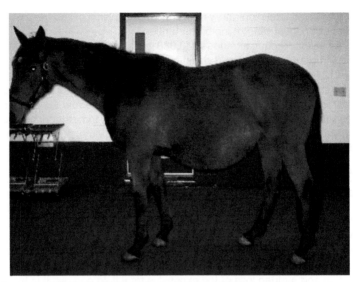

Fig. 7. Mare in month 6 of gestation, in early stage of hydrops allantois.

Diagnosis

Physical examination: Diagnosis of a hydropsic condition usually starts with visual recognition of marked abdominal distension. With increasing abdominal enlargement, mares become reluctant to move, move stiffly, and may spend more time lying down.

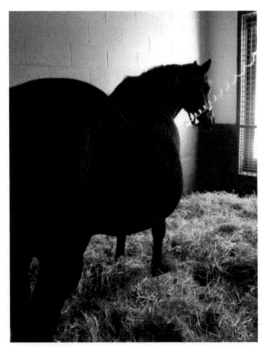

Fig. 8. Mare in month 10 of gestation with gross abdominal enlargement from hydrops allantois.

Heart rate and respiratory rate are usually high, as mares adopt a low-tidal-volume high-rate breathing pattern in response to the high abdominal pressure behind the diaphragm. The breathing quality may be labored as the hydraulic pressure in the abdomen progressively impairs diaphragmatic contraction. The skin along the caudal aspect of the ventral abdomen becomes palpably taut and may be highly sensitive to palpation. Edema often accumulates in a large ventral plaque along the abdomen. The excessive distension and weight can challenge body wall integrity, and the lateral and ventral abdominal walls should be carefully evaluated daily for regions of fascial separation and bulging of muscle into the subcutaneous layer of the skin, particularly in the mammary region, where the prepubic tendon attaches to the pelvic brim. When the excessive weight stretches and compromises the prepubic tendon, blood-tinged mammary secretions may be seen. Measuring abdominal circumference, distance from mammary gland to umbilicus, and distance from the umbilical scar to the ground can be objective ways of monitoring progression as abdominal contours grow.[71]

Ultrasound imaging: Upon transrectal palpation and ultrasonography, the uterus is grossly distended, taut, and often domes dorsally above the pelvic inlet to protrude into the pelvic canal. The contained fluid volume may be such that the fetus cannot be palpated or seen on ultrasonography (**Fig. 9**). The caudal area of the uterus and the cervix should be evaluated for placentitis, although the CTUP is often within normal limits with hydrops allantois.[67,70] In one case report, a mare with hydrops allantois had normal CTUP, but other areas of the chorioallantois were edematous, as was the amnion.[70]

Transabdominal ultrasonography can be performed to evaluate the depth of the amnionic and allantoic fluid compartments, character of the fluid, health of the placenta and fetus, and integrity of the abdominal wall; to gain a general assessment of the viewable abdominal contents; and to rule out some of the differential diagnoses. In a 1995 study[72] of 33 healthy mares that were scanned transabdominally within 2 months of parturition, the maximum vertical depth of amnionic fluid was 7.9 ± 3.5 cm and the maximum vertical depth of allantoic fluid was 13.4 ± 4.4 cm.

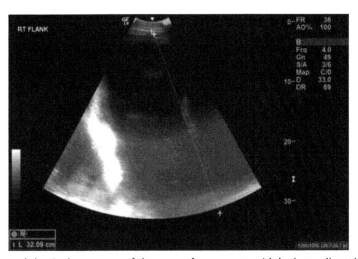

Fig. 9. Transabdominal sonogram of the uterus from a mare with hydrops allantois. Notice the fetus is not in view because of the extreme volumes of fetal fluids.

In another study of fetoplacental well-being in normal pregnancies, total fetal fluid depth was not significantly related to the gestational age in mares at 6 to 12 months' gestation, but the distribution of fetal fluid was related to the position of the fetus within the uterus.[73] Allantoic fluid depth greater than 18 cm is highly suggestive of hydrops allantois.[66]

Although it is not necessary for diagnosis, blood work, including serum chemistry, is recommended in the evaluation. Hypocalcemic mares may be more vulnerable to hypotensive shock on removal of the fetal fluids, and low blood calcium warrants intravenous calcium supplementation as preparations are made for reduction of the hydrops.[66] Hydrops is frequently followed by retained fetal membranes, and parenteral calcium may also help with the uterine atony after removal of the fetus. Findings of high creatine kinase, alkaline phosphatase, and serum amyloid A should point the veterinarian's attention to possible body wall compromise as a sequelae to the hydrops.[66,70]

Treatment

Intervention and treatment require a conversation with the client regarding the well-being and prognosis for both the mare and the fetus. Although there is one published report of a live foal birth following conservative management of a mare with hydrops amnion,[71] the more common hydrops allantois seems to confer a uniformly grave prognosis on foal survival. In nearly all instances of uterine hydrops of either type, the goal of intervention is to end the pregnancy to preserve the life of the mare.[62,67,70] The timing of and the method used to terminate the pregnancy have implications for the mare's well-being; it depends on factors such as the volume of fluid, compromise of the mare's body wall, the mare's gestational age, the mare's overall health, and the potential of a viable fetus.

If hydrops is diagnosed at an earlier stage of gestation or before the volume of the uterine fluid has become marked, elective termination of the pregnancy via routine protocols may be undertaken. Once the uterus has become grossly distended with a large volume of fluid, however, reduction of the hydrops should involve controlled removal of the allantoic fluid, over a period of one to several hours, before the fetus is removed. Rapid removal, even over a period of several hours, can induce hypovolemic shock and collapse or death, as the abrupt reduction in pressure in the abdominal cavity causes venous pooling in the splanchnic circulation with loss of effective circulating blood volume, blood pressure, and cardiac output. For these reasons, the mare should be prepared for the procedure. A large-bore intravenous catheter (10- to 14-gauge catheter) is placed in the jugular vein and an initial bolus of 10 L of a polyionic crystalloid fluid is administered. This step is followed by the continuous administration of fluids as the fluid is removed from the uterus, with the final administered volume of fluid measuring about one-fourth the volume of drained fetal fluid. The mare's heart rate, respiratory rate, and overall affect should be continuously monitored by a person assigned to that role, and if the mare becomes tachycardic (heart rate >56–60 beats/min), ataxic, or shaky, drainage of the fluid is paused and a colloid fluid or hypertonic saline is administered to correct hypotension.[66]

In preparation for intravaginal manipulation, the tail is wrapped, the perineum is cleansed, and the Caslick suture is removed if present. A cream containing hyoscine butylbromide, misoprostol, or prostaglandin E_2 can be applied to the cervix to induce cervical softening and facilitate intrauterine manipulations. The operator should prepare as for an aseptic procedure. Reaching through the softened cervix, the chorioallantois is identified. The chorioallantois at the internal os can be very thick, and an instrument such as a blunt scissor or an Argyle-type chest drain and trocar may be needed to penetrate it.[66,67,70] Use of a chest drain to pierce the chorioallantois enables attachment of sterile tubing to the drain once the trocar has been withdrawn, allowing better control of the rate of fluid drainage over 1 to 2 hours (**Fig. 10**). Because of the marked uterine distension and resulting myometrial flaccidity, fluid expulsion following rupture of the fetal membranes may not be explosive. After most of the fetal fluid has been removed, oxytocin can be administered to promote uterine contractility, delivery of the fetus, and expulsion of the placental membranes.[67] Manual extraction of the fetus is often necessary because of the vastly increased uterine size, inertia, and weakened abdominal musculature. Dystocia is common, and retention of the fetal membranes should be expected. The fetus is usually euthanized on delivery. The mare should continue to be monitored for hemodynamic stability multiple times daily for the next 1 to 2 days, with recording of the heart rate, respiratory rate, temperature, peripheral pulse quality, cutaneous temperature of the extremities, skin turgor, capillary refill time, and urine output.

Because of the prolonged cervical and uterine manipulations and frequent retained fetal membranes, broad-spectrum antimicrobials should be prescribed and routine postpartum care and monitoring provided. Application of abdominal support bandages or girdles likely gives the mare a degree of comfort and can continue to be provided as needed while the mare convalesces.

Subsequent Fertility

In a report of 5 mares, 1 of 2 mares with reported fertility data conceived during the same season in which an elective hydroallantois abortion was performed; the other mare in that report remained barren after several cycles of natural breeding.[67] In another report, one mare was used for breeding and became an embryo donor with successful embryo recovery.[70]

Summary: Use clinical signs and ultrasonography to diagnose and monitor abdominal enlargement. If the hydropsic fluid accumulation is severe enough to cause pain,

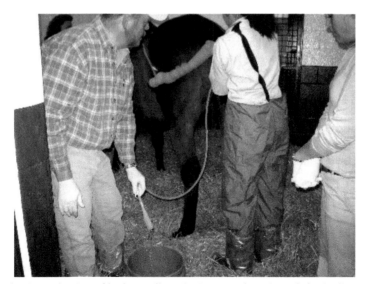

Fig. 10. Elective reduction of hydrops allantois. Operator has pierced chorioallantois transcervically with a 24F chest-tube trocar and is allowing controlled flow of allantoic fluid out of the uterus through Bivona tubing. The mare is being supported with IV fluids.

respiratory impairment, or challenge to the prepubic tendon attachments, consider elective removal of the fluid and induction of parturition to save the mare.

Prepubic Tendon Rupture and Abdominal Wall Hernia

Incidence

The prepubic tendon is composed of the tendons and aponeuroses of the muscles that make up the ventral and lateral body walls, including the rectus abdominis and abdominal oblique muscles. The prepubic tendon serves as the pelvic attachment of the linea alba.[74,75] Abdominal wall hernias and prepubic tendon rupture are emergencies because of the risk of evisceration. Prepubic tendon rupture is reported in draft mares and light breeds, typically in the last 2 months of pregnancy.[63,76,77] Predisposing factors to body wall defects include hydrops allantois, hydrops amnion, trauma, and twins.[63]

In one review of 13 cases of body wall defects, only 3 cases were associated with hydrops allantois or hydrops amnion, and no predisposing conditions were reported for 10 cases.[77] In that report, the median age at presentation was 13 years, all were light-breed mares, and all mares had produced at least one foal previously. The median time in gestation when naturally occurring body wall defects were diagnosed was 324 days.

Clinical signs

Clinical signs at initial evaluation of mares with body wall defects (either abdominal wall hernia or prepubic tendon rupture) included pitting ventral edema, pain on palpation of the abdominal wall, easily depressible abdominal wall tissue, colic, tachycardia, ventral displacement of the abdominal wall (**Fig. 11**), hemorrhagic mammary secretions, flattened mammary glands, reluctance to walk, abdominal enlargement, and sudden onset of lordosis.[77] Rupture of the prepubic tendon is associated with elevation of the tail head and ischial tuberosities, leading to a sawhorse stance and lordosis.[63,76]

Diagnosis

Abdominal wall defects may be unilateral or bilateral, and midline defects can extend into lateral abdominal musculature.[77] Rupture of the prepubic tendon should be distinguished from displacement or herniation of other abdominal musculature because prepubic tendon rupture implies loss of all ventral and lateral abdominal support.[76]

Clinical suspicion of abdominal wall defects can be confirmed with transabdominal ultrasonography. Ventral and ventrolateral abdominal wall muscles in pregnant and nonpregnant mares with and without abdominal wall disease were evaluated with transabdominal ultrasonography to establish normal ranges.[78] There were no significant differences between light and heavy mares and no effect of pregnancy status or age on measurements of muscle thickness. Two pregnant mares with abdominal wall disease were evaluated, and muscle measurements were similar to those of normal mares. However, echotexture changes with increased intramuscular edema and increased echogenicity consistent with hemorrhage were present.[78] Serum creatine kinase was high in 1 of 2 mares with abdominal wall disease[78] and was also high in hydrops allantois cases with abdominal wall disease.[66,70]

Management

Conservative management includes stall rest and abdominal support. Frequent or continuous fetal and mare monitoring, pain management, repeated ultrasonography, and treatment of placentitis if necessary were associated with a better outcome than interventional management for mares with body wall tears. One review (n = 13 with 10

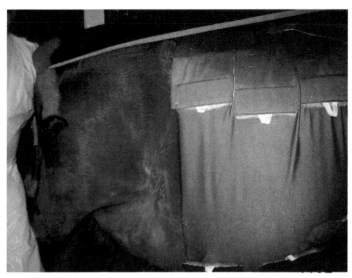

Fig. 11. Mare with ventrally displaced body wall secondary to failure of the prepubic tendon attachments at the pubic bone. This severity of structural failure predisposes the mare to body wall herniation and progression to rupture and evisceration.

mares surviving to discharge) found no difference in mare survival between mares with body wall hernia only and mares with prepubic tendon tear plus body wall hernia.[77] Others have stated the prognosis for mares with prepubic tendon rupture to be poor, with undefined end points.[77]

Foaling should be attended and assistance should be provided, although it is not always required.[77] Serial monitoring of mammary gland secretions can aid in predicting foaling or in timing induced parturition, although this can be complicated by placentitis. Changes to monitor include an increase in calcium to concentration > 40 ng/dL and inversion of the sodium and potassium concentrations. Elective cesarean delivery in mares with prepubic tendon rupture or significant body wall tears is typically terminal.[63] It is recommended that mares with body wall tears not be rebred with the intention of carrying a pregnancy to term.[63,76,77]

Summary: Some of the most noticeable signs in mares with a failing prepubic tendon are abdominal discomfort, colic, ventral edema, easily compressed areas of the body wall, flattened taut mammary glands, tachycardia, blood-tinged mammary secretions, reluctance to move, and a lordotic posture. Provision of abdominal support, an adequate analgesic protocol, stall confinement, and daily monitoring seem to yield better outcomes for the foal without compromising mare survival than does intervention by induced parturition or cesarean section surgery.

Uterine torsion

Torsion of the uterus is an uncommon problem in mares, but it is a significant risk to survival of both the fetus and the dam. Both nonsurgical and surgical methods of correcting the torsion have been described and will be discussed. Torsion of the uterus can affect mares of any age and parity and most frequently arises as an acute condition in the last 60 days of gestation, but it can also occur at the earlier and later stages of gestation.[79–81] Chronic torsion has also been reported.[82–84] Predisposing factors that set up the gravid uterus to rotate may include the mare falling, mare rolling, presence of a large fetus with a relatively small volume of fetal fluids, and vigorous fetal movement,[85,86] but in most instances no precipitating events or factors can be confirmed. Multiple studies have reported that the chance of survival in both mare and fetus is higher when torsion occurs earlier, rather than later, in gestation. A cutoff point of 320 days of gestation has been reported, with significantly higher survival percentages for cases occurring before that time, compared with mares in which uterine torsion happens greater than 320 days.[80,81]

Uterine torsion manifests in signs of depression and colic, which tends to be mild to moderate in severity and intermittent to persistent. The degree of colic has been likened to that seen with intestinal impaction,[86,87] but it is likely to be more severe if gastrointestinal segments are incorporated into the torsion. Routine colic treatment may yield transient improvement, but the signs of abdominal discomfort are usually not completely resolved, or they return. As the colic is often mild, and possibly intermittent, a period of several days may pass between the onset of abdominal discomfort and diagnosis of uterine torsion. Involvement of gastrointestinal tract structures in the uterine torsion elicit signs of abdominal pain commensurate with the type of gastrointestinal disease. In one retrospective study of 19 mares,[88] approximately 50% of the cases had concurrent gastrointestinal disease, including inflammatory bowel disease, impaction, large colon volvulus, right dorsal displacement of the large colon, and gastric rupture. In a 1995 case report[89] a mare at 126 days of gestation had the small intestine incarcerated in the uterine torsion, and in another report[87] mares with uterine torsion also had herniation of the jejunum through a broad ligament and incorporation of the small colon in the torsion. For these reasons, colic in the pregnant mare should prompt detailed examination of both the gastrointestinal and reproductive tracts. The pregnant uterus and broad ligaments should be palpated transrectally as part of the evaluation for colic.

Torsion is diagnosed by rectal palpation. The direction of the torsion, and the degree of rotation, vary. Although both directions have been reported as most frequent in different retrospective case series, rotation of the uterus in the clockwise direction is generally thought to be more frequent than counterclockwise rotation.[79–81,90,91] Rectal palpation reveals asymmetry in the broad ligaments.[86] With a clockwise rotation (with the mare being viewed from the rear), the left broad ligament can be palpated as a taut strap or band pulled horizontally and dorsally over the uterus, or less reliably, the right broad ligament being pulled more vertically and ventrally under the uterus. With counterclockwise rotation, the right broad ligament can be palpated being pulled dorsally toward the top of the uterus, and the left ligament will be pulled ventrally. The magnitude of torsion can vary from less than 180° to 540°, with most torsions diagnosed as less than or equal to 180°.[80,81] A torsion of 360° or more creates the most tension on the vascular structures in the broad ligaments and has greater potential to impair placental perfusion and fetal oxygen delivery. It has been posited by some investigators that torsions less than 180° may be within normal variation of uterine movement and may resolve spontaneously.[81] Once uterine torsion is diagnosed, a vaginal speculum examination adds additional information in indicating whether the cervix is open or closed, which can influence the choice of intervention.

If it is planned to attempt correction of the torsion on site and nonsurgically, it is necessary to correctly identify the direction of the rotation. If this cannot be done with certainty, nonsurgical correction should not be undertaken, as the corrective measures can exacerbate the torsion and cause uterine wall injury. The 2 nonsurgical methods of reducing uterine torsion are to manually rotate the uterus by manipulating the fetus per vaginum in the standing mare, or to roll the mare's body around the uterus while under general anesthesia.[92–96] In the few cases in which the mare is at term and the cervix is open, derotation may be possible by reaching a well-lubricated arm through the cervix, rupturing the chorioallantois and allowing the fetal fluids to drain, and grasping the foal on its ventrolateral aspects, optimally the forelimbs and some part of the body. Small arcs of rotation are begun, in the direction opposing the torsion. Wider and wider excursions are created, until the fetus and surrounding uterus have partially or fully derotated. It may require several cycles of the procedure before the uterus is restored to the normal position. This technique should be attempted only in torsions less than or equal to 270°.[90,97] Once the uterus is derotated, the foal should be delivered vaginally. If a term mare with torsion has a closed cervix, or uterine wall compromise is suspected, this technique cannot be used and the mare should be referred for ventral midline celiotomy.

The second nonsurgical correction method involves rolling the mare, and has been well described.[92,94–97] This maneuver exploits the mass and inertia of the pregnant uterus and aims to rotate the dam's body 360° over the stationary uterus. The technique is to roll the mare, while anesthetized, in the same direction of the torsion while a plank is placed on the abdomen directly over the uterus, and weighted. By rotating the mare in the same direction in which the uterus is rotated while holding the latter in place, the mare's body catches up with the uterus. Accurate determination of the direction of torsion is necessary before starting his procedure. For a clockwise torsion (uterus rotated toward the right when viewed from behind), the mare is anesthetized with routine intravenous anesthesia and positioned in right lateral recumbency. A long wooden plank is placed on the paralumbar fossa, running perpendicularly to the mare's long axis.[92,94,96] An assistant sits or stands on the plank, weighting and holding the uterus in place while ropes are used to pull the mare into dorsal recumbency, over into left lateral recumbency, into sternal recumbency, and back to right lateral recumbency. Rectal palpation with the mare pulled into sternal recumbency will indicate whether the uterus has returned to the normal position. For a counterclockwise rotation, the mare is positioned in left lateral recumbency and maneuvered through a 360° roll using the same technique. If torsion persists after rolling, the procedure can be repeated, but failure to correct the torsion with 2 attempts should prompt consideration of surgical methods of resolution.

The rolling technique necessitates general anesthesia of the mare, but has the advantages of being feasible to attempt at most farms, being associated with a reasonable to good chance of success, and being inexpensive, compared with the costs of hospitalization and surgery. The rolling technique is most appropriate for light-breed mares in months 7 through 10 of gestation in which the owners prefer not to pursue surgery and in which no concurrent gastrointestinal tract disease is suspected.[96] The technique is not without the potential for complications, including all the possible complications attending general anesthesia and recovery, plus uterine rupture, premature placental separation, and abortion.[79,90,95] Mares that are close to term are more likely to experience significant complications with the procedure and are better candidates for surgical resolution. Mares in which gastrointestinal disease is suspected should also be managed surgically to permit both reduction of the uterine torsion and evaluation of the gastrointestinal tract.

Surgical options for resolving uterine torsion include standing flank laparotomy, recumbent flank laparotomy, and ventral midline celiotomy. Standing flank laparotomy in mares that are less than 320 days gestation and that have no concurrent gastrointestinal involvement appears to yield the best outcome for mares and foals,[79–81] although recumbent flank laparotomy and ventral midline celiotomy can also resolve the torsion and result in delivery of a live foal. Uterine torsion in mares later than 320 days in gestation is likely to be met with more complications, irrespective of the method of resolution. After 320 days, the method of correction has less effect on outcome, and the risk of complications is higher. Foals delivered at the time of torsion correction should be managed as high-risk neonates for neonatal asphyxia syndrome or sepsis. Mares in which the fetus is alive at the time of correction have a good prognosis for delivering a live foal.[79–81,90,91] Future fertility in the mare is likewise favorable: stage of gestation, correction method, direction or degree of torsion, and postoperative wound complications had no influence on subsequent fertility.[79–81,92]

Surgical correction of uterine torsion is best done at a surgical facility. If the surgical expertise and technical assistance are available, standing flank laparotomy is possible at a farm with a dedicated area for veterinary work that is clean, has horizontal work surfaces, and includes stocks. The reader is referred to recent excellent descriptions for details of the surgical procedure.[92,93,96] In brief, the mare is restrained in stocks and started on standing intravenous sedation; a constant-rate infusion (CRI) of detomidine is useful for this purpose. A caudal epidural may also be placed but is typically not necessary. The lateral body wall on the side toward which the uterus is rotated is clipped and prepped for aseptic surgery. Local anesthesia is placed in a line block at the incision site, which will lie halfway between the last rib and the tuber coxa and follow a vertical line starting just above the dorsal margin of the internal oblique muscle and extending distad approximately 20 cm. The local anesthetic solution is infiltrated in the muscle and subcutaneous layers. Entry to the peritoneal cavity is made by a modified grid approach, in which, once the skin incision is made, the external abdominal oblique is incised vertically while a window is created through the internal oblique and transverse muscles by blunt separation of their fibers parallel to their orientation. The peritoneum is bluntly penetrated. The surgeon's hand is advanced into the abdominal cavity and placed underneath the gravid horn. With the surgeon lifting and pushing on the uterus rather than pulling on it, the uterus is rocked back and forth, until the uterus and fetus have flipped back to their normal position. Correction can be confirmed directly by palpation of the broad ligaments and by rectal palpation. Closure of the body wall is routine; the peritoneum is not typically closed, and the muscle layers opened during the approach are reapposed with #1 or #2 absorbable suture placed in a simple continuous pattern. The subcutaneous layer may be closed with the muscle layer or can be sutured in a separate layer, also in absorbable suture, whereas the skin is closed in nonabsorbable suture.[93,96]

Ventral midline celiotomy is the approach of choice if the uterus is ruptured, uterine wall compromise is suspected (eg, if the torsion is of several days' duration and congestion and edema of the uterus is likely, making it friable), degree of rotation is greater than or equal to 360°, the fetus is deceased and the mare is preterm, the mare has gastrointestinal tract, the mare is intractably painful, or if attempts at standing correction are unsuccessful.[93] Postoperative care of mares should include analgesics, antimicrobials, and meticulous incisional care. Mares that undergo surgery, especially ventral midline celiotomy, close to term should be considered a high-risk pregnancy, as the abdominal press recruited during active labor will challenge the sutures and/or staples used in the surgical closure and can result in catastrophic body wall failure and evisceration. Outfitting such a mare with an abdominal support wrap (nonstretching adhesive wrap or a commercially available abdominal girdle) before parturition starts is recommended. In one study of 7 mares with uterine torsion that underwent midline celiotomy, postoperative monitoring including assaying for progesterone (P4) and estradiol (E2), and mares with hormone profiles suggestive of inflammation or compromise were managed medically with a combination of a tocolytic, synthetic progesterone, and antimicrobial.[91] Fetal monitoring is also a part of postsurgical care in the pregnant mare.

Summary: Uterine torsion most frequently, but not exclusively, arises in mares in the last trimester of gestation and initially manifests as colic. The uterine torsion may incorporate gastrointestinal structures, in which case the colic will likely be more severe. The torsion should be corrected promptly for the best chance at mare and foal survival. Correction can be undertaken with nonsurgical means or with surgery. The prognosis for future fertility is good.

CLINICS CARE POINTS

- Injuries involving reproductive tract tissues are similar to those involving other body areas in that prompt recognition, thorough evaluation, and intervention underlie a favorable outcome
- In traumatic injuries, initial treatment to mitigate the peak severity and duration of inflammation and edema are particularly important in the external genitals of male horses
- Whether a practitioner will undertake full management of a reproductive tract emergency in the field or elects to evaluate and stabilize the patient and then refer, the first-line interventions provided can play the dominant role in outcome for the stallion, fetus, or mare
- Clear communications and management of client expectations are key skills for veterinarians managing reproductive emergencies

DISCLOSURE

The authors have nothing to disclose.

REFERENCES

1. Blue MG. Genital injuries from mating in the mare. Equine Vet J 1985;7:297–9.
2. Tulleners EP, Richardson DW, Reid BV. Vaginal evisceration of the small intestine in three mares. J Am Vet Med Assoc 1985;186:385–7.
3. Delling U, Stoebe S, Brehm W. Hand-assisted laparasocpic adhesiolysis of extensive small intestinal adhesions in a mare after breeding injury. Equine Vet Educ 2012;24:545–51.
4. Gomez JH, Rodgerson DH, Goodin J. How to repair cranial vaginal and caudal uterine tears in mares. In Proceedings. San Diego, CA: 54th Ann Conv Amer Assoc Equine Pract 2008; 54:295–7.
5. Zhang J, Ricketts SW, Tanner SJ. Antisperm antibodies in the semen of a stallion following testicular trauma. Equine Vet J 1990;22:138–41.
6. DeVries PJ. Diseases of the testes, penis, and related structures. In: McKinnon AO, Voss JL, editors. Equine reproduction. 1st edition. UK: Blackwell Publishing; 1993. 878–874.
7. Perkins NP, Frazer GS. Reproductive emergencies in the stallion. Vet Clin North Am Equine Pract 1994;10:671–83.
8. Kasaback CM, Rashmir-Raven AM, Black SS. Theriogenology question of the month. Septic orchitis-periorchitis and epididymitis. J Am Vet Med Assoc 1999; 215:787–9.
9. Estepa JC, Mayer-Valor R, Lopez I, et al. What is your diagnosis? Abscess developed as a result of scrotal and testicular lesions. J Am Vet Med Assoc 2006;228: 515–6.
10. Gonzales M, Tibary A, Sellon DC, et al. Unilateral orchitis and epididymitis caused by *Corynebacterum pseudotuberculosis* in a stallion. Equine Vet Educ 2008;20:30–6.

11. Beard W. Abnormalities of the testicles. In: McKinnon AO, Squires EL, Vaala WE, et al, editors. Equine Reprod. 2nd edition. West Sussex: Wiley-Blackwell; 2011. XX.

12. Da Silva Bonacin Y, des Santos Sousa S, Canola PA, et al. Haemoperitoneum secondary to testicular rupture caused by blunt trauma in a stallion. Equine Vet Educ 2020;32:622.

13. Papa FO, Leme DP. Testicular fine needle aspiration cytology from a stallion with testicular degeneration after external genitalia trauma. J Equine Vet Sci 2002;22: 121–4.

14. Brinsko SP, Blanchard TL, Varner DD. How to treat paraphimosis. In Proceedings. Orlando, FL: 53rd Ann Conv Amer Assoc Equine Pract, 2007;580–2.

15. Love CC. Ultrasonographic evaluation of the testis, epididymis, and spermatic cord of the stallion. Vet Clin North Am Equine Pract 1992;8:167–82.

16. Pozor MA, McDonald SM. Color Doppler ultrasound evaluation of testicular blood flow in stallions. Theriogenol 2004;61:799–810.

17. Turner RM, Dobbie T, Vanderwall DK. Stallion reproductive injuries. Acute paraphimosis. In: Orsini JA, Divers TJ, editors. Equine emergencies – treatment and procedures. 4th edition. St Louis (MO): Elsevier Saunders; 2014. p. 418–33.

18. Love CC, Kenney RM. Scrotal heat stress induces altered sperm chromatin structure associated with a decrease I protamine disulfide bonding in the stallion. Biol Reprod 1999;60:615–20.

19. Koch C, O'Brien T, Livesey MA. How to construct and apply a penile repulsion device (Probang) to manage paraphimosis. In Proceedings, Las Vegas, NV: 55th Ann Conv AAEP, 2009; 338–41.

20. Pozor MA. Ultrasonography of the penis. In: Kidd JA, Lu KG, Frazer ML, editors. Atlas of equine ultrasonography. West Sussex, UK: Wiley-Blackwell; 2014. p. 267–76.

21. Schumacher J. Penis and prepuce. In: Auer JA, Stick JA, editors. Equine surgery. 4th edition. St Louis (MO): Elsevier Saunders; 2012. p. 840–66.

22. Pauwels F, Schumacher J, Varner DD. Update on equine therapeutics: priapism in horses. Reprod Compend 2005;27:4.

23. Rezende ML, Ferris RA, Leise BS, et al. Treatment of intraoperative persistent penile erection in a stallion. J Equine Vet Sci 2014;4:431–5.

24. Wilson DV, Nickels FA, Williams MA. Pharmacologic treatment of priapism in two horses. J Am Vet Med Assoc 1991;199:1183–4.

25. Schumacher J, Hardin DK. Surgical treatment of priapism in a stallion. Vet Surg 1987;6:193–6.

26. Neely DP. Physical examination and genital diseases of the stallion. In: Morrow DA, editor. Current therapy in theriogenology. Philadelphia: Saunders; 1980. p. 694.

27. Simmons HA, Cox JE, Edwards GB, et al. Paraphimosis in seven debilitated horses. Vet Rec 1985;116:126–7.

28. De Lahunta A, Habel RE. Applied veterinary anatomy. Philadelphia: Saunders; 1986.

29. Vaughan JT. Examination of the stallion. In: Walker DE, Vaughan JT, editors. Bovine and equine urogenital surgery. Philadelphia: Lea & Febiger; 1980. p. 125.

30. Nie GI, Pope KC. Persistent penile prolapse associated with acute blood loss and acepromazine maleate administration in a horse. J Am Vet Med Assoc 1997;211: 587–9.

31. De Brauwer E, Ribera T, Climent F, et al. Alternative method to facilitate resolution of paraphimosis after penile trauma in the horse. Equine Vet 2017;9:655–8.

32. Hong CB, Donahue JM, Giles RC, et al. Etiology and pathology of equine placentitis. J Vet Diagn Invest 1993;5:56–63.
33. Giles RC, Donahue JM, Hong CB, et al. Causes of abortion, stillbirth, and perinatal death in horses: 3,527 cases (1986-1991). J Am Vet Med Assoc 1993; 203:1170–5.
34. LeBlanc MM. Ascending placentitis in the mare: an update. Reprod Dom Anim 2010;45(Suppl 2):28–34.
35. Timoney JF, Kalimuthusamy N, Velineri S, et al. A unique genotype of *Leptospira interrogans* serovar Pomona type Kennewicki is associated with equine abortion. Vet Microbiol 2011;150:349–53.
36. Erol E, Sells SF, Williams NM, et al. An investigation of a recent outbreak of nocardioform placentitis caused abortions in horses. Vet Microbiol 2012;58:425–30.
37. LeBlanc MM, Giguère S, Brauer K, et al. Premature delivery in ascending placentitis is associated with increased expression of placental cytokines and allantoic fluid prostaglandins E_2 and $F2\alpha$. Theriogenol 2002;8:841–4.
38. Calderwood Mays MB, LeBlanc MM, Paccamonti D. Route of fetal infection in a model of ascending placentitis. Theriogenol 2002;58:791–2.
39. LeBlanc MM, Giguère S, Lester GD, et al. Relationship between infection, inflammation and premature parturition in mares with experimentally induced placentitis. Equine Vet J 2012;44(Suppl 41):8–14.
40. Fedorka CE, Ball BA, Scoggin KE, et al. The feto-maternal immune response to equine placentitis. Am J Reprod Immunol 2019;2:e13179.
41. Fernandes CB, Ball BA, Loux SC, et al. Uterine cervix as a fundamental part of the pathogenesis of pregnancy loss associated with ascending placentitis in mares. Theriogenol 2020;145:167–75.
42. Renaudin CD, Troedsson MHT, Gillis CL, et al. Ultrasonographic evaluation of the equine placenta by transrectal and transabdominal approach in the normal pregnant mare. Theriogenol 1997;47:559–73.
43. Bucca S. Diagnosis of the compromised equine pregnancy. Vet Clin Equine 2006; 2:749–61.
44. Reef VB, Vaala WE, Worth LT, et al. Ultrasonographic assessment of fetal well-being during late gestation: development of an equine biophysical profile. Equine Vet J 1996;8:200–8.
45. Ousey JC, Houghten E, Grainger L, et al. Progestagen profiles during the last trimester of gestation in Thoroughbred mares with normal or compromised pregnancies. Theriogenol 2004;63:1844–56.
46. Ousey JC. Hormone profiles and treatments in the late pregnant mare. Vet Clin North Am Equine Pract 2006;22:727–47.
47. Morris S, Kelleman AA, Stawicki RJ, et al. Transrectal ultrasonography and plasma progestin profiles identifies feto-placental compromise in mares with experimentally-induced placentitis. Theriogenology 2007;67:681–91.
48. Coutinho da Silva MA, Canisso IF, MacPherson ML, et al. Serum amyloid A concentration in healthy periparturient mares and mares with ascending placentitis. Equine Vet J 2013;5:619–24.
49. Murchie TA, Macpherson ML, LeBlanc MM, et al. A microdialysis model to detect drugs in the allantoic fluid of pregnant pony mares. In Proceedings. San Antonio, TX: 49th Ann Conv Am Assoc Equine Pract 2006;49:118–21.
50. Rebello SA, Macpherson ML, Murchie TA, et al. Placental transfer of trimethoprim sulfamethoxazole and pentoxifylline in pony mares. Anim Reprod Sci 2006;94: 432–3.

51. Ellerbrock RE, Canisso IF, Roady PJ, et al. Diffusion of enrofloxacin to pregnancy fluids and effects on fetal cartilage after intravenous administration to late pregnant mares. Equine Vet J 2019;51:544–51.

52. D'el Rey Dantas FT, Canisso IF, et al. Doxycycline diffuses through the fetoplacental unit of late pregnant mares and accumulates in the joints of resulting foals. In Proceedings. Denver, CO: 65th Ann Conv Am Assoc Equine Pract 2019;65:61–2.

53. Bryant JE, Brown MP, Gronwall RR, et al. Study of intragastric administration of doxycycline: pharmacokinetics including body fluid, endometrial and minimum inhibitory concentrations. Equine Vet J 2000;32:233–8.

54. Macpherson ML, Giguère S, Pozor MA, et al. Pharmacokinetics of ceftiofur sodium in equine pregnancy. J Vet Pharmacol Ther 2017;40:656–62.

55. Macpherson ML, Giguère S, Hatzel JN, et al. Disposition of desfuroylceftiofur acetamide in serum, placental tissue, fetal fluids, and fetal tissues after administration of ceftiofur crystalline free acid (CCFA) to pony mares with placentitis. J Vet Pharmacol Ther 2013;36:59–67.

56. Bailey CS, Macpherson ML, Pozor MA, et al. Treatment efficacy of trimethoprim sulfamethoxazole, pentoxifylline and altrenogest in experimentally induced placentitis. Theriogenol 2010;74:402–12.

57. Christiansen D, Crouch J, Hopper R, et al. Experimentally induced placentitis in late gestation mares with *Streptococcus equi zooepidemicus*: therapeutic prevention of preterm birth. Clin Therio 2009;1:560–1.

58. Macpherson ML, Giguère S, Pozor MA, et al. Inflammatory mediator production in fetal fluids after firocoxib treatment in mares with experimentally-induced placentitis. J Equine Vet Sci 2018;6:227.

59. Macpherson ML. Treatment strategies for mares with placentitis. Theriogenology 2005;64:528–34.

60. Neuhauser S, Palm F, Ambuehl F, et al. Effects of altrenogest treatment of mares in late pregnancy on parturition and on neonatal viability of their foals. Exp Clin Endocrinol Diabetes 2008;116:423–8.

61. Curcio BR, Canisso IF, Pazinato FM, et al. Estradiol cypionate aided treatment for experimentally induced ascending placentitis in mares. Theriogenol 2017;102:98–107.

62. Vandeplassche M, Bouters R, Spincemaille J, et al. Dropsy of the fetal sacs in mares: induced and spontaneous abortion. Vet Rec 1976;99:67–9.

63. Roberts SJ. Veterinary Obstetrics and genital diseases (Theriogenology). 3rd edition. Woodstock, VT: Roberts; 1986.

64. Honnas CM, Spensley MS, Laverty S, et al. Hydramnios causing uterine rupture in a mare. J Am Vet Med Assoc 1988;193:334–6.

65. Morrow DA. Current therapy in Theriogenology 2. Philadelphia, PA: Saunders; 1986.

66. Slovis NM, Lu KG, Wolfsdorf KE, et al. How to manage hydrops allantois/hydrops amnion in a mare. In Proceedings. Nashville, TN: 59th Ann Conv Am Assoc Equine Pract 2013;59:34–9.

67. Govaere JLJ, De Schauwer C, Hoogewijs MK, et al. Hydrallantois in the mare – a report of five cases. Reprod Dom Anim 2013;48:e1–6.

68. Waelchli RO, Ehrensperger F. Two related cases of cerebellar abnormality in equine fetuses associated with hydrops of fetal membranes. Vet Rec 1988;123:513–4.

69. Shanahan LM, Slovis NM. Leptospira interrogans associated with hydrallantois in 2 pluriparous thoroughbred mares. J Vet Intern Med 2011;25:158–61.

70. Diel de Amorim M, Chenier TS, Card C, et al. Treatment of hydropsical conditions using transcervical gradual fetal fluid drainage in mares with or without concurrent abdominal wall disease. J Equine Vet Sci 2018;64:81–8.

71. Christensen BW, Troedsson MH, Murchie TA, et al. Management of hydrops amnion in a mare resulting in birth of a live foal. J Am Vet Med Assoc 2006;8: 1228–33.

72. Reef VB, Vaala WE, Worth LT, et al. Ultrasonographic evaluation of the fetus and intrauterine environment in healthy mares during late gestation. Vet Radiol Ultrasound 1995;36:533–41.

73. Bucca S, Fogarty U, Collins A, et al. Assessment of feto-placental well-being in the mare from mid-gestation to term: transrectal and transabdominal ultrasonographic features. Theriogeno 2005;64:542–57.

74. Habel RE, Budras KD. Anatomy of the prepubic tendon in the horse, cow, sheep, goat, and dog. Am J Vet Res 1992;53:2183–95.

75. Pasquini C, Spurgeon T, Pasquini S, et al. Anatomy of dmestic animals: systemic and regional approach. 10th edition. Minneapolis: Sudz; 2003.

76. Hanson RR, Todhunter RJ. Herniation of the abdominal wall in pregnant mares. J Am Vet Med Assoc 1986;89:790–3.

77. Ross J, Palmer JE, Wilkins PA. Body wall tears during late pregnancy in mares: 13 cases (1995–2006). J Am Vet Med Assoc 2008;232:257–61.

78. Card C, Dedden I, Ripley E, et al. Features of ventrolateral abdominal wall muscles in non-pregnant mares and pregnant mares with and without abdominal wall disease. J Vet Equine Sci 2014;34:229.

79. Pascoe JR, Meagher DM, Wheat JD. Surgical management of uterine torsion in the mare: a review of 26 cases. J Am Vet Med Assoc 1981;179:351–4.

80. Chaney KP, Holcombe SJ, LeBlanc MM, et al. The effect of uterine torsion on mare and foal survival: a retrospective study, 1985–2005. Equine Vet J 2007; 39:33–6.

81. Spoormakers TJP, Graat EAM, ter Braake F, et al. Mare and foal survival and subsequent fertility of mares treated for uterine torsion. Equine Vet J 2016;48:172–5.

82. Barber SM. Complications of chronic uterine torsion in a mare. Can Vet J 1995;36: 102–3.

83. Doyle AJ, Freeman DE, Sauberli DS, et al. Clinical signs and treatment of chronic uterine torsion in two mares. J Am Vet Med Assoc 2002;220:349–53.

84. Lopez C, Carmona JU. Uterine torsion diagnosed in a mare at 515 days' gestation. Equine Vet Educ 2010;22:483.

85. Taylor EL, Blanchard T, Varner D. Management of dystocia in mares: uterine torsion and cesarean section. Compend Contin Educ Pract Vet 1989;11:1265–72.

86. Barber SM. Torsion of the uterus – a cause of colic in the mare. Can Vet J 1979;20: 165–7.

87. Wheat JD, Meagher DM. Uterine torsion and rupture in mares. J Am Vet Med Assoc 1972;160:881–4.

88. Jung C, Hospes R, Bostedt H, et al. Surgical treatment of uterine torsion using a ventral midline laparotomy in 19 mares. Aust Vet J 2008;86:272–6.

89. Ruffin DC, Schumacher J, Comer JS. Uterine torsion associated with small intestinal incarceration in a mare at 126 days of gestation. J Am Vet Med Assoc 1995; 207:329–30.

90. Vandeplassche M, Spincemaille J, Bouters R, et al. Some aspects of equine obstetrics. Equine Vet J 1972;4:105–9.

91. Satoh M, Higuchi T, Inoue S, et al. Factors affecting the prognosis for uterine torsion: the effect of treatment based on measurements of serum progesterone and estradiol concentrations after surgery. J Equine Sci 2017;28:163-7.

92. Vasey JR, Russell T. Uterine torsion. In: McKinnon AO, Squieres EL, Vaala W, et al, editors. Equine reproduction. 2nd edition. West Sussex: Wiley-Blackwell; 2011. p. 2435-40.

93. Embertson R. Uterus and ovaries. In: Auer J, Stick JA, editors. Equine surgery. 4th edition. St Louis (MO): Elsevier Saunders; 2012. p. 883-92.

94. Riggs LM. How to perform non-surgical correction of acute uterine torsion in the mare. Proc 52nd Ann Conv Am Assoc Equine Pract 2006;52:256-8.

95. Wichtel JJ, Reinertson EL, Clark TL. Nonsurgical treatment of uterine torsion in seven mares. J Am Vet Med Assoc 1988;193:337-8.

96. Yorke EH, Caldwell FJ, Johnson AK. Uterine torsion in mares. Comp Cont Educ Vet Equine Pract 2012;E1-E5.

97. Turner RM, Dobbie T, Vanderwall DK. Mare reproductive injuries. Uterine torsion. In: Orsini JA, Divers TJ, editors. Equine emergencies – treatment and procedures. 4th edition. St Louis (MO): Elsevier Saunders; 2014. p. 433-49.

Managing Reproduction Emergencies in the Field

Part 2: Parturient and Periparturient Conditions

Kristina G. Lu, VMD[a], Kim A. Sprayberry, DVM[b],*

KEYWORDS

- Uterine • Hemorrhage • Shock • Prolapse • Dystocia • Retained membranes
- Metritis • SIRS

KEY POINTS

- Mares with pariparturient arterial rupture may bleed only into the broad ligament, or the bleeding can rupture the ligament and progress to hemoabdomen. With the former, mares usually manifest signs of colic, and with the latter, signs of hemorrhagic shock are dominant.
- Many cases of dystocia are amenable to intervention in the field, but the veterinarian should have access to a safe area for general anesthesia for controlled vaginal delivery and should follow the time-based guidelines for progressing from assisted delivery to controlled delivery.
- Uterine prolapse is amenable to management in the field but necessitates assistance and aftercare.
- The emergent problems arising in the pregnant mare usually have systemic ramifications and demand skilled monitoring and treatment.

In this second article on reproductive emergencies, conditions arising during parturition and in the periparturient period are discussed.

UTERINE ARTERY RUPTURE

Periparturient rupture of arteries supplying the uterus and ovaries is a significant cause of morbidity and fatality in broodmares.[1] Internal hemorrhage associated with the reproductive tract should be a common rule-out for any periparturient mare with abdominal discomfort. In a 1993 study[2] of 98 mares that died in the postpartum

Funded by: CSU2020.
[a] Hagyard Equine Medical Institute, 4250 Iron Works Pike, Lexington, KY 40511, USA;
[b] Department of Animal Sciences, Cal Poly University San Luis Obispo, 1 Grand Avenue, San Luis Obispo, CA 93407, USA
* Corresponding author.
E-mail address: kspraybe@calpoly.edu

Vet Clin Equine 37 (2021) 367–405
https://doi.org/10.1016/j.cveq.2021.04.008
0749-0739/21/© 2021 The Authors. Published by Elsevier Inc. This is an open access article under the CC BY-NC-ND license (http://creativecommons.org/licenses/by-nc-nd/4.0/).

period, 40 (41%) died of arterial rupture and internal hemorrhage. In a study of post-partum mares admitted to a referral hospital, urogenital tract hemorrhage was diag-nosed in 27 of 163 (16.6%) mares, and those mares had a significantly shorter time from parturition to hospital admission, compared with mares referred for other rea-sons.[3] Uterine artery rupture was the diagnosis in 9 of 67 (13%) horses evaluated for hemoperitoneum in another study.[4]

Arterial rupture has been diagnosed in younger mares and can affect mares of any parity, but multiparous older mares are most likely to be affected. In 3 retrospective studies,[3,5,6] the median ages were 13, 14, and 16.7 years; in one of those studies,[3] the odds of a mare having urogenital tract hemorrhage increased by 13.7% with each year of age. A necropsy study[6] revealed that 28% of mares older than 15 years died of periparturient artery rupture; when the subject mares were grouped as all ma-res older than 3 years, the percentage of those dying from arterial rupture was 9.9%. In 73 mares with periparturient hemorrhage that were admitted to a referral clinic, 10 ma-res (14%) had prepartum hemorrhage, whereas 63 (86%) had postpartum hemor-rhage.[5] In one of the studies previously cited,[6] 21 of 71 (29.6%) mares in a review of necropsy cases had hemorrhaged before parturition, 42 (59.1%) has hemorrhage during parturition, and 8 (11.3%) had hemorrhage after parturition. Arterial rupture is rarely seen at other times besides the periparturient period in mares. Not all cases of periparturient hemorrhage necessitate referral or even treatment: residual hema-tomas can be detected during routine transrectal palpation and ultrasonography of the reproductive tract in mares that never had signs of colic or hemorrhage after foaling.

Uterine Blood Supply

A review of urogenital tract blood supply is helpful in understanding the vascular injury. Arterial blood supply to the equine uterus is chiefly supplied by the uterine artery, which is a large branch of the external iliac artery, itself a part of the termination of the aorta. From the external iliac, the uterine artery (also called the middle uterine ar-tery) courses toward the uterine horn in the mesometrium, or broad ligament. At the uterine horn, the artery branches cranially and anastomoses with the uterine branch of the ovarian artery, and branches caudally to anastomose with the uterine branch of the vaginal artery. The vaginal artery arises from the internal pudendal artery, which is a branch of the internal iliac artery; the vaginal artery and other branches of the pu-dendal artery supply the caudal part of the uterus and more distal parts of the tract.[7] As the uterine artery runs longitudinally along the uterine body and horns in the broad ligament, it diverges into numerous tortuous small branches and anastomoses that meet on the dorsal and ventral aspects of the horn and enable vascular stretching to accommodate uterine engorgement and elongation (**Fig. 1**).

Serial Doppler monitoring of the uterine arteries has revealed that during the first half of gestation, the vasculature of the pregnant uterus undergoes transition from a high-resistance low-flow circulation to a low-resistance high-flow circulation accommoda-ting large volumes of blood flow.[8] In combination with degenerative histologic change that develops in arterial walls with age, senescence, and cyclic stretching and shear stress, the situation is set up for arterial wall failure to increase with age and parity.[9]

Upon arterial rupture, the extravasated blood can dissect along planes in the broad ligament, into the uterine or vaginal wall, into the space between the myometrium and serosal surface of the uterus, and occasionally into the uterine lumen. Arterial rupture can involve any of the arterial segments perfusing the reproductive tract, but most commonly involves the proximal segment of the uterine artery.[5,9–11] In a 2010 study of 31 mares with fatal broad ligament hematoma, 24 had uterine artery hemorrhage;

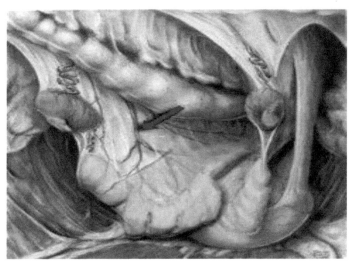

Fig. 1. Diagram of the uterus in situ, suspended by the broad ligaments. Arrow points to uterine artery. Notice how it communicates with the vaginal artery caudally and ovarian artery cranially as it supplies the length of the uterine horn. The small colon is seen suspended by mesocolon and lying dorsal to the uterine horns. (*Modified from*: "Equine Reproduction" McKinnon A.O. & Voss J.L., Lea & Febiger, 1993. Used with permission from Lippincott, Williams & Wilkens.)

in 18 of those the site of rupture was within 15 cm of the vessel's bifurcation from the external iliac.[9] Gross lesions in the affected vessels included longitudinal fissuring of the arterial wall or outright transection of the vessels. Detection of the site of arterial wall failure during necropsy can be difficult given the size of the broad ligament and the extensive hemorrhage, but the site of arterial wall failure is typically a partial-circumference tear with jagged dark red edges and covered by blood clot and fibrin.[12] Underlying histologic degenerative changes in the arterial wall include atrophy of the smooth muscle layer, fibrotic change in the tunica media, and disruption or mineralization of the internal elastic lamina.[9,13]

It has been reported that the right uterine artery is more often affected than the left,[13] and that the left is more frequently affected than the right.[2,9] With the former, it has been postulated that displacement of the uterus to the left by the cecum during gestation causes an added degree of tension on the right broad ligament and its vessels.[10] More recent studies have indicated no predilection for side and suggest that the left and right arteries rupture with equal frequency.[6] Mares that have hemorrhaged can successfully and uneventfully carry foals to term in successive pregnancies.

Clinical Signs

Arterial rupture quickly elicits signs of some combination of colic and hemorrhagic shock. Colic signs can range from mild to severe, including flank-checking, stretching, flehmen, and rolling. Signs of hypovolemic shock include tachycardia, flehmen, muscle fasciculations or trembling, sweating, depression, disorientation, undirected vocalization, and collapse.

The initial extravasation of blood into the broad ligament stretches the ligament and its dorsal attachments and creates tension and pressure within its planes; this usually causes acute colic pain, but the pressure contributes to staunching of the bleeding as long as the ligament remains intact. If the backpressure causes blood loss to cease at this point, signs of colic may persist for several hours but typically respond to analgesics. Depending on the volume of blood pulsing into the broad ligament, the severity of this colic can be mild to moderate. The owner or caretaker will see some combination of the mare pacing or pawing, lying down and getting back up, sweating, splinting the abdomen, flank-checking, and having steam rise from the back and flanks. One feature of pain from broad ligament stretching is raising of the upper lip typical of the flehmen response.

If hemorrhage escapes from the confines of the broad ligament, uncontrolled bleeding into the peritoneal cavity will commence, with rapid deterioration of hemodynamic status and signs of shock predominating over signs of colic. Death may ensue rapidly. If the mare has been observed from the beginning, signs of pain often abate, whereas depression, trembling, agitation, and weakness will progress, with continued sweating, steaming, and lip-lifting. The gingivae become noticeably pallorous, sometimes to the extent that they cannot be blanched with a thumb to check capillary refill. In the words of one experienced clinician, the gums take on the dry sheen of "an old white porcelain sink" (Byars TD, personal communication, April 2007). The pupils are usually dilated. High heart rate (60–80 bpm or higher) is invariably observed, and rectal temperature is usually low or normal. Internal exsanguination can take place rapidly or over a period of hours. The tachycardia, pupillary dilation, and sweating arise autonomically because the acute volume loss leads to activation of the sympathetic nervous system. In many instances, the mare is already in a state of hemodynamic shock at the time the problem is first recognized and a veterinarian summoned; absence of previous colic is not grounds for dismissing arterial rupture and hemorrhage from the top of a list of differential diagnoses in this scenario. It is important to remember that this reproductive emergency can happen days to weeks before parturition.

Diagnosis

Physical examination: Experienced owners can come to quickly recognize the signs of uterine artery rupture: a pawing, sweating postpartum (most frequently) mare with lifted lip. Nevertheless, the veterinarian's physical examination provides a database of findings that point to diagnosis and also provides the baseline values from which the patient can be seen to improve or worsen during serial monitoring. The examiner and holder should enter the stall with caution and with an assessing eye on the mare's mental state and physical stability. A mare can be depressed, painful, disoriented, comforted by human presence, agitated by the same, or on the verge of collapse and death. Grasping her foal and removing it from the mare's sight may cause a spike in anxiety that will upset a fragile stability and renew bleeding. During examination, the newborn foal should be quietly captured and held at the stall door, in close sight of the mare, but in a position to be removed from the stall quickly in the face of terminal excitation or abrupt collapse in the mare.

The examination must often be abbreviated in the interest of efficiency and safety; for instance, although rectal examination is part of full examination of a colicky animal and could confirm a hematoma in a broad ligament, in this situation it may not be advisable or safe for the mare or the examiner. Application of a nose twitch or other physical restraint can induce collapse, and advance of the examiner's arm into the rectum induces the mare to respond with abdominal press, which can disrupt an early or partial thrombus in the damaged artery. These adverse occurrences are not mere theoretic concerns, and in the authors' experience, it is possible to diagnose arterial internal hemorrhage without rectal palpation. Obtaining the temperature (often low or normal), heart rate (usually high but occasionally normal), and respiratory rate (usually high) can usually be accomplished. Physical parameters that serve as an index of circulatory status, such as skin turgor (often reduced), capillary refill (usually prolonged), arterial pulse quality (may be bounding but grows increasingly weak and "thready" as hypotension and hypovolemia approach the limits of compensation), jugular refill (usually prolonged), and the cutaneous temperature of the extremities (cool to cold) can usually be assessed quickly and without undue stress to the mare. Persisting tachycardia and the presence of vaginal hemorrhage have been significantly associated with outcome.[5]

Laboratory values: Blood should be collected and submitted for complete blood cell count (CBC) and serum chemistry. If full laboratory services are unavailable in the emergent field setting, a simple packed cell volume (PCV) and total protein analysis and possibly lactate are helpful, even if only for comparison in the ensuing hours to days. In the peracute phase of hemorrhage, PCV and protein values are normal,[5] as the blood remaining within the circulation to be sampled is unaltered until hemodilution occurs as a result of body mechanisms to preserve blood volume and pressure. Over a period of hours to days, water is pulled from the interstitial and intracellular spaces into the vascular space, plus the thirst response is induced. If the mare survives long enough for these mechanisms to bolster or replace plasma volume, or if veterinary intervention includes administration of intravenous (IV) fluids, serial blood sampling will show increasing hemodilution, with hypoproteinemia and anemia. Hypofibrinogenemia is also common.[3] Splenic contraction is also stimulated by the sympathetic nervous response to hemorrhage, ejecting erythrocyte mass into the circulation to support oxygen-carrying capacity. This effect may bolster PCV values, and serial blood monitoring may reveal nadir values of protein that are more markedly low than those of PCV. Assuming hemorrhage ceases, the lowest values for PCV and protein are usually seen at about 48 hours after the onset of bleeding.

Findings of leukopenia/neutropenia on the hemogram suggest that the systemic inflammatory response syndrome (SIRS) is in play. Sepsis from translocation of bacteria from the hypoperfused gastrointestinal tract into the lymph nodes, liver, and bloodstream is one sequela of severe hemorrhage and impaired perfusion of the gut mucosa.[14]

Increased values for serum urea nitrogen and/or creatinine are common in mares that are in the stages of surviving hemorrhagic shock. Decreased glomerular filtration and oliguria are common in hypovolemia. Liver values might also be high, reflecting hypoxic damage. Unlike with external hemorrhage, with internal hemorrhage icterus is common during convalescence because of heme recycling.

Normal blood lactate concentration in health is ≤ 2.0 mmol/L. When values increase in the setting of hemorrhage, it reflects a tissue shift to anaerobic metabolism and hence serves as an index of circulatory sufficiency. In hemorrhaging mares it is helpful to obtain an admission lactate level, and this can be run serially to determine the efficacy of resuscitation and maintenance support. When lactate values increase or remain high in the face of volume replacement with IV fluids, it is a useful indicator for blood transfusion. Mildly elevated values may be tolerated in the face of stabilization of other physical examination parameters.

Abdominocentesis is indicated when other differential diagnoses, such as uterine rupture or gastrointestinal disease, are suspected in place of or in addition to arterial hemorrhage.

Ultrasonography: Transabdominal ultrasonography is the quickest methodology for confirming hemoabdomen. Careful transrectal imaging can be useful when hemorrhage is suspected but confined to a site in the broad ligament. Transabdominal imaging can yield a wealth of information, even with a brief survey of the mare's abdomen. Whether hemoabdomen is present, whether bleeding is ongoing and active, an approximation of the volume of blood that has been lost to the abdominal third space, whether bleeding has stopped and then resumed, and if resorption of extravasated blood has begun, all can be determined easily and quickly. The best transducer to use for transcutaneous evaluation of the abdomen is a 2.5- to 5.0-MHz macroconvex probe, but nearly any transducer can yield useful images, including a linear rectal probe. The author (K.S.) finds that applying warmed rubbing alcohol (70% isopropyl) to the ventral abdomen and sides precludes the need to clip hair and elicits no signs of resentment from the mares.

The presence of free blood in the peritoneal cavity has a dramatic and unique sonographic appearance, and is not a subtle finding. When bleeding is active, it is usually possible to find an area where the pulsing blood enters the abdomen with smokelike swirling and formation of curlicues in the echogenic fluid (**Fig. 2**).

The sonographic appearance of the abdomen changes with the stage of bleeding. When there is echogenic fluid (blood) accumulated ventrally with viscera floating several to many centimeters above, even in the absence of curlicues or swirling appearance, this suggests that there is still active bleeding somewhere in the abdomen as once hemorrhage ceases, the third-space blood is resorbed fairly rapidly. Upon hemostasis, the cavitary blood rapidly separates into plasma and cellular components, and the fluid (serum) in this stage is hypoechoic to anechoic (**Fig. 3**). The plasma water is reabsorbed back into the circulation, proteins are returned to the liver for catabolism and recycling, and erythrocyte/hemoglobin Fe^{2+} and protein are also conserved and recycled. Scanning the mare in this stage as frequently as twice a day can reveal significant diminution of the abdominal fluid volume at every examination. After the acute phase of hemorrhage, when a mare has successfully been stabilized with volume replacement and analgesics, and is maintaining a stable if

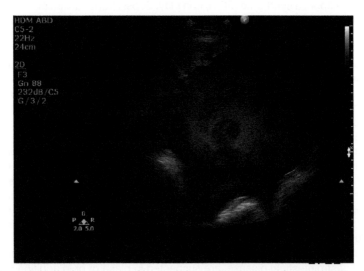

Fig. 2. Transabdominal sonogram of hemoabdomen in a mare with postpartum uterine artery rupture. Top of the image is ventral. The white curvilinear structures are colon segments buoyed in the free blood. The echogenicity of the gray fluid identifies it as highly cellular; the curlicue swirling pattern in the fluid and swirling motions seen in real time identify the fluid as blood with active arterial spurting.

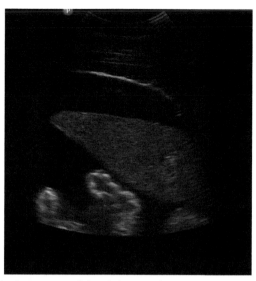

Fig. 3. Transabdominal sonogram of the abdomen of a mare with postpartum uterine artery rupture and hemoabdomen. Active hemorrhage has ceased, and resorption of the free abdominal blood is in process. The fluid remaining here is chiefly serum, which appears hypoechoic to anechoic. The spleen and several jejunal segments in cross section are seen buoyed in the fluid.

persistently high heart rate, bleeding may continue for several days as seen by persisting swirling in the abdominal blood, but the volume of blood loss will come to be offset by a commensurate rate of resorption, such that the mare's vital signs and comfort level remain stable. Once active bleeding ceases, resorption commences and is fairly rapid.

Treatment

Concepts
Systemic mean arterial pressure (MAP; 90–120 mm Hg in a healthy adult horse) drives rapid, voluminous extravasation through the ruptured vessel wall, and the drop in pressure is detected by arterial baroreceptors in the aortic arch and carotid bodies. Afferent neurons carry this information to the autonomic control centers in the brainstem, and this elicits a state of sympathetic nervous system outflow.[15] Fear, pain, exercise, and acute blood loss are all potent activators of the sympathetic fight-or-flight response. For clear reasons it is better to manage uterine hemorrhage at the farm and avoid trailering. However, if provision of the care and monitoring needed to manage this type of emergency is not available at the farm, transporting the mare to a hospital is warranted. Because of the unpredictability and sporadic nature of these cases, much of the information available to guide management of mares with uterine hemorrhage has been derived from retrospective case series involving hospitalized mares rather than from controlled studies.

The first step in providing care to an internally bleeding mare is to provide a quiet, low-stress space in which to work. This step means keeping the foal in immediate view or contact with the mare, yet close enough to the stall exit so that it can be removed if the mare becomes terminally agitated or collapses. Other horses should be kept away to avoid the mare taking up protective maneuvers that will increase blood pressure and disrupt initial coagulation.

The paradigm of intervention for trauma and massive hemorrhage in human medicine consists of would damage-control resuscitation, which consists of permissive hypotension, hemostatic restoration and blood product transfusion, and damage-control surgery. The concept originated in military medicine, and has progressed to also become the current management paradigm for massive bleeding in civilian settings.[16] Damage control surgery refers to initial laparotomy in a field setting to achieve vascular ligation and hemostasis, with temporary closure techniques used to close the abdomen. The patient undergoes blood transfusion and low-volume crystalloids for physiologic stabilization while being transferred to another location, where the abdomen is reopened and definitive laparotomy is undertaken. These methods yield higher survival rates than in patients in whom definitive laparotomy was the first-line intervention.[17,18] Although these measures were developed in human patients with internal hemorrhage from traumatic injury, and these types of studies have not been and likely will not be performed in horses, there is rationale for drawing on these concepts to treat horses with uncontrolled internal hemorrhage.

Arterial ligation during open-abdomen surgery is not feasible in the postpartum mare because of the poor anesthetic candidates represented by anxious, painful, hypovolemic, hypotensive, thousand-pound patients. Even if the mare survived anesthetic induction and the positioning into dorsal recumbency, the sheer volume of free blood in the peritoneal cavity, volume of the broad ligaments, and complex anatomy of the vasculature collectively make detection of the site of rupture difficult and time consuming at best. Therefore, the big picture for the veterinarian undertaking care of the internally bleeding mare is one of being limited to medical management of what is essentially a surgical problem, with an inability to use even the basic first-aid measure of applying pressure to the wound. Understanding this is important in managing client expectations and in implementing and revising interventions as patient status stabilizes or worsens.

Analgesics

For mares in which hemorrhage is contained in the broad ligament or pelvic canal, the treatment aims are to control pain and monitor serially to ensure the situation does not progress to hemoabdomen. In a retrospective study cited earlier in this article,[5] 72 of 73 mares with periparturient hemorrhage required pain management. Providing analgesia and offering a laxative diet to avoid the need for gastric intubation may be all that is required in some mares. Common treatments include flunixin meglumine (1.1 mg/kg, IV), xylazine (0.2–0.5 mg/kg, IV or intramuscular [IM]), and detomidine (0.01–0.02 mg/kg, IV or IM). Alpha-2 agonist drugs have significant cardiac and vasomotor effects, including bradycardia and first- and second-degree atrioventricular block, together with a sustained period of increased peripheral vascular resistance.[19] These effects decrease cardiac output. These effects are well tolerated by healthy horses, but given the labile, sympathetic-dominated state of a hemorrhaging horse, the author (K.S.) finds it useful to use alpha-2 agonist drugs at lower dosages that may be a fraction of published formulary dosages. Butorphanol, a mixed mu agonist opioid, is also helpful; some twitching may be seen, but in painful horses the analgesic and sedative effects predominate and butorphanol provides significant analgesia when paired with an alpha-2 agonist. Dosage range is 0.01 to 0.03 mg/kg, IV or IM. Similar to the alpha-2 drugs, butorphanol given IM can be helpful in providing analgesia with less noticeable sedation. When opioids are administered several times a day, constipation should be anticipated, and the mare should be given a laxative diet. Restraining a hemorrhaging or newly stabilized mare with a nose twitch for nasogastric intubation should be avoided if possible. A useful approach is to give an initial combination of flunixin plus an alpha-2 agonist and butorphanol IV to gain a level of analgesia, then give additional doses of the latter two drugs IM at intervals thereafter if needed.

Fluids

The aims in stabilizing the mare with hemoabdomen and shock are more complex. The treatment goals are to provide partial volume replacement to a state of permissive hypotension, promote coagulation or impede clot lysis, control pain, and support oxygen-carrying capacity with blood transfusion if necessary and possible. The concept of permissive hypotension means providing sufficient perfusion to support vital functions but not restore normal MAP values and threaten a fragile thrombus at the site of arterial rupture. Volume support can be provided in the form of hypertonic saline, polyionic crystalloid fluids, plasma, and whole blood. Synthetic colloids such as hetastarch are useful in rapid expansion of intravascular volume but should be avoided in this scenario because of its potential negative impact on coagulation and the potential for renal tubular injury in the volume-contracted state. Some practitioners find careful use of synthetic colloids useful, but administration of these fluids have come under scrutiny and questioning recently.[20]

In a mare that is unstable and near collapse from shock at initial evaluation, resuscitation is required. A bolus of hypertonic saline (7.2%; 2–4 mL/kg, IV) can be given, followed by balanced polyionic crystalloids. The optimum volume of fluids to administer in this setting has not been established by evidence-based medicine. With the goal of supporting circulation and critical functions, there is rationale in adopting commonly used resuscitation strategies but stopping short of using full attainment of euvolemia as the targeted endpoint. One method of providing resuscitatory support is to give a 20 mL/kg bolus of IV fluids and assess heart rate and other vital signs. Sequential boluses are given until indices of volume repletion are seen. In an internally hemorrhaging horse that presents in shock, an initial dose of hypertonic saline can be given, followed with an initial slow bolus of polyionic fluids. If the mare's affect improves, heart rate stabilizes, and perfusion of peripheral tissues improves, this could be followed by no additional fluids, additional slow boluses at scheduled intervals, or a constant infusion of fluids at maintenance or submaintenance volumes. In addition to the risk of restored arterial blood pressure disrupting or dislodging a developing thrombus at the site of vascular rupture, overzealous administration of IV fluids also dilutes clotting factors, platelets, and oxygen-carrying capacity. Constant infusions are not always possible in the field setting, but can be useful for delivering antimicrobials and antifibrinolytic drugs. Indices to monitor for sufficiency of organ perfusion include heart rate, comfort level/affect, blood lactate, and urine output. The maintenance fluid requirement in healthy adult horses is 40 to 60 mL/kg/d,[21,22] and water consumption would be taken into account with this calculation.

Once hypertonic saline has been given and crystalloids have been started, if heart rate remains at or near the value before the hypertonic saline was given, there is continued sweating or signs of distress, gums are pallorous, or lactate is high or increasing (reference range, <2.0 mmol/L); these collectively suggest that increased tissue oxygen delivery is needed in addition to volume improvement. In this instance, transfusion of fresh whole blood transfusion (4–8 L, given over 1–4 hours) is warranted. Blood is an effective colloid that not only supplies plasma proteins and oncotic pressure but also erythrocytes and oxygen-carrying capacity. There is no single value for PCV that can be used as a trigger for blood transfusion in all cases. However, a steadily falling value, in conjunction with signs of unabated severe tachycardia, increasing blood lactate, and visual confirmation of continued bleeding on ultrasound, do provide grounds for transfusion. The decision is not a trivial one: fresh whole blood transfusions cost well upward of $1000 in many practices, and the exogenous blood administration can set the mare up for developing antibodies against future fetuses. Sometimes multiple transfusions will be needed over the course of several days. Packed cell volume and protein values usually reach their nadirs in 36 to 48 hours as bleeding slows and ceases while IV fluids and body fluid shifts dilute the remaining intravascular red cell mass and protein. The reader is referred to other texts for details of fresh whole blood transfusion and donor compatibility testing.[23,24]

Antifibrinolytics

Administration of an antifibrinolytic or clot-stabilizing drug is also warranted in the mare with uncontrolled internal hemorrhage. A large meta-analysis of antifibrinolytics in acute severe hemorrhage in human patients revealed that administration of tranexamic acid within 3 hours of onset of bleeding improved overall survival in trauma and postpartum hemorrhage.[25] The natural balance of procoagulant and anticoagulant processes that are ongoing in the vasculature in health can be tipped toward clot preservation during uncontrolled hemorrhage by administration of tranexamic acid (5–25 mg/kg IV every 12 hours) given as a slow IV bolus or ε-aminocaproic acid (40 mg/kg [20 g for an adult light-breed mare] diluted in 1 L saline and given over 30 to 60 minutes, followed by 20 mg/kg [10 g] given the same way every 6 hours). Both drugs are synthetic lysine analogs that slow fibrinolysis by competitively and reversibly binding to the lysine active site on the plasminogen molecule.[26] This action prevents activation to plasmin and thwarts the lytic action of plasmin on fibrin, stabilizing a polymerized clot and prolonging its duration. These drugs are usually given for 1 to 2 days, or as indicated by ongoing or resumed hemorrhage. Tranexamic acid has other properties that have been demonstrated experimentally that may have relevance in hemorrhagic shock. In addition to its antifibrinolytic properties, it is also a serine protease inhibitor, one action of which is to inhibit gut epithelial sheddases. Sheddases are activated by shock-mediated hypoxia, and attack syndecan-1, breaking down the mucosal barrier function. In one study,[27] intraluminal tranexamic acid mitigated intestine and lung injury secondary to hemorrhagic shock in rats. Also interestingly, administration of tranexamic acid is a known cause of nausea and emesis in humans and dogs, and of nausea in experimental rodents such as rats, which, like horses, are nonvomiters.[28,29] An IV infusion of tranexamic acid has even been used to induce emesis in dogs that ingested foreign substances.[30] To the authors' knowledge, this has not been reported in horses, but it is reasonable to observe mares receiving IV infusions of this drug for signs of discomfort or distress.

During the first 24 hours, heart rate and physical status should be frequently monitored. The mare is encouraged to consume a laxative meal and some hay, and analgesics are usually continued. Flunixin, butorphanol or another opioid, and alpha-2 receptor agonists all have a place in controlling pain. In the first one to several hours from the initial evaluation, most mares will respond to these measures with a decreasing heart rate (although usually not to normal range) that remains steady, a state of less distress and controlled pain, and evidence of improving hemodynamic stability. However, it is not unusual for a mare to appear improved for a period of time but then resume signs of decompensation and shock.

Antimicrobials

Antimicrobials are indicated in mares with hemoabdomen and shock. Hemorrhagic shock is an innately inflammatory condition, with cellular hypoxia resulting in accumulation of lactic acid and oxygen radicals and eliciting release of danger-associated molecular proteins (DAMPs). These mediators activate the SIRS response, and multiple organ failure occurs in many tissues, including the intestinal mucosal barrier.[17,27,31–33] Hypoxia during shock has a quick-onset permissive effect on microbial translocation across the intestinal mucosal barrier. This can manifest in serial blood monitoring as a developing leukopenia/neutropenia, although hemodilution from IV fluids also contributes to this effect. Another reason for antimicrobial support is that hemorrhaging mares cannot be turned out to exercise, depriving them of one of the most important mechanisms supporting uterine clearance and involution: normal physical activity. These mares are also usually not candidates for uterine lavage or administration of oxytocin to help remove luminal blood and residual fluids, at least initially. In select cases, a sterile tube can be inserted into the uterus and used to siphon fluids, but typically this is not resorted to until several days have passed.

Other Treatments

Prednisolone sodium succinate (500–1000 mg per adult mare, IV) is given by some veterinarians to mitigate the effects of shock.

Naloxone is a pure narcotic antagonist that targets all subclasses of opiate receptors (μ, κ, and δ) but has the highest affinity for μ receptors. In studies in both animals and humans, it increased MAP in both endotoxic and hemorrhagic models of shock.[34] Naloxone application in the shock patient is thought to derive from the assumption that endogenous opiates such as endorphins contribute to the pathophysiology of shock and the antagonizing action of naloxone mitigates these effects.[35,36] The effects of naloxone in models of acute hemorrhage in dogs yielded no discernible hemodynamic benefit.[37] IV infusion of naloxone has anecdotally been observed to have a calming, anxiolytic effect in bleeding mares,[38] but it is not thought likely to provide a significant hemodynamic benefit. The interplay between naloxone and butorphanol (which is a mixed μ agonist/antagonist) in horses when given concurrently is unknown.

Yunnan baiyao is a Chinese herbal preparation that is used as an adjunctive treatment of bleeding in veterinary and human medicine. In human and laboratory animal studies, it has been reported to decrease intraoperative blood loss, stimulate platelet function, and quicken clotting times as measured by the buccal mucosa bleeding test. In one study, it decreased template bleeding time in healthy anesthetized ponies.[39] The place of this herb in the treatment of uncontrolled hemorrhage in peripartum mares may find rationale in the results of these studies and by anecdotal observations of effect. Recent studies in healthy cats,[40] dogs,[41] and horses,[42] in which the hemostatic effects of the herb were evaluated with traditional coagulation tests, tests for von Willebrand factor (vWF) and platelet function, and thromboelastography, revealed no significant differences between treated animals and controls. The herb is purchased in powder form, and the published dosage is 8 mg/kg, given as an oral suspension made by adding water to the powder in which the product is supplied, every 6 to 12 hours.

Formalin has been used as a procoagulant treatment in the setting of uncontrolled peripartum hemorrhage. One controlled study[43] revealed no effect of formalin administration on hemostasis, and a case study[44] involving postcastration hemorrhage in one horse reported no benefit from IV formalin administration. Given the lack of evidence for any benefit and the availability of other methods of supporting the hemorrhage patient, it is hard to recommend this treatment, particularly if the hemorrhage is occurring in the prepartum mare. A published dosage is 30 to 150 mL of 10% buffered formalin in 1 L isotonic fluids.[45]

Supplemental O_2 provided by nasal insufflation at a rate of 10 to 15 L/min significantly increases Pao_2 and arterial oxygen saturation[46] and may be particularly indicated to support oxygen delivery in mares hemorrhaging during the prepartum period.

Summary: mares with life-threatening hemorrhage and shock can be stabilized and managed to survival and a good outcome, including future production of foals, although there may be increased risk of a second hemorrhagic event.

DYSTOCIA

Dystocia is a significant problem at the equine industry level, ranking high on the list of parturition-associated deaths.[47,48] Advances in neonatology and critical care have improved the outcome for compromised foals after delivery through even severe dystocia,[49] but parturition remains an event with a narrow window for successful intervention when it is needed. Normal parturition in the horse is a rapid event, the successful outcome of which results in the fetus exiting the uterus in an orchestrated sequence of events that has been characterized as explosive. Once the chorioallantois ruptures, the allantoic fluid exits and the fetus and amnion move into the birth canal. About 30 minutes is allotted for normal passage and transition of the fetus from residing in an aqueous environment and depending on placentally delivered oxygen to becoming a terrestrial animal dependent on a functioning pulmonary system. At 40 minutes from the time of chorioallantois rupture, the prognosis for survival of the foal decreases sharply.[48,50] Thus difficulties in any aspect of this parturitional process, or dystocia, constitutes a bona fide emergency. The emergent nature of dystocia has been underscored many times by the finding that the single most important factor determining whether the foal will survive or be lost is minimizing the duration of stage II labor.[48,50,51]

Parturition can be considered as consisting of 3 stages: stage I refers to the premonitory hours to minutes when coordinated uterine contractions are beginning and intensifying, but the mare is not yet recruiting abdominal press in active labor and the chorioallantois has not ruptured. This stage may be recognized by signs of restlessness and mild colic: pawing, pacing, flank-checking, sweating, lying down and standing back up, urinating, and defecating. Some mares may show no signs of restlessness or discomfort. During stage I, the fetus, which has spent much of gestation in a dorsopublic position (foal lying nearly on its back, head toward the mare's pelvis), is being rotated around on its longitudinal axis by myometrial contractions and the mare's physical movements into a dorsosacral position commonly called the diver's position. Getting the body rotated and the limbs extended requires both the myometrial contractions and a requisite level of viability in the fetus.[52] Once the fetus' neck and forelimbs are extended so that the foal enters the pelvis and contacts the cervix, contractions are intensified and the chorioallantois ruptures, releasing the light-colored allantoic fluid from the reproductive tract. This water breaking denotes the beginning of stage II. During stage II, the mare usually lies down and begins bearing down with abdominal press to augment the uterine contractions. During passage through the birth canal, the foal is still dependent on the interdigitation between chorionic villi and endometrial crypts for placental oxygenation. The length of the birth canal in mares is only a few feet long, but traversing it can be the most dangerous journey a horse ever takes and the process is unforgiving when there is failure or significant delay at any point. Stage III begins once the foal has been delivered, and is a period of continued uterine contraction that results in expulsion of the chorioallantois and initial uterine involution. A combination of pharmaceuticals for sedation and general anesthesia plus equipment for fetal manipulations and resuscitation should be kept assembled in the veterinarian's toolkit for dystocia (**Box 1**).

Examination of the Mare

When a client first calls with a dystocia, it is helpful to have them make some important observations while the veterinarian is traveling to the site. The clients should make

---

Box 1
Equipment and pharmaceuticals needed for equine obstetric interventions

obstetric (OB) chains or straps

Foal snare

Stainless-steel buckets

Sterile lubricant

Nonsterile lubricant—carboxymethylcellulose

Pump—sterilized

Sterile nasogastric tube—optimally reserved for obstetric use

Fetotomy wire

Xylazine

Detomidine

Butorphanol

Diazepam or midazolam

Ketamine

Banamine

Epinephrine and/or vasopressin

Ventipulmin oral gel

Self-inflating Ambu-type bag

Cuffed endotracheal tubes for nasotracheal intubation of fetus/foal- keep several sizes, ranging from 7- to 10-mm internal diameter for light horse breeds

Clean towels

Sterile OB sleeves

Optional: E cylinder tank of oxygen with demand valve

---

note of the time at which the mare's water broke and watch for any progress in the foal's position relative to the vulva and any movement in the foal. Upon arrival, a brief history should be obtained while physical evaluation of the mare is begun. Chemical restraint should be provided if needed (xylazine or detomidine, with or without butorphanol), and the mare is examined with a scrubbed, disinfected, and lubricated bare arm and hand or with a sterile lubricated obstetric sleeve, with the aim of expeditiously determining what is preventing the foal's progression through the canal. As much chemical restraint needed to facilitate safely working with the mare in the stall should be provided; because of the chance that the mare will abruptly go down during a contraction, the use of stocks is dangerous to the mare and examiner alike and is contraindicated in this situation. The foal's presentation (normal is anterior longitudinal), position (normal is dorsosacral), and posture (normal is forelimbs, neck, and head extended) should be determined.

Abnormal presentations include posterior presentation and transverse presentation. Posterior presentation of the fetus may result in the hind limbs preceding the fetus into the birth canal. If the hind limbs are extended, the foal can be delivered without complication. However, posterior presentations are often complicated by flexion of the hips at the pelvic inlet, in which case the foal's buttocks, tail, and possibly the hocks, but no extremities, will be palpated; this is a breech presentation. A transverse ventral presentation will result in an abnormal combination of hooves or extremities in the birth canal, and the fetus's abdomen may be palpated. With a dorsal transverse presentation, no hooves or limbs will be in the birth canal, and the fetus' dorsum may be palpated.

Postural abnormalities involve flexion of the limbs (all 4 should be in extension during birth), shoulders, neck, or head. Limbs may be flexed as a result of faulty placement upon entry into the birth canal (**Fig. 4**), or may be caused by congenital contracture, for instance, of the carpi or hocks. Although large fetal size relative to mare size can cause birthing difficulty, most cases of dystocia confronted by veterinarians at the farm are caused by postural abnormalities: flexion at the carpus or elbow joints, flexion of the shoulder joints, and flexion of the head or neck are all common postural abnormalities that cause dystocia.

Not all dystocias involve abnormalities in the foal's positioning; in one study of 517 on-farm parturitions,[53] 58 (11.2%) were dystocias, and of those 58 cases, 22.6% had body malpositioning, 41% had malposturing, and 31% had no abnormal positioning but required traction.

Evaluation of Fetal Viability

The next step is to determine whether the fetus is alive. Even if the head is still within the birth canal, this can be done by checking for a corneal reflex, withdrawal reflex of a limb, an anal pinch reflex in a posteriorly presented fetus, detection of peripheral pulses in any available body part, a pulse in the umbilicus, or a heartbeat. The fetal response to hypoxia is to reduce cardiac output and motor activity, an adaptive reflex that minimizes oxygen requirement. A hypoxic fetus may have sluggish pulses and absent reflexes, and in these instances it is not always straightforward to determine whether the fetus is alive or has expired.

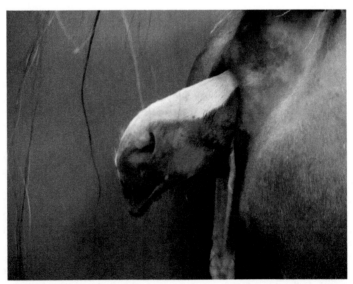

Fig. 4. Foal with muzzle exiting the vulva unaccompanied by extended forelimbs or front hooves. Palpation of the birth canal revealed both forelimbs in carpal flexion, wedged at the pelvic inlet. After a brief attempt at controlled vaginal delivery, a cesarean delivery was required to deliver the foal.

Correction of the Dystocia

Once the nature of the problem and the status of the fetus have been established, the options for resolving the dystocia should be explained to the owner. Assisted vaginal delivery, controlled vaginal delivery, and cesarean section surgery are the options by which a viable foal can be delivered; fetotomy and euthanasia of the mare are the remaining options for resolution.

Assisted vaginal delivery refers to manipulation of the fetus to correct abnormal presentation, position, or posture with the mare sedated and standing or lying down. *Controlled vaginal delivery* refers to inducing general anesthesia and hoisting the hindquarters to facilitate repulsion and manipulations of the fetus (**Fig. 5**). With either assisted or controlled vaginal delivery, use of obstetric chains or straps will likely be helpful for forced fetal extraction. Taking into account how much time has elapsed since the water broke, the nature of the dystocia, the availability of a safe place for general anesthesia and sufficient equipment and help to hoist the mare, and the likelihood of resolving the malpositioning, the decision must be made whether to undertake correction of the problem on site or refer the mare to a hospital.[48,50,51,54] The decision should be made promptly, with referral being elected as an early option, not an endgame capitulation.

Often a timed period of assisted delivery is attempted, followed by either induction of general anesthesia for controlled vaginal delivery or referral. For purposes of managing the case at the farm, if the mare's hindquarters cannot be hoisted, there is little to no benefit from general anesthesia. If the foal cannot be delivered vaginally, cesarean delivery or fetotomy are the remaining options. Cesarean delivery should be done at a referral center.

For assisted vaginal delivery (AVD), because some degree of repulsion of the fetus back toward the uterus is nearly always necessary to correct limb or body position, preventing straining is helpful. In addition to sedation, 10 mL clenbuterol (Ventipulmin)

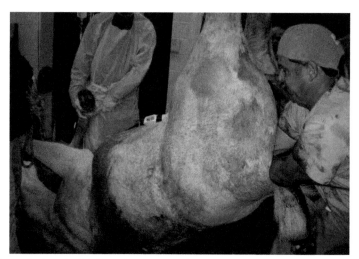

Fig. 5. Controlled vaginal delivery in a mare with dystocia. The mare is hoisted into the Trendelenburg position to facilitate displacement of viscera toward the diaphragm and better enable attempts at fetal repositioning. If the mare has the option of cesarean delivery, personnel will be clipping the abdomen and beginning aseptic skin preparation while the operator is still in the process of attempting to deliver the foal.

syrup given orally will provide tocolytic effect. An epidural can also be administered. Administration of a caudal epidural will not terminate uterine contractions, but it induces anesthesia of the perineal region and will reduce the mare's urge to strain in response to vaginal manipulations.[55] In addition, administration of epidural anesthesia may complicate recovery from general anesthesia, either at the farm if controlled vaginal delivery (CVD) on site is elected or at the referral hospital if referral is a possibility. Epidural anesthesia can be provided with a combination of lidocaine, carbocaine, or xylazine. Even with these aids, pushing the fetus backward into the tract is inherently risky for contusion, laceration, or rupture of the tract wall. Plenty of lubrication should be used. Carboxymethycellulose-based lubricant is preferred over polyethylene polymer powder, if possible, as leakage of the latter into the peritoneal cavity through tears or lacerations in the tract wall can cause severe peritonitis and death.[56] Inadequately diluted povidone solution can do the same.[54] Once fetal manipulations are underway, a bystander should be tasked with monitoring the time that has passed. If significant progress has not been made after 15 to 20 minutes of effort, controlled vaginal delivery or referral are indicated. It must be kept in mind that survival of the foal is related to the length of stage II labor, and for a mare that has the option of referral the transport time must be figured into the 30 to 40 minutes (from the rupture of the chorioallantoic membrane) inside of which the foal's chances are optimum. For a farm that is far from a referral center, the superior option is for prompt transport after a few minutes if fetal manipulations do not meet with success.

Hoisting the anesthetized mare's hindquarters for CVD is helpful in several ways. The myometrial tone and abdominal wall contractions are relaxed by the anesthetic drugs, and the head-down positioning causes the abdominal viscera to fall toward the diaphragm, which creates more room in the abdomen for repulsion of the foal and fetal manipulation. It should be remembered that this positioning is unfavorable for the mare with regard to ventilation, and one person should be tasked with monitoring the mare's respiratory rate and mucus membrane color while the foal is being extracted.

Posterior presentation dystocias can be very difficult to resolve, and certain types of malpostures are also notoriously difficult to correct. Ventral flexion of the neck, such that the neck and head are beneath the forelimbs; lateral flexion of the neck; and bilateral shoulder flexion can be particularly difficult to resolve without cesarean delivery. If 15 minutes of working to manipulate fetus does not yield progress and referral to a hospital is an option, the mare should be tranquilized and transported.

The reader is referred to detailed guides for correcting specific malpositions or malpostures.[52]

EXIT Technique for Fetal Support During Dystocia

EXIT is an acronym for ex utero intrapartum treatment during a prolonged stage II and refers to supporting the foal in the birth canal with oxygen while efforts are being made to accomplish its delivery. First reported in humans around 1989[57] the procedure has been adapted for use in equine dystocias,[58] although the objectives in human dytocias are different.[59] In brief, the foal is nasotracheally intubated and ventilated while it remains in the birth canal. Having several sterilized tubes, ranging from 7 to 10 mm in internal diameter and 55 cm in length, will accommodate most light-horse foals. The technique is relatively straightforward if the foal's head is exteriorized; the extended posture of the head and neck facilitate advancement of a tube into the airway rather than the esophagus, and the upper part of the neck can be palpated during the procedure to help ensure proper placement. The procedure can require technical skill and necessitates cooperation between the person or persons working on fetal mutations and those providing ventilations. Although it is not necessary for support of the fetus, the EXIT technique's usefulness can be enhanced by inserting a capnograph between the nasotracheal tube and self-inflating bag used to provide breaths. Monitoring end-tidal CO_2 ($ETCO_2$) is useful because the first few lung inflations induce conversion of placental circulation to pulmonary circulation,[60] and CO_2 is delivered to the lungs for removal. In a healthy neonate or one that is responding favorably to cardiopulmonary resuscitation, $ETCO_2$ levels are in the range of 40 to 60 torr. Readings in the range of 8 to 20 torr indicate severe compromise and reduced cardiac output, and deceased foals will have no $ETCO_2$. The benefit of supporting the foal with ventilation lies in removing some of the need for haste, and turns an emergent situation into a more controlled event. However, although the procedure provides oxygen across the blood-alveolar interface, placental oxygen transfer is permanently reduced, so ventilation should be continued until the foal is delivered. Attaching the breathing bag to an oxygen line is helpful, but not necessary.

Postdelivery Care

Once the foal has been delivered, resuscitation should be provided as needed. Specifics or neonatal foal resuscitation are beyond the scope of this article. The reader is referred to other publications for details of advanced resuscitation.[61] The mare should be carefully examined internally and allowed to investigate and bond with the foal. Depending on the rigor of the efforts to reduce the dystocia, the length of time manipulations were being performed, and resulting abrasions or other injury to the reproductive tract, antimicrobials along with a nonsteroidal anti-inflammatory drug (NSAID) for comfort are often warranted. Dystocia is a risk factor for retention of the fetal membranes, and the mare should be monitored for this complication.

SUMMARY

Overview of principles useful in attending the mare with delayed stage II labor:
1. The situation is emergent: examine mare, determine the problem preventing delivery, assess the premises and assistance available
2. Explain options to owners: AVD, CVD, or cesarean delivery for a live foal; fetotomy if foal is deceased.
   a. Commence AVD, allow 15 to 20 minutes for successful delivery or significant progress
   b. If AVD unsuccessful, CVD is the next step. If mare has a referral option, refer for CVD at hospital so can proceed to cesarean delivery if unsuccessful. Otherwise commence CV at farm.
   c. If CVD on site is unsuccessful, refer for surgery or perform fetotomy.
3. Manage expectations, explain the range of possible outcomes and costs, communicate with clinicians at referral facility.
4. If dystocia resolved and foal delivered at farm, tend to foal resuscitation needs, especially if mare was anesthetized for CVD. Examine mare's reproductive tract for vaginal and uterine trauma. Prescribe antimicrobials and NSAIDs. Monitor for retained fetal membranes, and plan intervention beginning around 3 hours postpartum if indicated.
5. Evaluate placenta for completeness once passed.

UTERINE PROLAPSE

Prolapse of the uterus following parturition is an infrequent but dramatic emergency that can lead quickly to shock and fatality if movement of the uterus out of the abdominal cavity causes vascular rupture in the broad ligaments. The marked relaxation of the uterus' supporting structures and all the structures in the pelvis, including the bladder, urinary sphincter, rectum, vulva, and pelvic musculature, is an adaptation for parturition, but facilitates prolapse if there is excessive straining or tension. Reported implicating factors include dystocia, retained fetal membranes, excessive oxytocin administration, abortion, straining because of other causes, colic, and cribbing.[62–66] The extent of prolapse can vary: the uterus may evert through the cervix only into the vagina, or may exit the vulva completely (**Fig. 6**). Rarely, the cervix also prolapses. The greater the degree of prolapse, the greater the tension on the broad ligaments and the chance of vascular rupture. Prolapse of the uterus from the abdominal cavity is occasionally complicated by accompanying prolapse of the bladder. If the uterus had a full-thickness rent in the wall, it is possible that intestinal segments will be exteriorized with the uterus. The relentless straining occasionally everts the bladder through the urethra such that the bladder will be seen in the vestibule or hanging from the vulva along with the uterus.

If appropriate in light of the owners' or caretakers' experience level, when the veterinarian is summoned for a prolapse (client photographs sent via text are helpful), he or she can give instructions for a clean sheet or a large plastic bag to be procured and placed underneath the exteriorized tissues, whether the mare is standing or recumbent. The caretakers can start surface irrigation of the uterus with warm water or dilute povidone solution to remove gross contamination while the veterinarian is in transit. Elevating the uterus to the level of the pelvis by placing it on a clean sheet or plastic

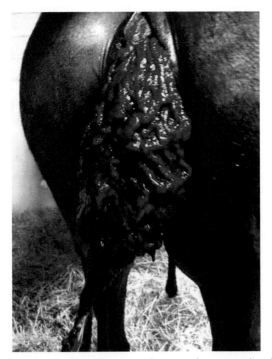

Fig. 6. Prolapsed uterus in a postpartum mare. The organ has everted and exited the vulva, and the endometrial surface is exposed. (*Courtesy of* Dr. Peter Morresey, *BVSc MVM MACVSc DipACT DipACVIM CVA, Kentucky.*)

and supporting it on a cart or table, if the situation allows, removes the tension on the uterus and broad ligaments and will give the mare immediate comfort.

Upon arrival, the physiologic state of the mare should quickly be assessed and analgesia and adequate sedation provided. Antimicrobials should also be given. Taking the time to administer an epidural anesthetic will help reduce straining and facilitate working with the exteriorized tissue. However, anesthesia of the hindquarters is contraindicated if general anesthesia is needed. If there is an option to refer the mare to a surgical facility if standing correction is not successful, sedation and a tocolytic may be given, but the referral surgeon should be consulted before an epidural is given. In addition, securing venous access with a catheter will make it easier to extend the sedation or have an assistant administer other medications at the veterinarian's direction.

Although time is of essence in replacing the uterus, it is important to examine all the exteriorized tissue for a laceration or rent, and to rule out exteriorization of any extra-uterine structures such as the bladder and intestinal segments. The exposed tissues should be lavaged with sterile saline to remove blood and surface contaminants, and this also helps enable identification of the various structures that have prolapsed. The straining can also cause the bladder to evert through the urethra and exit the vulva, with the everted mucosal surface and ureteral openings seen. If the prolapse has been in place long enough for venous congestion and edema to develop, differentiating between the engorged endometrium and rectal prolapse, or identifying eviscerated intestine or bladder, is not always straightforward. A prolapsed bladder should be rinsed with saline and protected from injury during the manipulations to replace the uterus, and carefully replaced through the urethra after the uterus has been replaced. Appearance of the noneverted bladder into the vestibule or outside the vulva indicates extrusion through a full-thickness rent in the vagina or perineum.[67] Retention of fetal membranes (RFM) is common with uterine prolapse, and the weight of the membranes exacerbates (and may have precipitated) the prolapse and will complicate the efforts to replace the uterus. If they cannot be removed with gentle tension, the bulk of the membranes can be trimmed with a scissor, leaving a long enough tag to enable detection of the stub of retained membranes once the uterus is back *in situ*. If tears in the uterus are detected, they should be closed with absorbable suture material in a double-layer inverting pattern before beginning reduction of the prolapse.[66]

With the cleansed uterus supported at the level of the pelvis, the tip of the uterus is identified. Using the flat of the fingers or softly rounded fists for even distribution of pressure, the tip of the uterus is pressed into the vagina and through the cervix. As the tip of the uterus reenters the abdominal cavity, the organ's weight will help retract the remaining portions by gravity. Congestion and edema make the uterine tissue more friable, and great care and patience must be used. Keeping the uterus inside a plastic bag and manipulating it through the bag can help reduce the likelihood of perforating the wall with hands or fingers.

Once the organ is replaced, it is important to ensure that both horns are fully everted; intussusception of a horn tip will lead to renewed straining, colic, and possible reprolapse of the entire uterus. Palpation and ultrasonograohy can be used to appreciate the status of the horn tips, but it can be difficult or impossible to manually evaluate the full extent of the horns, particularly when the uterus is flaccid. Once the uterus is back in place, the mare can be given 3 to 5 L of a crystalloid fluid with 250 to 500 mL of 23% calcium gluconate, and a low dose (10–20 units) of oxytocin IV or IM to promote myometrial tone. If the extent of the horns cannot be palpated to confirm they are fully everted, a well-lubricated sterile speculum can be advanced into each horn and used as an extension of the operator's arm to gently push against the horn tips.

Glass beverage bottles can serve the same function, as can a rectal sleeve, tightly distended with fluid or air and covered with sterile lubricant, and advanced into each horn. Uterine lavage with a high volume (3–10 L) of sterile warmed fluids can also be used to reexpand the uterine body and horns while also diluting and carrying out contaminants; this can be followed with antibiotic infusion into the uterine lumen and serial dosing with oxytocin to help maintain tone and prevent sequestration of fluids. Until it is certain that straining can be controlled, it is advisable to place retaining sutures in the vulva with umbilical tape or heavy suture material; the suture should leave the ventral aspect of the vulva open so as not to impair urination.

If the uterus is found to have a full-thickness laceration or rent, once the prolapse has been reduced, the mare must be evaluated for peritonitis, on site and over the ensuing few days. Similarly, if any intestinal structures are involved with the prolapse and replaced into the peritoneal cavity, once the uterine prolapse has been reduced, the mare is a candidate for referral to a hospital.

Barring complications that warrant referral, the mare's treatment regimen for the days following prolapse should include NSAIDs, systemic antimicrobials, a laxative diet, and close monitoring. The attending veterinarian should be vigilant for signs of uterine artery hemorrhage and peritonitis following correction of the prolapse. A protocol for retained fetal membranes is necessary if tags of placental tissue were bound to the endometrium. Ultrasonography and palpation of the reproductive tract per rectum enable confirmation that the uterus is involuting, rather than remaining flaccid and sequestering luminal fluid. Uterine lavage should be withheld if the uterine wall was sutured, but luminal fluid can be siphoned. Some veterinarians give intrauterine infusions of antimicrobials. A daily CBC for several days will facilitate monitoring of the white cell count as an indicator of systemic inflammation and the SIRS response that could arise with endometritis, metritis, or peritonitis.[68] Any of these complications can be anticipated to result in the downstream complications of hypogalactia, laminitis, and founder. Digital pulses should be closely monitored as part of serial daily physical examinations.

Summary: Examine mare to determine physiologic status, and administer sedation, analgesia, an NSAID, and antimicrobials. Elevate the uterus and irrigate with warm water or dilute povidone in saline to remove surface contamination, and inspect the prolapsed tissue to determine whether the bladder or intestine is incorporated. Suture rents in the uterine wall before beginning replacement. Have assistants hold the uterus elevated to the level of the pelvic brim while it is methodically replaced, tip first, through the vagina and cervix. General anesthesia and hoisting the hindquarters as for controlled vaginal delivery will facilitate replacement of the prolapse if standing correction was not successful. Ensure the position of the horn tips by palpation or ultrasonography. Prolapse may cause broad ligament vasculature to rupture, leading to a clinical picture of internal hemorrhage in addition to the prolapse. Peritonitis complicates the convalescent period if a full-thickness rent was found.

POSTPARTUM COLIC

Signs of colic in a recently foaled mare can be normal and self-limiting, as with third-stage labor contractions or mild postpartum constipation. However, colic in the postpartum period can persist and develop into an emergency clinical entity. Signs of abdominal pain in this setting warrant thorough evaluation of the gastrointestinal tract and the urogenital tract, as the clinical signs can be similar. Moreover, mares with postpartum colic do not infrequently have problems requiring attention in both tracts. Particularly in a mare that had recent dystocia, injuries in the reproductive tract, intestinal tract, or both may manifest in the hours to several days following parturition. The most common serious conditions causing colic in a postpartum mare include uterine artery rupture and bleeding into a broad ligament, bleeding into the abdomen, uterine atony with gross fluid distension, intussuscepted uterine horn tip, metritis-sepsis-SIRS complex, intestinal tract injury, uterine rupture and peritonitis, and intestinal displacement or volvulus.[69,70]

All of these conditions have a high potential to trigger activation of the systemic inflammatory response and culminate in multisystem tissue injury, particularly laminitis. Therefore, mares with any of these problems merit a full clinicopathologic database, setup of a hospital-level treatment regimen if they will be managed at the farm, and close monitoring for multiple days after the primary problem has been resolved.

The authors approach first evaluation of an uncomfortable postpartum mare with a comprehensive physical examination, including palpation of both the gastrointestinal structures and the urogenital tract per rectum, and speculum examination of the birth canal. If signs of toxemia are observed (any combination of fever, hypothermia, tachycardia, altered mucus membrane color, bounding digital pulses, and indicators of compromised circulatory status such as low skin turgor, poor jugular refill, poor peripheral arterial pulse quality, and cold extremities) in the physical examination, ultrasound imaging and blood work are also performed.

Arterial rupture with hemorrhage into a broad ligament or into the abdomen has been discussed. With the former, diagnosis is based on rectal palpation and detection of the enlarged broad ligament, with ultrasound imaging confirming the problem if helpful. Affected mares can be quite painful. The author (K.S.) finds multimodal analgesia helpful in mares with severe or persistent discomfort, based on a combination of flunixin meglumine, butorphanol, and an alpha-2 agonist at routine dosages given IV initially and followed up with serial doses of butorphanol and the alpha-2 drug given IM afterward to maintain a reasonable level of comfort. Serial monitoring is indicated to ensure that bleeding into the broad ligament does not proceed to uncontrolled bleeding into the abdomen. The mare should be offered a laxative diet for 2 to 3 days to minimize the need for straining to defecate while the hematoma organizes and matures.

Intussusception of the tip of a uterine horn should be considered if the mare has or recently had retained placental membranes. Signs of colic may be accompanied by repeated tenesmus. The straining response to the inverted horn tip can result in prolapse of the uterus, bladder, rectum, or small colon. The uterine lumen should be examined manually and the endometrial surface of each horn palpated. If the extent of the horns can be reached, an inverting horn tip can be felt telescoping into the lumen of the horn. In the immediate postpartum period when the uterus is still dilated, it can be beyond the examiner's reach to digitally evaluate the full length of the horns. The uterus should also be palpated and imaged transrectally. The sonographic view of an inverted horn is the well-described target lesion or image of 2 concentric circles of tissue as is seen with intestinal intussusception. Retained tags of fetal membranes may also be seen in the inverting horn. If the uterus has not involuted and the horn is too long for the examiner's fingers to reach to the tip, a well-lubricated glass speculum, glass bottle, or palpation sleeve filled and distended with air or fluid can gently be advanced into each horn and used as an extension of the arm. The uterus can also be lavaged with a moderate volume of sterile saline (3–10 L) to distend and evert the horn tips. Resolution of the intussuscepted tip should be confirmed with palpation and/or ultrasound. Failure to restore the horn tip to its proper everted state elicits continued straining, which can result in consequences that become the new emergency, in particular prolapsed uterus or rectum. Rectal prolapse that progresses to small colon prolapse is usually fatal because of tearing of the mesocolon, abdominal hemorrhage, and disrupted blood supply to the lower small colon (**Fig. 7**).

Uterine atony and sequestration of luminal fluid is common following dystocia, hydrops, and in any postpartum scenario when a mare is not allowed free movement following parturition, including mares that are stalled with a hospitalized foal; those with uterine artery hemorrhage, in which restriction of movement is an important part of management; or mares that underwent peripartum surgery. Whatever the cause, mares with accumulation of large volumes of fluid in the uterine lumen usually have signs of vague malaise, mild colic, and lethargy. Rectal palpation or transabdominal ultrasonography easily reveals the fluid-distended uterus, with fluid that is echogenic. Treatment consists of removing the fluid by sterile uterine lavage or careful siphoning. Serial doses of oxytocin (10–20 units, IV or IM, every 6 hours or according to veterinarian preference) will help maintain myometrial tone, which prevents further sequestration of fluid. Some veterinarians administer an antibiotic infusion into the uterine lumen following uterine lavage or siphoning, as adjunctive treatment. Mares will likely already be receiving a broad-spectrum antimicrobial regimen because of dystocia or other problems, and this should be continued until uterine tone improves to a normal postpartum state and the mare can be hand-walked or turned out for exercise. NSAIDs should also be given for the same duration. Digital pulses should be monitored closely during the treatment interval. A CBC performed during this time may reveal leukopenia with neutropenia, a finding that points to activation of the systemic inflammatory response to translocating bacteria. At the authors' practice, low white blood cell count in a postpartum mare being treated for periparturient complications of any etiology may prompt prophylactic measures for laminitis, including immersion of the front feet in ice boots several times daily and application of sole support pads and bandages between icing treatments, in addition to addressing the source of sepsis.

Metritis/sepsis/SIRS complex is a serious complication of parturition that can lead to life-threatening complications in the affected mare. This complication can arise as an extension of postpartum uterine atony and fluid sequestration as mentioned

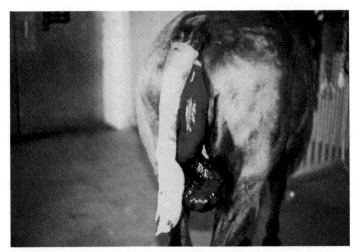

Fig. 7. Postpartum mare in which continuous straining led to rectal and small colon prolapse. Sonographic imaging of the mare's abdomen revealed hemorrhage from mesenteric vessel tearing.

previously. Colic is not the primary clinical sign, but the inappetance, depression, and vague appearance of abdominal malaise can mimic gastrointestinal colic, and presumed colic may be what prompts the client's call. One of the most common postpartum diseases,[3] metritis refers to infection of deep layers of the uterine wall, not just the endometrial surface, and is most frequently seen in the aftermath of dystocia and retained fetal membranes.[3,71] Other scenarios that have been reported in mares with metritis are uterine trauma, autolysis of residual placental tissue, uterine inertia, excessive lochial accumulation, abortion, normal foaling in unsanitary conditions, and fetotomy.[11,72] Delayed involution and uterine atony allow accumulation of lochial fluid, which, together with autolyzing debris from retained fetal membranes or inflammatory fluid from uterine injury, creates an incubation environment for bacteria. Translocation of bacteria and toxins across the uterine wall leads to sepsis and activation of the SIRS, with the attendant downstream complication of laminitis. Clinical signs of depression, inappetance, and fever show up in the first 7 to 10 days following parturition.[3,73] In some instances, lameness is the first clinical sign noticed.[74] If strands of residual fetal membranes are protruding from the vulva, the association is straightforward. With or without retained tissues, vulvar discharge is often present, may or may not be voluminous, and may have a fetid odor.[72] Digital pulses may already be abnormally strong at the time of initial examination.

Metritis is diagnosed by physical examination, ultrasound imaging, and culture of uterine fluid. Both transabdominal and transrectal ultrasonography will reveal fluid-filled uterine body and horns, sometimes with edema and thickening in the uterine wall, and careful imaging of the horns may show tags of retained fetal membranes (**Fig. 8**). A sample of the uterine fluid submitted for aerobic and anaerobic culture will identify organisms present and aid in making antimicrobial selections, but an empirical broad-spectrum regimen with activity against gram-positive and gram-

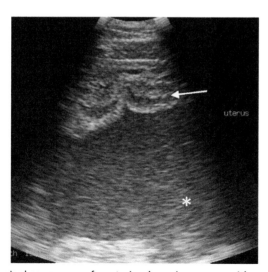

Fig. 8. Transabdominal sonogram of a uterine horn in a mare with metritis and uterine atony approximately 60 hours after foaling. The uterine wall is thickened (*arrow*), and edema can be seen in its layers. The luminal fluid (*) is echogenic, indicating high cellularity, but is not swirling, indicating that it is not active hemorrhage. The clinical picture was one of lethargy, fever and other signs of systemic inflammation, and abdominal malaise rather than of hemorrhagic hypovolemia and shock.

negative bacterial species should be started immediately even before culture and sensitivity results are available. *Streptococcus* spp and *Escherichia coli* are frequently isolated, along with the anaerobic species *Bacteriodes fragilis* and *Clostridium* spp.[72] In a recent study[73] of bacterial isolates from 45 mares with metritis, the most frequent gram-negative pathogens were *E coli*, *Klebsiella* spp, and *Enterobacter* spp, and the most frequent gram-positive pathogens were *Streptococcus zooepidemicus*, other *Streptococcus* spp, *Enterococcus* spp, *Citrobacter* spp, and *Staphylococcus* spp. Strains of *E coli* were the most common pathogen isolated. In that study, there were more (28%; 62%) mixed infections than single-growth infections (17%; 38%). Interestingly, the penicillin + gentamicin combination was only appropriate for 65% of the mares and a trimethoprim-sulfonamide combination was only appropriate for 49%. Given that these are among the most common first-pick empirical treatments, culturing the uterine fluid is probably worthwhile. The pillars of treatment of metritis and the sepsis/SIRS complex are antimicrobials, uterine lavage, NSAIDs, and oxytocin. A parenteral combination of a β-lactam antibiotic with an aminoglycoside usually covers the mixed population of bacteria, and the possibility of anaerobes' presence merits addition of oral metronidazole to the regimen, at least until culture results are known. Some veterinarians also add intrauterine antibiotic infusions to the parenteral drugs.[72] Oxytocin is helpful in providing myometrial tone so that luminal fluid is expelled and further accumulation is minimized. It may also help release remaining fetal membrane tags. Other important components of treatment are aimed at the systemic inflammatory response driving organ injury and laminitis. The laminitis associated with metritis and with peritonitis from uterine rupture can be exceptionally rapid and devastating,[75] with rotation and sinking of the distal phalanx already developed at the time of initial examination. Therefore, many veterinarians include plasma known to contain anti-endotoxin antibodies, IV polymyxin B, IV or oral pentoxifylline, and IV lidocaine infusions as adjunctive anti-inflammatory treatment measures. In addition, the veterinarian should consider incorporating icing of the feet and applying sole-supporting hoof wraps or pads into the management protocol immediately, even prophylactically, if digital pulse quality is normal at the time of examination. Frequent checking of digital pulse quality, hoof wall warmth, and the coronary band area for softening or depression is an important part of the daily physical examination. CBC can be monitored daily during the first part of treatment for ensuring the leukopenia/neutropenia associated with the endotoxemia is responding to treatment. Uterine lavage should continue for as long as retained tissue tags are present, as lavage dilutes and carries out the inflammatory fluid and bacterial load. When retained tissue is no longer evident and peripheral blood white blood cell count returns to reference range, it is usually safe to taper off the laminitis-protective treatments in mares that did not develop digital pain. Mares that did sustain laminar injury as a complication of metritis/sepsis/SIRS are likely to be orthopedic patients and require treatment of laminitis for some time after resolution of the metritis. In some instances rotation and sinking are so rapid and severe that the mare is a euthanasia candidate even if the metritis resolves.

Uterine laceration and rupture are thought to arise from fetal limb movements, the mare straining against a fetus with impaired movement through the birth canal, or as an accident of manipulations in an assisted birth. It is not surprising when uterine injury is a sequela of dystocia, but uterine rupture or tear also happens in mares that had apparently normal parturitions. In a 2003 retrospective study[76] of 33 mares with postpartum uterine rupture, only 10 had had dystocia or an assisted delivery; the other tears had occurred spontaneously during apparently normal parturitions. History of recent foaling, signs of peritonitis, and results of abdominocentesis are the basis of diagnosis; palpating the uterus per vaginum is unsuccessful at revealing the rent more often that it is successful.[76] Rents in the uterine body are more likely to be detectable by palpation, but rents in the horns are significantly more frequent and are not frequently detected by palpation.[3,76,77] Although not borne out by all studies, the 2 recent large retrospective surveys both reported a strong preponderance of tears in the right uterine horn, compared with the left.[76,77]

Diagnosis is typically made on days 1 through 3 following parturition, as the mare develops the clinical features of peritonitis. Depression, tachycardia, and leukopenia on blood work were the most common signs in the 2003 report; across the collection of retrospective reports, the most common presenting signs are some combination of depression, inappetence, reduced borborygmus, ileus, congested or toxic mucus membranes, hypogalactia, mild colic, and fever.[3,76–79] A frequent presentation is a mare that appeared clinically normally for an initial period after foaling, and then is presented 24 to 48 hours after foaling with depression, low-grade fever, toxic mucus membranes, mild colic, and a hungry foal. Leukopenia on an admission CBC in mares evaluated at a hospital is common.[3]

The rents can be small or large, and varied from 2 to 15 cm in one study.[77] Transmural diapedesis and leakage of uterine fluids with life-threatening peritonitis can also occur with severe bruising injury[80,81] or infarction and necrosis of the uterine wall,[3] in the absence of true perforation. Prepartum uterine rupture is also reported, in association with hydropsic conditions and uterine torsion.[79,82,83] In one mare with signs of peritonitis and azotemia, the uterus was perforated by the sharp end of a fetal long bone with a compound fracture, diagnosed on exploratory celiotomy.[84] The possibility of uterine laceration or perforation should be considered in any peripartum mare with signs of peritonitis. Chronic postpartum uterine rupture has also been reported, in which the clinical signs were referable to infertility rather than peritonitis.[85]

The clinical signs seen in any given postpartum mare with a uterine tear depend on when the mare is being examined. With a large uterine rent, signs of abdominal hemorrhage may be seen initially. Although a perforated uterine wall does not bleed as severely as a ruptured uterine artery, mares may still have significant blood loss, both into the abdomen and into the uterine lumen, and the clinical picture of hemorrhage can mask the signs of uterine wall injury. Transabdominal ultrasound may reveal a pattern consistent with hemorrhage early after the injury, but by days 1 to 3 after foaling, usually reveals nonswirling echogenic (cellular) fluid in the ventral abdomen. A fluid sample obtained by abdominocentesis will reveal hemorrhagic, septic, suppurative characteristics, with high protein, nucleated cell count, and lactate. Bacteria may or may not be seen.

If uterine rupture is suspected, no fluids should be introduced into the uterus. Despite the fact that manual evaluation of the endometrial surface may not reveal a tear, it is part of a complete examination, and tears in the uterine body are amenable to detection. The luminal surface of the body and horns should be examined digitally per vagina. Polyethylene polymer lubricant should not be used.[86] In the immediate postparturient period, the endometrial surface is highly folded and engorged, which contributes to the difficulty in detection. When a perforation is suspected but not found with digital palpation, a technique of transmural palpation has been described[70] that may enable detection of hard-to-find tears in the caudal part of the uterus. In some cases, laparoscopy[81] or celiotomy[3,76] is required to locate the injury. A 2010 study comparing outcomes between uterine tears managed medically versus surgically reported a favorable outcome with either approach, with a survival rate of about 75% in both populations.[77] Medical management involves allowing the injury to heal by secondary intention. Treatment would usually include broad-spectrum antimicrobials including metronidazole, oxytocin at modest doses to maintain uterine tone and prevent sequestration of fluids, placement of a drain and lavage of the peritoneal cavity with warmed crystalloid fluids, NSAIDs, antiendotoxin measures, and prophylaxis for laminitis and founder.

Peritoneal lavage and drainage is an important part of treatment of peritonitis, as mares that do not survive uterine tear frequently are lost to complications of peritonitis, such as extensive adhesions[2] and founder. Several techniques are used for peritoneal lavage in standing horses. In brief, one technique involves placing a lavage tube in one or both paralumbar fossae and a drainage tube on or to the right side of ventral midline. Warmed crystalloid fluids are infused in the flank tube/s and drain through the ventral tube. Another technique involves placing a single drain, often a ballooned Foley catheter or a chest drain with a trocar, ventrally. With that system, the fluids are infused into and drained from the same drain. Both methods have been used successfully in the treatment of peritonitis. The reader is referred to previously published reports for practical details of inserting abdominal drains.[87–90] Many clinicians are of the opinion that larger tears or tears not limited to the dorsal aspect of the tract are best managed with surgical closure, which gives primary closure of the defect and removal of the source of contamination and sepsis. Surgery also enables effective peritoneal lavage and evaluation of surrounding visceral structures. Laminitis associated with uterine rupture and peritonitis can be particularly fulminant and progress rapidly to founder; prophylactic measures for laminitis should be started as soon as uterine rupture is identified or suspected.

Visceral injury or rupture is an occasional cause of postpartum colic. The small intestine, cecum, large colon, small colon, and bladder can all be directly injured by fetal positioning during gestation or fetal movements during parturition.[3,91–94] Segmental ischemic injury from mesenteric tears and disruption of blood supply can also occur, leading to intestinal rupture and fulminant peritonitis.[92,93,95,96] Clinical signs from this type of injury generally manifest in the 1 to 3 days after parturition and initially start as colic, depression, inappetence, and reduced manure output. With failure of the bowel wall, signs of septic shock predominate: fever or hypothermia, tachypnea, tachycardia, toxic-appearing mucus membranes, hypovolemia, and trembling. The clinical signs seen in any given mare may reflect any of these stages. In the early stages, this cause of colic in a postpartum mare can be difficult to pinpoint, and may be a diagnosis reached by exclusion of other causes of colic or by exploratory laparoscopy[93] or laparotomy. Blood work usually reveals severe leukopenia and neutropenia. In mares that have signs of peritonitis, the uterus and vagina should be carefully palpated digitally, to search for a rent. Small lacerations or rents can be challenging to find, especially if they are located near the tip of a horn or if the endometrium is edematous and engorged. If no such injury can be identified in the reproductive tract in a mare that has sonographic and clinicopathologic evidence of peritonitis, injury of the intestinal tract should be suspected and investigated.

As seen sonographically, free peritoneal fluid in the ventral aspect of the abdomen or pockets of free fluid at other, more dorsal, areas of the abdomen may reflect a segment of bowel injury. With intestinal wall failure, abdominocentesis will reveal fecal contamination, with intracellular and extracellular bacteria, although these changes may not be seen initially. With laceration or rupture of the bladder wall, the serum biochemistry changes classically associated with uroperitoneum, including high serum urea nitrogen and creatinine, hyperkalemia, hyponatremia, and hypochloremia, will be seen. Free peritoneal fluid can be identified as urine if the creatinine concentration is ≥ 2 times that in peripheral blood. In the early stages of postpartum visceral injury, exploratory laparotomy or laparoscopy may be necessary to identify the site and precise nature of the injury and to resect the injured segment if indicated. If abdominocentesis confirms intestinal rupture, euthanasia is indicated.

Recent studies on the intestinal microbiome have revealed that there are differences in the microbiota of colicky postpartum mares, versus noncolicky postpartum mares.[97]

Large colon volvulus: This strangulating displacement of the large colon is one of the most devastating of all equine diseases. From onset of clinical signs, without intervention it runs a fulminant course of pain and shock and results in death in a matter of hours. This condition accounts for 10% to 20% of colic surgery cases[98,99] and is not limited to broodmares, but broodmares accounted for 91% of large colon surgical cases in central Kentucky over a 16-year period in one study.[100]

Recent parturition is a known risk factor for this emergency condition in mares, along with recent increase in dietary concentrates and recent exposure to lush pasture. The most common presentation in broodmares is that of a postpartum mare within 90 days of foaling that has acute onset of severe, intractable pain.[101] Occasionally, mares are presented with a history of having been mildly uncomfortable for the preceding day or two but then becoming acutely more painful.[102] With either history, once the large colon has become rotated in a strangulating volvulus, the clinical picture is one of intractable pain and rapid systemic deterioration into hypovolemic and septic shock.

Rotation of the large colon along its long axis that involves the mesentery between the ventral and dorsal segments is most correctly termed a volvulus, rather than a torsion, but both terms are commonly used. The site of twisting is most frequently between the right ventral and right dorsal colons, near where the cecocolic ligament ends on the lateral wall of the right ventral colon.[102,103] Most commonly the twisting occurs with the right ventral colon migrating medially and dorsally, so that in a 180° twist the large colon segments distal to the volvulus are oriented with the ventral colon lying dorsal to the dorsal colon. The degrees of volvular rotation reported range from 180° to 720°.[103] The area where the duodenum, cecal base, and origin of the ascending colon are in proximity is tethered to the dorsal body wall by a short mesentery, and this is the only fixed point in the entire large intestine. With the site of fixation restricted to only the beginning of the large colon and the considerable length (around 25 ft) and mobility of the colon segments distal to that point, it is perhaps understandable why gaseous distension or motility alterations can lead to their rotation and migration. Less understood is the predilection of periparturient broodmares for this problem.[104,105] It has also been observed that Thoroughbred broodmares are over-represented in populations of horses that develop large colon volvulus.[103,106,107] Recent studies of Thoroughbred mares on farms in central Kentucky suggest that developing large colon volvulus may be a moderately heritable trait.[108] It is likely that the main risk factors for volvulus are all in play in the recently foaled mare: in many regions where there are high numbers of broodmares, mares reside in rich pasture during the spring and high-energy concentrate feeds are given to support the dual aims for the professional broodmare—lactation for the present foal and efficiently conceiving and beginning the next gestation—and these could contribute to changes in the microbiome and fermentative environment of the cecum and ventral colons. It has also been conjectured that there is more room for migration of the large colon segments in the abdomen of a recently foaled mare. This migration may play a role, but large colon volvulus is also seen in prepartum mares and nonpregnant horses. Recent studies have shed light on the problem of large colon volvulus by characterizing the fecal microbiome in pregnant and postpartum mares. In one study, the large colon microbiome and metabolome of foaling mares were evaluated by quantifying volatile organic compounds (VOC) produced by the resident microbes. In healthy mares sampled from 3 weeks prepartum through 7 weeks postpartum, there was little change in the fecal microbiota: the microbiome and VOCs were remarkably stable with no significant change associated with parturition.[109] However, significant differences in the fecal microbiome were seen between postpartum mares that developed colic and those that did not.[97]

Acute onset of severe colic pain in a peripartum mare is the hallmark of large colon volvulus and should incite expedited examination and referral if it is an option. Colon volvulus is a surgical disease and not amenable to resolution in the field, but the actions of the veterinarian attending the mare at the farm will play an important role in the mare's prognosis for survival, as minimizing the length of time to surgery is the single most important determinant of survival.[110,111] The time taken for examination in the field and transport to a referral center are the main components of this time interval; therefore it is incumbent on the attending veterinarian to conduct an expedited evaluation that either rules out or confirms large colon volvulus as the chief differential. As would be expected, mares that undergo surgery promptly have fewer complications and a better prognosis for life and future fertility.

Physical examination of a colicky mare in the early stages of volvulus may reveal a normal heart rate, depressed intestinal motility, and few signs of endotoxemia, but within a short period of time increasingly violent pain, hypovolemia, tachycardia, tachypnea, and toxic mucus membranes become prominent. Palpation per rectum reveals progressively severe gas distension of the large colon. Mares may have significant volumes of gastric reflux from occlusion of the duodenum on the right side of the abdomen.[103] The fluid should be removed, but the gastric decompression will not result in relief as it would in a case of simple obstruction. Ultrasonography of the colon segments on the right side of the abdomen, especially in intercostal spaces 12 to 15, often reveals engorgement of mesenteric vessels and edematous thickening of the large intestinal wall,[112,113] (**Fig. 9**) a result of venous and lymphatic engorgement secondary to the strangulation. Abdominocentesis is usually not needed for diagnosis and

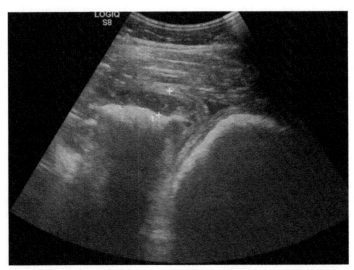

Fig. 9. Transabdominal sonogram of a large colon segment on the right side of the abdomen in a postpartum mare with large colon volvulus. The image was obtained in right intercostal space #14. Notice the grossly increased mural thickness (between the asterisks).

can be dangerous to attempt. If peritoneal fluid is obtained well into the course of a volvulus ≥360°, the color is usually serosanguinous and will have high protein, nucleated cell count, and lactate, reflecting colon ischemia and necrosis. Irrespective of the type and location of the intestinal lesion, severe intractable pain is an indication for exploratory celiotomy. If a mare has signs of significant hypovolemia, it may be prudent to place an IV catheter and administer a bolus of resuscitative fluids (hypertonic saline at 4 mL/kg, IV, followed by 3–5 L crystalloid fluids if they can be administered rapidly) before transporting. If gastric reflux was obtained on passage of a nasogastric tube, the tube should be capped, affixed to the halter, and left in place during transit. With severe gaseous distension of the colon segments, the diaphragm's ventilatory excursions are impaired, which can cause death during transit. Trocarization to decompress the colon segments pressing against the diaphragm should be considered in preparing for transporting a mare with severe abdominal tympany and tachypnea, dyspnea, or cyanotic mucus membranes. All medications and fluids given should be written down and sent with the horse. In addition to the role of conducting an expedited examination and facilitating the decision to refer, the veterinarian is also a critical element in communications between the client and referral center and should play a key role in managing expectations with regard to outcomes and costs. Timely communication with insurance professionals is also an important part of the veterinarian's service to the client in this emergency scenario.

The prognosis for survival and future fertility has improved significantly over the past decade and presently is good for mares that are promptly diagnosed and referred.[104,105,110,111] In fact, repetitive postpartum volvulus is a problem encountered in some mares.[114–116] Colopexy refers to fixation of the one of the colon segments to the body wall, and the resulting permanent adhesion is a method of preventing colon volvulus in successive pregnancies. Some surgeons recommend colopexy after a single episode of colon volvulus, whereas at other practices colopexy is performed after the second volvulus.[114–118] In one recent report, dehiscence of a previous colopexy led to repeat volvulus, and repeat colopexy, in 3 mares.[115] Colopexy generally resolves the problem of future volvuli but does have known possible complications, some of which can be fatal. Mares that have undergone celiotomy to correct large colon volvulus, either with derotation or colon resection, can survive and bear live foals.

Summary: postpartum mares may have simple constipation and respond to routine administration of an analgesic plus mineral oil and water to ease defecation. However, persistent colic with clinical signs of inflammation and activation of the SIRS should prompt a search for injury to the reproductive tract or GI tract with ultrasound imaging and blood work. Large colon volvulus is a devastating condition of colic in which signs of pain progress along with fulminant hypovolemic and septic shock and should be recognized and the mare referred as quickly as possible. All the conditions causing serious colic in the peripartum mare can cause systemic inflammation and culminate in laminitis, even when the primary condition is addressed.

RETAINED FETAL MEMBRANES

RFM is thought to be the most common postpartum problem in mares and may have an incidence as high as 10%.[119–121] Certain subpopulations of mares and peripartum situations, including draft breeds,[122,123] Friesian mares,[124,125] mares that had dystocia,[80,121] prolonged gestation, a previous episode of retained membranes,[120] uterine hydrops, fetotomy,[80,121] and cesarean section surgery,[11,126] are associated with higher incidences of retention. An investigation of draft breed mares, in which the incidence of RFM is approximately 50%, has recently revealed a significantly decreased density of oxytocin receptors in placental membranes, explaining the uterine atony and poor response to oxytocin seen in those breeds.[122] Up to 54% of foalings in Friesian mares result in RFM, attributed in part to the effects of inbreeding.[125] Friesian mares appear to be unique in their response to retained membranes, as they do not frequently develop the sepsis, metritis, and laminitis that affect other mares, and the reproductive performance of Friesian mares that had RFM is not different from those that did not have retained membranes, including likelihood of conceiving on a foal-heat breeding.[124]

Release of the chorioallantois from the endometrium after birth normally takes place during third-stage labor contractions, when the trophoblastic cells of the chorionic villi separate from the endometrial epithelium. When the umbilical cord ruptures following delivery of the foal, it is thought that the fetal placental vessels collapse, causing shrinkage of the chorionic villi and facilitating release of their interdigitations with the endometrial crypts.[127,128] The myometrial contractions, which originate at the horn tips and migrate caudally through the uterine body, expel the released membranes. Although one can find a range of published time intervals said to be normal, many practitioners consider membranes still attached after 3 hours to be retained.[127,128] Most mares release the membranes within an hour of parturition.[129] Failure of the membranes to be released expelled promptly usually results in a cascade of severe complications, such as metritis, sepsis, endotoxemia, hypogalactia, and laminitis,[11,127] although there are exceptions.[54,127] The point of retention is usually near the tip of the nongravid horn. Several observations explain this finding. The chorionic microvilli are longer and have more extensive branching in this area, and the endometrial and placental folding is more extensive in the nongravid horn. Uterine involution also takes place more slowly in the nongravid horn.[121,127,128] For these reasons, among others, separation of the chorion from the endometrium may be slower in the nongravid horn.

Clinical signs: diagnosis is straightforward when placental membranes are seen protruding from the vulva. If no retained tissues are seen at the vulva and RFM is not suspected, the first clinical signs may not be seen until a day or more after parturition and will likely be those of lethargy, inappetence, colic, fever, and injected mucus membranes. The uterine interior should be palpated digitally (with the examiner donning a sterile sleeve or using a bare, scrubbed, disinfected, and lubricated arm) for any adherent tags of membrane. If the extent of the horns cannot be reached, common in an atonic, flaccid postpartum uterus, the horns can be imaged sonographically to search for retained tissue. Manual palpation repeated after a dose of oxytocin (10–20 IU, IV or IM) has induced myometrial contraction may improve the examiner's ability to reach the tips of the horns. Membranes hanging at the level of the mare's hocks or lower should be tied up to avoid being kicked or stepped on. Stepping on the placenta can evert the horn tip where it is attached or tear it from the endometrium.

By the time a mare has clinical signs of fever and lethargy, bacterial or endotoxin translocation, sepsis, and activation of the SIRS are under way. As discussed previously, the sepsis-associated systemic inflammatory response represents a global, overzealous immune response to a local infection, which proceeds to generalized host tissue injury. The laminae of equidae are a unique site of tissue injury among animals, and laminitis and life-threatening loss of architectural integrity in the horse's digit is the common end point of severe inflammation incited by a multitude of causes. For this reason, mare owners or farm employees can be instructed on how to evaluate a newly passed placenta for completeness or to make a routine of placing placentas in a clean bucket or plastic bag for veterinary inspection. Retention of even a small portion of fetal membranes can be as lethal as retention of a large mass. A missing horn tip in the chorioallantois alerts to the possibility of RFM, even if no membranes are externally visible. The placenta contains a wealth of information about the gestation and health of the neonate, and the reader is referred to excellent practical articles on evaluation of the placenta.[128,130]

Treatment of RFM usually begins with oxytocin administration. The doses given and frequency of administration are subject to veterinarian experience and preference, but in brief, a common regimen is to give 10 to 20 units of oxytocin, as an IV or IM bolus, every 1 to 2 hours up to 24 hours.[127] In many cases, a single dose of oxytocin elicits expulsion of the membranes within minutes. Higher doses have been used, but bolus doses greater than 20 units are associated with colic secondary to excessive uterine cramping that can lead to other complications.[11,126] Alternatively, oxytocin can be given as an IV infusion. Most veterinarians who work with broodmares have a preferred protocol, but published doses include adding 80 to 100 units of oxytocin to 500 mL saline and infusing over 30 minutes,[131] adding 10 to 20 units to I L of saline and giving over 1 hour,[132] and adding 30 to 60 units to 1 to 2 L saline and infusing over 30 to 60 minutes.[121] Supplementing calcium by giving 50 units of oxytocin in 450 mL calcium borogluconate solution and infusing over 15 minutes in Friesian mares has also been described.[133] Failure of oxytocin to induce expulsion of the membranes within 12 to 24 hours may be an indication that the retained tissue is not going to be released spontaneously, and the problem will have to be resolved by necrosis of the retained microvilli and cellular clearance mechanisms over a period of time.[70]

Whether retained membranes should be manually removed meets with different opinions among veterinarians. Several methods and techniques for manually separating the chorionic and uterine surfaces at the site of adherence have been described and used with success,[127] but the decision should be tempered by the known potential complications. Subendometrial hemorrhage, luminal hemorrhage, absorption of bacterial toxins, invagination of the horn tip, pulmonary embolism, delayed involution, and permanent endometrial damage and impaired fertility have all been reported.[127,134] Irrespective of the method used, it seems likely that manual shearing of the chorioallantois from its site of retention leaves at least some microvilli embedded in the endometrium, which will be cleared by liquefaction and passage as particulate debris into the uterine lumen. That said, in some instances manual removal is an acceptable management choice, for example, when other methods of resolving RFM have failed[135] or the veterinarian is ambulatory and must limit the number of visits to the farm.[134]

Several reports support the quick resolution of RTM by manual removal.[123,124] Another method of detaching the membranes involves introducing fluid (water, saline, and povidone iodine in saline have all been used) into an intact allantochorionic space and retaining the fluid by tying off the membranes at the vulva. This technique stretches the uterus, inducing oxytocin release, and causes the chorionic microvilli to release their attachment.[136] Alternatively, water or saline can be infused into the uterine lumen, between the chorion and uterus, which may aid expulsion by separating the chorionic and endometrial surfaces. Infusion into the uterine space has the added benefit of diluting and carrying out inflammatory debris and bacteria.[70,134]

If these techniques do not elicit release of the membranes, the mare should be treated with continued oxytocin injections (less frequently than the original 24 hours), systemic antimicrobials, an NSAID drug, daily uterine lavages to remove the source of sepsis, tetanus toxoid, and prophylaxis for laminitis and founder. Intrauterine infusion of antimicrobials is also commonly used.[72,127] Retained placenta and metritis are associated with clinical tetanus in cattle; to the authors' knowledge there are no published reports of tetanus in mares with RFM, but given that anaerobes, including

Bacteroides and *Clostridium* spp, are cultured in some cases,[72,75,127] administering a dose of tetanus toxoid is merited. It is common practice to tie a 250- to 500-mL bag of fluids to the external part of the retained membranes to provide a tonic, mild level of tension.[70] As normal release of the fetal membranes results from both expulsive actions by smooth muscle contraction and the traction exerted by the weight of the initial portions of placenta to pass,[127] some believe there is rational for this practice. However, the same caveats pertaining to manual disruption of the connection apply to affixing weights to the placenta, and it should be undertaken carefully. The practice is avoided by some veterinarians.[127]

A technique for intraumbilical injection of a collagenase solution to aid in breaking down the connections between microvilli and endometrium has been used in cows[137] and was described in a 1998 study of 4 mares.[138] In that study, 200,000 units of bacterial collagenase diluted in 1 L saline was infused into 2 of the 3 umbilical vessels in 4 mares with RFM. In all cases, retained membranes were passed within 6 hours, with no adverse effects. The procedure would not be feasible in retained membranes that are internal to the vulva or that are shredded and autolyzing. To the authors' knowledge, this technique is not frequently practiced.

Even in mares in which efforts to remove the retained membranes is not successful, attentive management with a regimen of systemic antimicrobials, daily uterine lavage, oxytocin, intrauterine antimicrobials, NSAIDs, and prophylactic measures for laminitis usually return the mare to health and with the potential to carry a foal in the future. Mares that have had RFM are at risk for the problem in future pregnancies.

CLINICS CARE POINTS

- Injuries involving reproductive tract tissues are similar to those involving other body areas in that prompt recognition, thorough evaluation, and intervention underlie a favorable outcome
- Because of the episodic, unpredictable incidence of uterine artery rupture, randomized controlled clinical trials to evaluate treatments are infeasible, and most interventions are based on experience rather than being evidence-based
- Nevertheless, treatment of mares with internal hemorrhage and shock is justified and often rewarding
- Controlled reduction of the voluminous fetal fluids in hydropsic conditions necessitates monitoring and support for hypovolemic shock
- Uterine prolapse can lead to shock and endotoxemia after replacement of the organ
- Dystocia necessitating anesthesia and controlled vaginal delivery yields 2 postintervention patients in need of monitoring for complications
- Clear communications and management of client expectations are key skills for veterinarians managing reproductive emergencies

DISCLOSURE

The authors have nothing to disclose.

REFERENCES

1. Dolente B, Sullivan E, Lundberg S. Postpartum complications in the mare, in Proceedings: 8th International Veterinary Emergency and Critical Care Society Symposium, San Antonio, 2002:790.

2. Dwyer R, Harrison L. Postpartum deaths of mares. Equine Dis Q 1993;2:5.

3. Dolente BA, Sullivan EK, Boston R, et al. Mares admitted to a referral hospital for postpartum emergencies: 163 cases (1992-2002). J Vet Emerg Crit Care 2005; 15:193–200.

4. Dechant JE, Nieto JE, Le Jeune SS. Hemoperitoneum in horses: 67 cases (1989–2004). J Am Vet Med Assoc 2006;229:253–8.

5. Arnold CE, Payne M, Thompson JA, et al. Periparturient hemorrhage in mares: 73 cases (1998–2005). J Am Vet Med Assoc 2008;232:1345–51.

6. Williams NM, Bryant UK. Periparturient arterial rupture in mares: a postmortem study. J Equine Vet Sci 2012;32:281–4.

7. Nickel R, Schummer A, Seiferle E. Female genital organs, general and comparative. In: Schummer A, Nickel R, Sack WO, editors. The viscera of the domestic animals. 2nd ed. Berlin and Hamburg: Verlag Paul Parey; 1979. p. 351–92.

8. Ousey JC, Kolling M, Newton R, et al. Uterine haemodynamics in young and aged pregnant mares measured using Doppler ultrasonography. Equine Vet J 2012;44(Suppl 41):15–21.

9. Ueno T, Nambo Y, Tajima Y, et al. Pathology of lethal *peripartum* broad ligament haematoma in 31 Thoroughbred mares. Equine Vet J 2010;529–33.

10. Pascoe RR. Rupture of the utero-ovarian or middle uterine artery in the mare at or near parturition. Vet Rec 1979;104:77.

11. LeBlanc M. Common peripartum problems in the mare. J Equine Vet Sci 2008; 28:709–15.

12. Toro Mayorga AG, 2015. Uterine artery rupture, an angiopathy of the reproductive system of the mare: occurrence and potential effects. Theses and dissertations – Veterinary Science. 24. Available at: https://uknowledge.uky.edu/gluck_etds/24.

13. Rooney JR. Internal hemorrhage related to gestation in the mare. Cornell Vet 1964;54:11–7.

14. Koyluoglu G, Bakici MZ, Elagoz S, et al. The effects of pentoxifylline treatment on bacterial translocation after hemorrhagic shock in rats. Clin Exp Med 2001; 1:61–6.

15. Wohl JS, Clark TP. Pressor therapy in critically ill patients. J Vet Emerg Crit Care 2000;10:21–34.

16. Chovanes J, Cannon JW, Nunez TC. The evolution of damage control surgery. Surg Clin North Am 2012;92:859–75.

17. Cannon JW. Hemorrhagic shock. N Engl J Med 2018;378:370–9.

18. Duchesne JC, McSwain NE, Cotton BA, et al. Damage control resuscitation: the new face of damage control. J Trauma 2010;69:976–90.

19. Wagner AE, Muir WW, Hinchcliff KW. Cardiovascular effects of xylazine and detomidine in horses. Am J Vet Res 1991;52:651–7.

20. Fielding L. Crystalloid and colloid therapy. Vet Clin Equine 2014;30:415–25.

21. Schott HC. Fluid therapy: a primer for students, technicians, and veterinarians in equine practice. Vet Clin North Am Equine Pract 2006;22:1–14.

22. Corley K. Fluid therapy. In: Corley K, Stephen J, editors. The equine hospital manual. West Sussex: Blackwell Publishing; 2008. p. 364–92.

23. Mudge MC. Acute hemorrhage and blood transfusions in horses. Vet Clin Equine 2014;30:427–36.

24. Divers TJ. Liver failure, anemia, and blood transfusion. In: Orsini JA, Divers TJ, editors. Equine emergencies – treatment and procedures. 4th edition. St Louis (MO): Elsevier Saunders; 2014. p. 268–88.

25. Gayet-Argeron A, Prieto-Merino D, Ker K, et al. Effect of treatment delay on the effectiveness and safety of antifibrinolytics in acute severe hemorrhage: a meta-analysis of individual patient-level data from 40,138 bleeding patients. Lancet 2018;391:125–32.

26. Fletcher DJ, Brainard BM, Epstein K, et al. Therapeutic plasma concentrations of epsilon aminocaproic acid and tranexamic acid in horses. J Vet Intern Med 2013;27:1589–95.

27. Peng Z, Ban K, LeBlanc A, et al. Intraluminal tranexamic acid inhibits intestinal sheddases and mitigates gut and lung injury and inflammation in a rodent model of hemorrhagic shock. J Trauma Acute Care Surg 2016;81:358–65.

28. Kantyka ME, Meira C, Bettschart-Wolfensberger R, et al. Prospective, controlled, blinded, randomized crossover trial evaluating the effect of maropi-tant versus ondansetron on inhibiting tranexamic acid-evoked emesis. J Vet Emerg Crit Care 2020;30:436–41.

29. Kakiuchi H, Kawarai-Shimamura A, Kuwagata M, et al. Tranexamic acid induces kaolin intake stimulating a pathway involving tachykinin neurokinin 1 receptors in rats. Eur J Pharm 2014;723:1–6.

30. Orito K, Kawarai-Shimamura A, Ogawa A, et al. Safety and efficacy of intrave-nous administration for tranexamic acid-induced emesis in dogs with accidental ingestion of foreign substances. J Vet Med Sci 2017;79:1978–82.

31. Shi HP, Deitch EA, Da Xu Z, et al. Hypertonic saline improves intestinal mucosal barrier function and lung injury after trauma-hemorrhagic shock. Shock 2002;17:496–501.

32. Moore FA. The role of the gastrointestinal tract in post-injury multiple organ fail-ure. Am J Surg 1999;178:449–53.

33. Glover LE, Lee JS, Colgan SP. Oxygen metabolism and barrier regulation in the intestinal mucosa. J Clin Invest 2016;126:3680–8.

34. Weld JM, Kamerling SG, Combie JD, et al. The effects of naloxone on endotoxic and hemorrhagic shock in horses. Res Commun Chem Pathol Pharmacol 1984;44:227–38.

35. Salerno TA, Milne B, Jhamandas KH. Hemodynamic effects of naloxone in hem-orrhagic shock in pigs. Surg Gynecol Obstet 1981;152:773–6.

36. Schadt JC. Sympathetic and hemodynamic adjustments to hemorrhage: a possible role for endogenous opioid peptides. Resuscitation 1989;18:219–28.

37. Gin SL, Dronen SC, Syverud SA, et al. Naloxone does not improve hemody-namics following graded hemorrhage in a canine model. Am J Emerg Med 1987;5:478–82.

38. Scoggin CF, McCue PM. How to assess and stabilize a mare suspected of periparturient hemorrhage in the field. In Proceedings. Am Assoc Equine Pract, Orlando, FL, 2007:342–8.

39. Graham L, Farnsworth K, Cary J. The effect of yunnan baiyao on the template bleeding time and activated clotting time in healthy halothane anesthetized ponies, in Proceedings. 8th Intl Vet Emer Crit Care Soc Symposium, San Anto-nio, 2002;790.

40. Patlogar JE, Tansey C, Wiebe M, et al. A prospective evaluation of oral Yunnan Baiyao therapy on thromboelastographic parameters in apparently healthy cats. J Vet Emerg Crit Care 2019;29:611–5.

41. Lee A, Boysen SR, Sanderson J, et al. Effects of Yunnan Baiyao on blood coag-ulation parameters in beagles measured using kaolin activated thromboelastog-raphy and more traditional methods. Int J Vet Sci Med 2017;5:53–6.

42. Ness SL, Frye AH, Divers TJ, et al. Randomized placebo-controlled study of the effects of Yunnan Baiyao on hemostasis in horses. Am J Vet Res 2017;78: 969–76.

43. Taylor EL, Sellon DC, Wardrop KJ, et al. Effects of intravenous administration of formaldehyde on platelet and coagulation variables in healthy horses. Am J Vet Res 2000;61:1191–6.

44. Trumble TN, Ingle-Fehr J, Hendrickson DA. Laparoscopic intra-abdominal ligation of the testicular artery following castration in a horse. J Am Vet Med Assoc 2000;216:1596–8.

45. Jones W. IV formalin to control hemorrhage. J Equine Vet Sci 1998;18:581.

46. Wilkins PA, Seahorn TL. Intranasal oxygen therapy in adult horses. J Vet Emerg Crit Care 2000;10:221.

47. Giles RC, Donahue JM, Hong CB, et al. Causes of abortion, stillbirth, and perinatal death in horses: 3,527 cases (1986–1991). J Am Vet Med Assoc 1993;203: 1170–5.

48. McCue PM, Ferris RA. Parturition, dystocia, and foal survival: a retrospective study of 1047 births. Equine Vet J Suppl 2012;41:22–5.

49. Wilkins PA. Prognostic indicators for survival and athletic outcome in critically ill neonatal foals. Vet Clin North Am Equine Pract 2015;31:615–28.

50. Norton JL, Dallap BL, Johnston JK, et al. Retrospective study of dystocia in mares at a referral hospital. Equine Vet J 2007;39:37–41.

51. Byron CE, Embertson RM, Bernard WV, et al. Dystocia in a referral hospital setting: approach and results. Equine Vet J 2009;35:82–5.

52. Frazer G. Dystocia management. In: McKinnon AO, Squires EL, Vaala WE, et al, editors. Equine reproduction. 2nd edition. West Sussex: Wiley-Blackwell; 2011. p. 2479–96.

53. Ginther OJ, Williams D. On-the-farm incidence and nature of equine dystocias. J Equine Vet Sci 1996;16:159–64.

54. Freeman DE, Hungerford LL, Schaeffer D, et al. Caesarean section and other methods for assisted delivery: comparison of effects on mare mortality and complications. Equine Vet J 1999;31:203–7.

55. Frazer GS. Fetotomy. In: McKinnon AO, Squires EL, Vaala WE, et al, editors. Equine reproduction. 2nd edition. West Sussex: Wiley-Blackwell; 2011. p. 2497–504.

56. Frazer GS, Beard WL, Abrahamson E, et al. Systemic effects of a polyethylene polymer-based obstetrical lubricant in the peritoneal cavity of the horse. In Proceedings. 50th Ann Conv Am Assoc Equine Pract, Denver, 2004;50:484–7.

57. Norris MC, Joseph J, Leighton BL. Anesthesia for perinatal surgery. Am J Perinatol 1989;6:39–40.

58. Palmer JE, Wilkins PA. .In Proceedings. 51st Ann Conv Am Assoc Equine Pract, Seattle, 2005;51:281–3.

59. Subramanian R, Mishra P, Subramamiam R, et al. Role of anesthesiologist in *ex utero* intrapartum treatment procedure: A case and review of anesthetic management. J Anaesthesiol Clin Pharmacol 2018;34:148–54.

60. Adamson SL, Myatt L, Byrne MP. Regulation of umbilical blood flow. In: Polin RA, Fox WW, Abman SH, editors. Fetal and neonatal physiology, vol. 1, 3rd edition. Philadelphia: Saunders; 2004. p. 748–58.

61. Corley KT. Foal resuscitation. In: Orsini JA, Divers TJ, editors. Equine emergencies – treatment and procedures. 4th edition. St Louis (MO): Elsevier Saunders; 2014. p. 509–19.

62. Slack A. Uterine prolapse in a mare. J Am Vet Med Assoc 1973;162:780.

63. Pascoe J, Pascoe R. Displacements, malpositions, and miscellaneous injuries of the mare's urogenital tract. Vet Clin North Am Equine Pract 1988;4:439–50.

64. Frazer GS. Postpartum complications in the mare: Part 1. Conditions affecting the uterus. Equine Vet Educ 2003;15:45.

65. Schambourg MA. Idiopathic prolapse of 1 uterine horn in a yearling filly. Can Vet J 2004;45:602–4.

66. Spirito MA, Sprayberry KA. Uterine prolapse. In: McKinnon AO, Squires EL, Vaala WE, et al, editors. Equine reproduction. 2nd edition. West Sussex: Wiley-Blackwell; 2016. p. 2431–4.

67. Schott HC. Urinary tract infection and bladder displacement. In: Sprayberry KA, Robinson NE, editors. Current therapy in equine medicine. 7th edition. St Louis (MO): Elsevier Saunders; 2015. p. 448–50.

68. Hewes CA, Johnson AK, Kivett LE, et al. Uterine prolapse in a mare leading to metritis, systemic inflammatory response syndrome, septic shock and death. Equine Vet Educ 2011;23:273–8.

69. Dolente BA. Critical peripartum disease in the mare. Vet Clin North Am Equine Pract 2004;20:151–65.

70. Turner R. Post-partum problems: the top ten list. In Proceedings. 53rd Ann Conv Am Assoc Equine Pract, Orlando, 2007;305–19.

71. Frazer GS. Postpartum complications in the mare. Part 2: fetal membrane retention and conditions of the gastrointestinal tract, bladder, and vagina. Equine Vet Educ 2002;14(Suppl 5):50–9.

72. Blanchard TL. Postpartum metritis. In: McKinnon AO, Squires EL, Vaala WE, et al, editors. Equine reproduction. 2nd edition. West Sussex: Wiley Blackwell; 2011. p. 2530–3.

73. Ferrer MS, Palomares R. Aerobic uterine isolates and antimicrobial susceptibility in mares with post-partum metritis. Equine Vet J 2018;50:202–7.

74. Blanchard TL, Varner DD, Scrutchfield WL, et al. Management of dystocia in mares: retained placenta, metritis, and laminitis. Comp Cont Educ Pract Vet 1990; 12:563–71.

75. Blanchard TL, Vaala WE, Straughn AJ, et al. Septic/toxic metritis and laminitis in a postpartum mare: case report. J Equine Vet Sci 1987;7:32–4.

76. Sutter WW, Hopper S, Embertson RM, et al. Diagnosis and surgical treatment of uterine lacerations in mares (33 cases). In Proceedings. 49th Ann Conv Amer Assoc Equine Pract, New Orleans, 2003;357–9.

77. Javsicas LH, Giguere S, Freeman DE, et al. Comparison of surgical and medical treatment of 49 postpartum mares with presumptive or confirmed uterine tears. Vet Surg 2010;39:254–60.

78. Fischer AT, Phillips TN. Surgical repair of a ruptured uterus in five mares. Equine Vet J 1986;18:153–5.

79. Hooper Rn, Schumacher J, Taylor TS, et al. Diagnosing and treating uterine rupture in the mare. Vet Med 1993;88:263–70.

80. Blanchard TL, Bierschwal CJ, Youngquist RS, et al. Sequelae to percutaneous fetotomy in the mare. J Am Vet Med Assoc 1983;182:1127.

81. Hassel DM, Ragle C. Laparoscopic diagnosis and conservative treatment of uterine tear in a mare. J Am Vet Med Assoc 1994;205:1531–6.

82. Wheat JD, Meagher DM. Uterine torsion and rupture in mares. J Am Vet Med Assoc 1972;160:881–4.

83. Honnas CM, Spensley MS, Laverty S, et al. Hydramnios causing uterine rupture in a mare. J Am Vet Med Assoc 1988;193:334–6.

84. Sprayberry KA. Personal case files. 2003.

85. McNally TP, Rodgerson DH, Lu KG. Infertility in a mare with a chronic uterine tear: diagnosis and successful hand-assisted laparoscopic repair. Equine Vet Educ 2012;24:439–43.
86. Frazer G, Beard WL, Abrahamsen E, et al. Systemic effects of peritoneal instillation of a polyethylene polymer based obstetrical lubricant in horses, in Proceedings. Society for Theriogenology Annual Meeting, Lexington, KY, 2004;93–7.
87. Rowe E. Peritoneal lavage. In: Corley K, Stephens J, editors. The equine hospital manual. West Sussex: Wiley Blackwell; 2008. p. 18–21.
88. Nieto JE, Snyder JR, Vatistas NJ, et al. Use of an active abdominal drain in 67 horses. Vet Surg 2003;32:1–7.
89. Lepage OM, Monteiro S, Desmaizieres LM. Peritoneal drainage of fenestrated balloon catheters in standing horse: a comparative study. In Proceedings. 55th Ann Conv Am Assoc Equine Pract, Las Vegas, 2009;487–91.
90. Hardy J, Rakestraw PC. Postoperative care, complications, and reoperation. In: Auer J, Stick JA, editors. Equine surgery. St Louis (MO): Elsevier Saunders; 2012. p. 514–29.
91. Platt H. Caecal rupture in parturient mares. J Comp Pathol 1983;93:343–6.
92. Dart AJ, Pascoe JR, Snyder JR. Mesenteric tears of the descending (small) colon as a postpartum complication in two mares. J Am Vet Med Assoc 1991;199:1612–5.
93. Ragle CA, Southwood LL, Galuppo LD, et al. Laparoscopic diagnosis of ischemic necrosis of the descending colon after rectal prolapse and rupture of the mesocolon in two postpartum mares. J Am Vet Med Assoc 1997;210:1646–8.
94. Rodgerson DH, Spirito MA, Thorpe PE, et al. Standing surgical repair of cystorrhexis in two mares. Vet Surg 1999;28:113–6.
95. Zamos DT, Ford TS, Cohen ND, et al. Segmental ischemic necrosis of the small intestine in two postparturient mares. J Am Vet Med Assoc 1993;202:101–3.
96. Livesey MA, Keller SD. Segmental ischemic necrosis following mesocolic rupture in postparturient mares. J Am Vet Med Assoc 1986;10:763–8.
97. Weese JS, Holcombe SJ, Embertson RM, et al. Changes in the faecal microbiota of mares precede the development of postpartum colic. Equine Vet J 2015;47:641–9.
98. Moore RM. Equine large colon volvulus. In Proceedings. Amer Coll Vet Surg Ann Symp, San Francisco, 1996;236–7.
99. Proudman CJ, Smith JE, Edwards GB, et al. Long-term survival of equine surgical colic cases. Part 1: Patterns of mortality and morbidity. Equine Vet J 2002;34:432–7.
100. Moore JN, Dreesen DW, Boudinet DF. Colonic distension, displacement, and torsion in Thoroughbred broodmares: results of a two-year study. In Proceedings. 4th Equine Colic Symposium. Athens: Univ of Georgia, 1991;23–5.
101. Suthers JM, Pinchbeck GL, Proudman CJ, et al. Survival of horses following strangulating large colon volvulus. Equine Vet J 2013;45:219–23.
102. Rakestraw PC, Hardy J. Large intestine. In: Auer JA, Stick JA, editors. Equine surgery. 4th edition. St Louis (MO): Elsevier Saunders; 2012. p. 454–94.
103. Harrison IW. Equine large intestine volvulus. A review of 124 cases. Vet Surg 1988;17:77–81.
104. Snyder JR, Pascoe JR, Olander HJ, et al. Strangulating volvulus of the ascending colon in horses. J Am Vet Med Assoc 1989;195:757–64.

105. Ellis CM, Lynch TM, Slone DE, et al. Survival and complications after large colon resection and end-to-end anastomosis for strangulating large colon volvulus in 73 horses. Vet Surg 2008;37:786–90.
106. Barclay WP, Foerner JJ, Phillips TN. Volvulus of the large colon in the horse. J Am Vet Med Assoc 1980;177:629–30.
107. Suthers JM, Pinchbeck GL, Proudman CJ, et al. Risk factors for large colon volvulus in the UK. Equine Vet J 2013;45:558–63.
108. Petersen JL, Lewis RM, Embertson RM, et al. Preliminary heritability of complete rotation large colon volvulus in Thoroughbred broodmares. Vet Rec 2019; 185:269.
109. Salem SE, Hough R, Probert C, et al. A longitudinal study of the faecal microbiome and metabolome of periparturient mares. PeerJ 2019;7:e6687.
110. Leahy ER, Holcombe SJ, Hackett ES, et al. Reproductive careers of Thoroughbred broodmares before and after surgical correction of ≥ 360° large colon volvulus. Equine Vet J 2018;50:208–12.
111. Hackett ES, Embertson RM, Hopper SA, et al. Duration of disease influences survival to discharge of Thoroughbred mares with surgically treated large colon volvulus. Equine Vet J 2015;47:650–4.
112. Abutarbush SM. Use of ultrasonography to diagnose large colon volvulus in horses. J Am Vet Med Assoc 2006;228:409–13.
113. Busoni V, Busscher V, Lopez D, et al. Evaluation of a protocol for fast localised abdominal sonography of horses (FLASH) admitted for colic. Vet J 2011;188: 77–82.
114. Hance SR, Embertson RM. Colopexy in broodmares: 44 cases (1986–1990). J Am Vet Med Assoc 1992;201:782–7.
115. Hall MD, Rodgerson DH. Colopexy dehiscence preceding an episode of large colon volvulus, followed by repeat colopexy, in three Thoroughbred broodmares. Equine Vet Educ 2020;32:407.
116. Broyles AH, Hopper SA, Woodie JB, et al. Clinical outcomes after colpexy through left ventral paramedian incision in 156 Thoroughbred broodmares with large colon disorders (1999–2015). Vet Surg 2018;47:490–8.
117. Hunt RJ, Spirito MA. Ventral midline colopexy as a prevention of large colon volvulus. In Proceedings. Am Assoc Equine Pract 41st Ann Conv. Lexington, KY. Dec 2-5, 1995;202.
118. Markel MD. Prevention of LC displacements and volvulus. Vet Clin North Am Equine Pract 1989;5:395–405.
119. Blanchard T, Varner D. Therapy for retained placenta in the mare. Vet Med 1993; 88:55–9.
120. Provencher R, Threlfall WR, Murdick PW, et al. Retained fetal membranes in the mare: a retrospective study. Can Vet J 1988;29:903–10.
121. Vandeplassche M, Spincemaille J, Bouters R. Aetiology, pathogenesis and treatment of retained placenta in the mare. Equine Vet J 1971;3:144–7.
122. Rapacz-Leonard A, Raś A, Całka J, et al. Expression of oxytocin receptors is greatly reduced in the placenta of heavy mares with retained fetal membranes due to secondary uterine atony. Equine Vet J 2015;47:623–6.
123. Cuervo-Arango J, Newcombe JR. The effect of manual removal of placenta immediately after foaling on subsequent fertility parameters in the mare. J Equine Vet Sci 2009;29:771–4.
124. Sevinga M, Hesselink JW, Barkema HW. Reproductive performance of Friesian mares after retained placenta and manual removal of the placenta. Theriogenology 2002;57:923–30.

125. Sevinga M, Vrijenhoek T, Hesselink JW, et al. Effect of inbreeding on the incidence of retained placenta I Friesian horses. J Anim Sci 2004;4:982–6.
126. Canisso IF, Rodriguez JS, Sanz MG, et al. A clinical approach to the diagnosis and treatment of retained fetal membranes with an emphasis placed on the critically ill mare. J Equine Vet Sci 2013;3:570–9.
127. Threlfall WR. Retained fetal membranes. In: McKinnon AO, Squires EL, Vaala WE, et al, editors. Equine reproduction. 2nd edition. West Sussex: Wiley Blackwell; 2011. p. 2520–9.
128. Pozor M. Equine placenta – a clinician's perspective. Part 1: normal placenta – physiology and evaluation. Equine Vet Educ 2016;28:327–34.
129. Rosales C, Krekeler N, Tennent-Brown B, et al. Periparturient characteristics of mares and their foals on a New Zealand Thoroughbred stud farm. N Z Vet J 2017;65:24–9 [95% of mares expelled FM by 4 hours; 2/3 within 1 hour].
130. Morresey PR, Lu KG. Placental evaluation for assessment of foal problems and maternal reproductive health. In: Robinson NE, Sprayberry KA, editors. Current therapy in equine medicine. 6th edition. St Louis (MO): Elsevier Saunders; 2009. p. 851–7.
131. Held JP. Retained placenta. In: Robinson NE, editor. Current therapy in equine medicine. 2nd edition. Philadelphia: WB Saunders Co; 1987. p. 547–50.
132. Arthur GH. Wright's veterinary obstetrics. 3rd edition. Baltimore: Williams and Wilkins Co; 1964. p. 341–4.
133. Sevinga M, Barkema M, Hesselink JW. Serum calcium and magnesium concentrations and the use of a calcium-magnesium-borogluconate solution in the treatment of Friesian mares with retained placenta. Theriogenology 2001;57:941–7.
134. Samper J, Plough T. How to deal with dystocia and retained placenta in the field. In: Proceedings. 58th Ann Conv Amer Assoc Equine Pract. Anaheim, CA, 2012;359–61.
135. Neely DP, Liu IKM, Hillman RB. Equine reproduction. Nutley (NJ): Veterinary Learning Systems; 1983. p. 87–8.
136. Burns SJ, Judge NG, Martin JE, et al. Management of retained placenta in mares. In: Proceedings. 23rd Ann Conv Am Assoc Equine Pract, 1977;381–90.
137. Eiler H, Hopkins FM. Successful treatment of retained placenta with umbilical cord injections of collagenase in cows. J Am Vet Med Assoc 1993;203:436–43.
138. Haffner JC, Fecteau KA, Held JP, et al. Equine retained placenta: technique for and tolerance to umbilical artery injections of collagenase. Theriogenology 1998;49:711–6.

Emergency Management of Equid Foals in the Field

Elsbeth A. Swain O'Fallon, DVM, DACVIM

KEYWORDS

- Foal • Emergency • Field • Neonatal • Equid • Critical

KEY POINTS

- Early intervention and prevention are crucial factors for successful outcomes for foals.
- Intravenous fluid bolus (20 mL/kg; 1 L of crystalloid fluids for a 50 kg foal) provides appropriate initial volume replacement support and can be repeated if necessary.
- Lameness, heat, and effusion palpated in a foal suggests a septic synovial structure until proved otherwise and emergency intervention is recommended.
- Many emergent conditions of foals can be successfully managed in the field.

INTRODUCTION

Equid foal emergencies require quick decision-making and therapeutic intervention, especially when involving neonates. The foal's condition can change rapidly from appearing clinically normal to progression to obtundation or recumbency depending on the severity of the underlying condition. Swift and appropriate initiation of therapy is imperative for this population. One of the most challenging aspects of managing foal emergencies in the field is the decision to treat on the farm versus the referral to a specialty hospital. This decision is influenced by the foal's response to initial triage, treatment, and diagnostic options available from the field truck or the farm facility, monitoring capabilities on the farm, proximity to a referral facility, and financial considerations. When referral is possible, then the goal of the field practitioner is stabilization of the foal before transport.[1]

When referral is not an option or if management in the field is preferable, the objective becomes achieving the best outcome for the foal using what supplies and assistance are available. Foals can decline rapidly without appropriate support. With early intervention many conditions are possible to treat successfully with field care (**Table 1**).

Because early intervention and prevention are crucial factors in the successful treatment of foals, client education during gestation is recommended. The following are the

Department of Clinical Sciences, James L. Voss Veterinary Teaching Hospital, Colorado State University, 300 W. Drake Road, Fort Collins, CO 80523, USA
E-mail address: eswain@colostate.edu

Vet Clin Equine 37 (2021) 407–420
https://doi.org/10.1016/j.cveq.2021.04.009
0749-0739/21/© 2021 Elsevier Inc. All rights reserved.

Table 1
Recommended field truck supplies for foal emergencies

Obstetric Chains	50% Dextrose	Foal-Sized Nasogastric Tubes
Umbilical tape	1 L isotonic fluids	Red rubber tubes
IgG testing	Foal catheters	Di-tri-octahedral smectite
Stall-side lactate	Stall-side serum amyloid A	± Stall-side glucometer
Towels	Knee pad/foal mat	± Electrocardiogram (ECG)
± Oxygen	± Foal resuscitator kit[a]	± Foal-sized endotracheal tube
± Vitamin E/selenium	± Blood culture bottles	± Fetotomy equipment

simple client guidelines to recommend even for apparently healthy foals that target the goal of early recognition of an emergent condition:

- Follow recommended timelines for normal foaling.
- Dip the umbilicus using dilute chlorhexidine following foaling. Monitor the umbilicus for signs of moisture, discharge, or swelling.
- Have the foal examined within the first 24 hours by a veterinarian and have blood tested for passive transfer/immunoglobulin G (IgG) assessment at the least.
- Monitor the foal's attitude and playfulness, manure production, and appetite.
- Monitor for lameness or joint swelling; this is considered an emergency.
- Pay close attention to *subtle* changes and call your veterinarian with any concerns.

DISCUSSION
Diagnostic Approach in the Field

Risk factors
Maternal, placental, and fetal/foal risk factors[2] influence neonatal emergencies. Maternal factors include dystocia, dam illness or concurrent conditions, genetic conditions, gestation length/premature delivery, mare-foal bonding, parity, and if they have previously had mule foals.[3] Placentitis or other forms of placental insufficiency, such as fescue toxicity, influence placental factors; these can disrupt the fetal development and predispose to fetal infection in utero.[4,5]

Foal risk factors include failure of passive transfer, omphalitis, sepsis, postpartum maladjustment including pharyngeal weakness, congenital defects, genetic inheritance, and traumatic injury. The geographic region influences the risk for many infectious agents,[6] with examples including *Rhodococcus equi*,[7] clostridial enteritis, *Lawsonia intracellularis*, antibiotic-associated changes in microbiota and dysbiosis,[8] and mare reproductive loss syndrome. The geographic region also can predispose to deficiencies such as selenium.[9]

Handling and restraint of foals in the field
Restraint of neonatal equid foals can be much easier to handle when compared with the strength and size of older foals. Most compromised neonatal foals do not require sedation for noninvasive procedures. When using sedation, special considerations include the risk of alpha-2 agonist use in foals younger than 4 weeks. Neonates depend on heart rate to maintain perfusion and blood pressure.[10] The bradycardic effects of alpha-2 agonists alter the cardiovascular protective balance and place even healthy foals at risk for complications.[10,11] An effective alternative for sedation in neonates are midazolam or diazepam (0.05–0.1 mg/kg intravenously [IV]). These benzodiazepines can be used in combination with butorphanol (0.01–0.05 mg/kg IV or

intramuscularly [IM]) for additional sedation and analgesia effects in neonatal foals. Another option for short-term restraint in a healthy neonate can be performed using squeeze-induced somnolence with the Madigan squeeze technique.[12]

Foals older than 4 weeks can safely be sedated with an alpha-2 agonist for minor procedures or for induction for anesthesia (xylazine 0.5–1 mg/kg; detomidine 0.005–0.01 mg/kg; preanesthetic dexmedetomidine 0.005 mg/kg IV).[13] Anesthesia is frequently used in foals to facilitate short-term, minimally invasive procedures in the field.[10,14,15]

Physical examination

Examination of a foal encompasses unique differences when compared with adult equids. Weakness, obtundation, and recumbency are common and nonspecific signs of a compromised foal. Hypovolemia, septic shock, and hypoglycemia are examples of conditions that can result in these clinical signs.[16] If a neonatal foal is weak and not nursing, then hypoglycemia will quickly develop due to their lack of glycogen stores. Milk staining or crusting on a foal's face is an early indicator of a foal that has lost interest in nursing (**Fig. 1**).

Guidelines for approaching the differences when examining foals compared with adults:

- Cardiac auscultation: arrhythmias are common in the first few hours of life and then should resolve into normal sinus rhythm. The rule of thumb for cardiac murmurs: if greater than II/VI with no resolution by 1 to 2 weeks of age, recommend an echocardiogram.[16]
- Respiratory auscultation and rib palpation: airflow should be equal bilaterally. Auscultation of the trachea postnursing should be clear and free of fluid. Friction

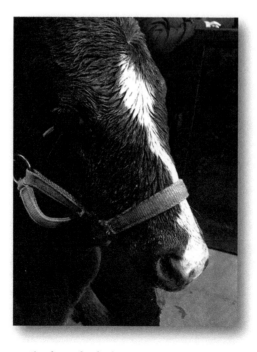

Fig. 1. Milk staining on the face of a foal.

rubs or clicks may indicate a rib fracture. Rib fractures are identified by local edema, pain on palpation, or by using diagnostic imaging. Milk visualized from the nostrils may indicate pharyngeal paresis, dysphagia, or a cleft palate.[1]

- Urinary and umbilical examination: umbilicus should feel dry, small, and have no pain response to palpation. Inguinal and umbilical hernias can be palpated, and ultrasound may aid diagnosis. Umbilical hernia of size greater than 3 or more fingers are at risk for complications.[17] Colts usually urinate by 8 to 10 hours and fillies by 10 to 12 hours. The first urine-specific gravity is concentrated and quickly progresses to hyposthenuria as the foal nurses. Foals frequently cycle between nursing, urination, play, and sleep.
- Mucous membranes include the third eyelid and vulva. Petechial hemorrhages indicate a coagulopathy and/or sepsis and can also be identified on the inner pinna surfaces (**Fig. 2**). Hyperemic mucous membranes and a capillary refill time of 1 second suggests sepsis, systemic inflammatory response syndrome (SIRS), or anaphylaxis.
- Ocular examination: menace response is absent in first few weeks of life. Uveitis, hypopyon, and scleral injection are signs of sepsis. Hyphema is a sign of trauma. Entropion and ulcerative keratitis are common. Evaluate for congenital cataracts.
- Musculoskeletal: palpate all synovial structures on every foal examination. Lameness, heat, and effusion suggest a septic synovial structure until proved otherwise and is considered an emergency. There are synovial structures that cannot be palpated and require diagnostic imaging to diagnose sepsis. Hyperemic coronary bands are a sign of sepsis. Angular and flexural deformities are common and may require intervention.
- Signs of hypovolemia[16] include cold extremities, sunken eyes, poor pulse quality, obtundation, pale mucous membranes, and tachycardia.
- Gastrointestinal: gentle digital rectal examination can be performed. Tail flagging or swishing can be a sign of meconium impaction or a sign of developing enterocolitis.

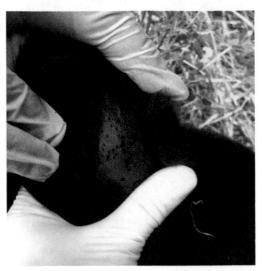

Fig. 2. Petechiae visible on the inner pinna of a foal. (*Courtesy of* Dr Diane Rhodes, DVM, DACVIM, California.)

Box 1
Ultrasound of a foal in the field

- Any equine transducer (frequencies 2–12 MHz) can be used to image a foal. The various transducer types may yield optimal imaging of different regions.[20,21]

- Obtain videos in addition to saving still images, and these can be used for consultation with a referral practice. Video conferencing is also possible as the ultrasound is being performed.

- Ultrasound can be used to image the following regions: thoracic organs including the lungs and heart, abdominal organs, bladder, umbilicus, musculoskeletal structures, and ocular structures.

- Umbilical structures[20,21]
  - Urachus: abnormal if it is filled with fluid; should be collapsed.
  - Umbilical stump (urachus and umbilical arteries combined): less than 2.5 cm in size if normal
  - Umbilical arteries: paired; vessel width less than 1.3 cm if normal; as they diverge into the bladder: less than 1.0 cm in width.
  - Umbilical vein: vessel width less than 1.0 cm if normal; courses toward the liver.

Diagnostic testing

Diagnostic imaging can be easily performed in the field for foal emergencies (**Boxes 1–3**). The size of the foal increases the usefulness of field abdominal and thoracic radiographs. In addition to imaging, additional testing is easily performed in the field setting (**Box 4**). Point-of-care testing, or stall-side testing, can help direct rapid therapeutic decision-making and can be performed for tests including IgG, lactate, glucose, and serum amyloid A. Many of these tests are useful for monitoring response to treatment when used with serial sampling.[18,19]

Therapeutic Options in the Field

Initial triage of the foal in the field

The compromised foal requires efficient and thorough examination to determine the degree of compromise and the body systems affected. Status of passive transfer should be confirmed. Establishing the client's goals of treating the foal on the farm versus referral to a hospital is essential. The most common conditions causing weakness and the inability to rise or nurse are sepsis, neonatal maladjustment, trauma, and prematurity/dysmaturity.[1] Specifically, hypovolemia and dehydration, hypoperfusion associated with SIRS/septic shock, hypothermia, hypoglycemia, and hypoxemia can be the contributing factors.[2,16] Simple approaches to supportive care can be lifesaving in the face of these conditions.

- Assess respiratory and cardiovascular status and intervene as indicated. Cardiopulmonary resuscitation may be warranted.[1,37] Foal resuscitation kits[a] are easily transported. An average-sized foal weighs 45 to 50 kg. A size 9 to 12 mm inner diameter nasotracheal tube works well for average-sized foals.[15]
- Jugular or cephalic veins are the easiest to access for catheter placement and venipuncture in a foal.
- Resuscitation includes administration of an initial 20 mL/kg IV bolus of crystalloid fluids and allows time to reassess the foal (**Box 5**); this can be repeated up to 3

---

[a] McCulloch Medical™ Foal Resuscitator Kit; 3A Marken Place, Wairau Valley, Auckland 0627, New Zealand.

Box 2
Digital radiography of a foal in the field

- Premature foals are at risk of incomplete ossification. Carpal and tarsal lateromedial and dorsopalmar/plantar views are indicated.
- Radiographs can define the location and severity of the deformation of an angular limb deformity.
- Radiographs are indicated to aid in diagnosis of septic arthritis/physitis/osteomyelitis.[22]
- Thorax and abdominal radiography are possible on a foal in the field.
- Indwelling feeding tubes and over-the-wire catheters are radiopaque and may be visualized in thoracic views if placed.

---

times as the foal's condition indicates. If improvement is not observed, then continuous fluids and further supportive care are recommended.

- Dextrose supplementation should be avoided in bolus fluids if possible. If hypoglycemia is suspected, no more than a 0.5% to 1% dextrose may be added to the initial fluids[1] and the rate can be adjusted for a slower bolus. Avoid iatrogenic hyperglycemia caused by excessive dextrose administration.
- Antimicrobials are warranted for many conditions; this is essential when sepsis is suspected.[38]
- Butorphanol is an effective analgesic alternative if the foal is hypovolemic and dehydrated to avoid renal insult from nonsteroidal antiinflammatory drug (NSAID) use.
- Passive warming via use of a towel and massage can improve hypothermia without causing harm by other reheating methods.[1,39]
- Field diagnostics for a colic in a foal are very similar to an adult horse with the addition of abdominal radiographs and therapeutic enema administration.

Catheter placement can be performed in a standing foal and in a recumbent foal. Sedation can be helpful in older foal catheter placement, although should be avoided in a compromised neonate. The recommended size of an IV catheter for a foal is 14 or 16 gauge and 3.25 inch in length for short-term use. In the field, an over-the-wire catheter can be maintained for longer periods of time. Only one port is necessary because most often fluid pumps will not be used for field care. When placing the catheter in a recumbent neonate, place a small stack of towels or gauze 4 × 4 squares (4 inches thick) underneath the foal's neck to improve visualization of the jugular vein. After aseptic preparation, a small amount of a local anesthetic can be infused subcutaneously over the intended catheter site. It is recommended to use a stab incision by tenting the skin away from the foal and using a No. 15 blade to decrease the skin drag against the catheter.[40,41] If venous access is not possible, then sterile intraosseous

---

Box 3
Endoscopy of a foal in the field

- Endoscopy is indicated in cases of dysphagia and upper airway obstruction.
  - May aid in diagnosis of congenital defects such as a cleft palate or choanal atresia.
- Gastroduodenal ulcers are common in foals.[23]
- Indicated in cases of *Streptococcus equi* spp *equi* infection where guttural pouch involvement is suspected.

Box 4
Additional testing in the field

- Stall-side IgG kits are readily available and guide recommendations for therapy to achieve greater than 800 mg/dL IgG for adequate passive transfer.

- Serum amyloid A is a nonspecific acute phase protein with a rapid increase in response to inflammation and a rapid decrease with resolution.[19] Stall-side testing is readily available. Serial testing can be helpful to monitor changes in clinical condition including worsening inflammation and response to therapy.

- Lactate[24] is also available with stall-side testing. Normal postpartum foals have higher lactate levels compared with adult horses (range <1.0–4.0 mmol/L). After 3 days foals return to adult values. Serial lactate measurements can be useful when assessing the foal's response to therapy or predicting the outcome compared with a single point in time measurement.[18]

- Complete blood count and serum biochemistry analysis in foals can differ from adult values.[25–27] Use foal reference ranges for interpretation.

- Blood cultures are recommended when septicemia is suspected.[28–34] Human neonatal blood culture tubes can increase the yield of isolate growth. Foal blood, synovial fluid, or cerebrospinal fluid can be used in these tubes. Aseptic preparation of the vein is required for sample collection and can be immediately obtained following sterile placement of a catheter.

- Immunotesting and surface immunoglobulin testing for erythrocyte and platelet surfaces are commercially available[35,36] (Clinical immunology laboratory of Kansas State Veterinary Diagnostic Laboratory, Manhattan, KS). These tests can confirm neonatal isoerythrolysis or neonatal alloimmune thrombocytopenia.

- Enteric pathogen testing is easily collected in the field: parasitic fecal testing, commercial foal/equine diarrhea polymerase chain reaction (PCR) panels for bacterial, viral and protozoal pathogens, and fecal culture for bacteria such as *Salmonella* spp. Field fecal floatation for sand can be helpful.

- Respiratory pathogen testing: transtracheal aspirates can be safely performed in the field and may guide diagnosis of viral, bacterial, aspiration, or fungal pneumonia or characterize the sensitivity pattern of a *R equi* isolate. Commercial equine respiratory pathogen PCR panels are available using nasal secretions.

---

delivery of fluids can be performed using the access point of the medial/proximal tibia and a 14 gauge, 1.5 inch needle.[42]

Stabilization before transport

When referral to a hospital is possible, the mare can be transported separately from the foal if this allows for a quicker or safer transport. The mare may require sedation if transported separately. Early intervention by providing initial IV fluid therapy and dextrose supplementation (see **Box 5**) with antimicrobial support can positively influence the outcome for the foal. In more intensive situations, the IV fluids can be continued in the car during the transport of the foal. Therapy before transport is recommended when hypovolemia, hypoglycemia, and sepsis are suspected. The referral hospital can consult on the recommended antimicrobial for the condition suspected. The longer the time before receiving antimicrobials in a septic patient, the more the risk for progression toward septic shock.[38,43]

Field treatment of nonreferral cases

Many conditions can be successfully managed with on-farm supportive care. A section of a large stall can be arranged by use of hay or shavings bales to allow delivery

---

Box 5
Foal fluid therapy in the field

- Emergency fluid bolus:
  ○ Example: 50 kg foal at 20 mL/kg IV fluid volume = 1 L (L)
- Estimating fluid deficit in Liters = percent dehydration x body weight
  ○ Example 50 kg foal is 10% dehydrated = 5 L fluid deficit
- Maintenance fluids for a foal:
  ○ Administer ~100 mL/kg/d (4–6 mL/kg/h) for maintenance fluid support without significant ongoing losses. With ongoing losses, could consider "twice maintenance" dosing.
  ○ Example of intermittent/bolus delivery: 50 kg foal receiving maintenance fluids with the goal of administering fluids every 6 hours.
    100 mL × 50 kg = 5000 mL (5 L) for a 24-h period required volume for maintenance.
    5000 mL ÷ 6 hours = ~833 mL volume delivered every 6 hours meets maintenance requirements (or could round up to 1 L every 6 hours).
- Hypoglycemia:
  ○ Conservative therapy adequate to increase glucose without causing hyperglycemia: add 0.5% dextrose (10 mL dextrose/L of isotonic fluids), up to 1% dextrose (20 mL dextrose/L of isotonic fluids) delivered using intermittent/bolus fluid administration at a slower rate.
  ○ Maintenance glucose supplementation can be achieved with a continuous rate infusion dose 4 to 8 mg/kg/min.
- Plasma transfusions: use a filter infusion set.
  ○ Treat/prevent failure of passive transfer in neonates, prevention against *R equi* in endemic regions or for treatment of hypoproteinemia (eg, *L intracellularis*).
  ○ Monitor for signs of a transfusion reaction: hyperthermia, tachypnea, tachycardia, and hyperemic mucous membranes. Stop the transfusion and administer: an antihistamine (eg, hydroxyzine 1 mg/kg PO) and flunixin meglumine (1 mg/kg IV or PO). If signs resolve after 30 min then the transfusion can begin again *slowly*.

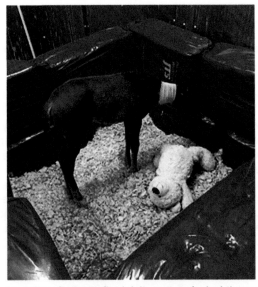

Fig. 3. Sectioning of a stall to facilitate fluid delivery to a foal while temporarily separating from the dam.

of IV fluids without interference from the dam, although they can still see and touch each other (**Fig. 3**).

If the foal requires additional fluid support following the initial triage volume replacement, then intermittent or continuous are 2 methods of delivering maintenance fluids in the field. Intermittent/bolus IV fluid therapy every 4 to 6 hours is often more manageable in the field setting compared with continuous delivery of fluids unless the foal will have constant monitoring (see **Box 5**). Although the goal of fluid therapy is to treat dehydration and hypovolemia and to support against ongoing losses, it is also important to avoid fluid overload in foals. Balanced electrolyte fluids are recommended unless the foal has specific electrolyte abnormalities suspected or confirmed such as hyperkalemia in the case of a ruptured bladder, then 0.9% sodium chloride would be preferred.

Antimicrobial selection can be guided by culture and sensitivity, although empirical selection should be initiated due to the importance of coverage in this susceptible population. When sepsis is suspected, the selection of intravenous antimicrobials is preferred because intestinal or muscle absorption may be delayed.[38] Beta lactams (ampicillin, 20 mg/kg IV q 6–8 h or potassium penicillin, 22,000–44,000 U/kg IV q 6 h, slowly) with an aminoglycoside (amikacin, 25 mg/kg IV q 24 h) remain the ideal selection for initial treatment of a septic foal.[28,38] Third-generation cephalosporins (ceftiofur sodium; 5 mg/kg IV is the author's preferred field dose) can be used in cases of sepsis or pneumonia where renal injury or other compromise prohibits the use of amikacin. Failure of passive transfer and omphalitis should be considered and monitored in all cases of sepsis for young foals.

Continuing antimicrobial support once a patient is stabilized or if its condition does not warrant the use of IV antimicrobials is often necessary. Trimethoprim sulfadiazine (24 mg/kg PO q 12 h) and the long-acting third-generation cephalosporin (ceftiofur crystalline free acid, 13.2 mg/kg IM or SQ q 48 h) are 2 field options for continued support, especially in the case of susceptible bacteria.

Treatment of failure of passive transfer in the field depends on the timing postparturition. Complete failure is immunoglobulin G (IgG) less than 400 mg/dL, and partial failure occurs where IgG is greater than 400 mg/dL and less than 800 mg/dL. A foal less than 24 hours of age requires 1 to 2 L of good-quality colostrum (specific gravity $\geq$1.060 using a colostrometer) for adequate passive transfer. If a foal is not nursing, this volume has to be given via nasogastric intubation in increments of 250 to 500 mL delivered by gravity flow. The volume will depend on the size of the foal. Even a poor-quality colostrum can be protective for a neonatal foal aged 12 to 24 hours because it triggers the closure of the specialized enterocytes in the foal's gastrointestinal tract, which will protect against bacterial translocation.[42] For foals older than 24 hours, IV commercial plasma is required to improve a foal's IgG level due to the closure of the enterocytes and inability to absorb colostral antibodies. At least one unit of plasma (20 mL/kg) is indicated in cases of failure of passive transfer, although the volume and dosage are variable depending on the product used and foal's response measured by repeated IgG assessment to ensure IgG greater than 800 mg/dL.[2,44] Plasma administration requires a blood filter administration set (10 drop per ml). The frozen plasma should be thawed in a lukewarm water bath. Administration should begin slowly with monitoring for adverse reaction by assessing the foal's vital parameters every 5 min for the first 25 to 30 min. Some foals will tolerate a faster rate at that point, although continue to monitor for signs of anaphylaxis. If a plasma reaction occurs (hyperemic membranes, tachypnea, hyperthermia) then stop the transfusion at the earliest sign. Administration of an antihistamine (hydroxyzine, 1 mg/kg, PO) and flunixin (1 mg/kg, IV) may mitigate the signs observed. Once signs subside, the transfusion can begin again at a slower rate. Severe cases may require epinephrine (1 mL per 45 kg foal of 1:1000 or 1 mg/mL).

When *R equi* is suspected and the foal's clinical condition warrants therapy, then microbial cultures obtained by transtracheal wash may help guide antimicrobial selection in the face of growing resistance patterns. Frequently a macrolide combined with rifampin is the first line of antimicrobial defense. In some cases, doxycycline may be preferable.

Colic and diarrhea[45–47] are common causes for foal emergencies in the field. Gastrointestinal support for foals (**Box 6**) depends on the underlying condition,[1,16,42,45] including colic, infectious/noninfectious enteritis, meconium impaction, sand enteropathy, congenital atresia ani/coli, and genetic conditions. When treating foals for enteritis where *Clostridium* spp are suspected, the use of the penicillin class and metronidazole[38] (10–15 mg/kg PO or IV, q 12 h for neonatal foals) is recommended.[48]

Box 6
Gastrointestinal therapy in the field

- Enteral (nasogastric) and IV fluid support
  Check for reflux first before administering enteral fluids.
  - Use gravity flow for enteral fluids for all foals because stomach volume is difficult to estimate. An average size neonate usually comfortably tolerates 350 to 500 mL.

- Analgesia: similar to adult gastrointestinal pain management
  - Avoid NSAIDs if the foal is hypovolemic/dehydrated.
  - Opioids and alpha-2 agonists (foals > 1 month of age) may be used as alternatives.

- Enema administration for treatment of meconium retention
  - Can be given prophylactically post partum. Trauma from client-administered enemas may be observed; therefore client education is important.
  - Options include soapy water (500 mL–1 L) or glycerine enemas administered via a soft red rubber or Foley catheter delivered by gravity flow.
  - Acetylcysteine Retention enema (4% solution) can be performed using a Foley catheter (30 French) if the meconium impaction does not resolve.[1,16,42]

- Laxatives including mineral oil (50–100 mL) or psyllium may be indicated depending on the cause of an impaction.

- Gastroprotectants in foals: sucralfate (10–20 mg/kg, PO q 6–8 h) is a safe mucosal protectant and will not alter the protective barrier of normal gastric pH. Use of proton pump inhibitors and histamine-2 receptor antagonist may support the healing of gastroduodenal ulcers, although their use in foals is controversial.

- Broad spectrum antimicrobial use is recommended in foals with enteritis due to the risk of translocation of bacteria.[46,47]

- Nutritional management
  - Oral lactase supplementation (Lactaid 3000–6000 U, PO q 4–8 h[46,47]) can support the breakdown of lactose in milk when the brush border has been disrupted in cases of enteritis.
  - Milk restriction or reduction in volume may benefit a foal that becomes colicky after nursing; this can be combined with lactase supplementation and IV fluid therapy.
  - Probiotics or transfaunation have controversial benefit, although they are used to support a healthier microbiome.
  - Enteral or parenteral nutrition support[1,16] are indicated in orphan foals, when a foal cannot nurse adequately on its own, or in some cases of diarrhea.[46,47] An indwelling feeding tube can be placed in the field with radiographic confirmation of correct placement.

Initiating early therapy is especially important in regions where clostridial enteritis is common even while test results are pending.

In neonatal foals, seizures can be related to neonatal maladjustment/perinatal asphyxia syndrome and sepsis. A manageable genetic condition called juvenile idiopathic epilepsy in Egyptian Arabian foals older than 1 month has been described.[49] With appropriate anticonvulsant support, foals will outgrow this condition with age. Head trauma may lead to development of seizures. Repeated musculoskeletal trauma can be an early sign of seizure activity before a seizure is witnessed. Anticonvulsants such as diazepam or midazolam in foals can be successfully used in the field setting to control seizure activity.[1]

In cases of synovial sepsis, diagnostic arthrocentesis or synoviocentesis can be combined with a therapeutic needle lavage of the synovial structure. Total nucleated cell count greater than 30,000/μL with a neutrophil percentage greater than 80% to 90% and a fluid protein greater than 4 g/dL[22] strongly indicates synovial structure sepsis. Ideally bacterial culture and sensitivity testing of the synovial fluid can help guide antimicrobial therapy. If the cell count or the synovial protein is equivocal, then a physitis, osteomyelitis, or trauma to the region may be suspected as the origin of lameness and or synovial effusion. Radiographs and ultrasound can help diagnose these conditions.

Antimicrobials and needle lavage are the pillars of treatment of a septic arthritis[22] in the field. Intrasynovial infusion of antimicrobial such as amikacin is performed before removal of the last needle from the lavage. Daily lavage can be performed until the cytology seems improved. Stall-side general anesthesia is frequently indicated for safe completion of the needle lavage. Systemic antibiotics should be administered concurrently, with consideration of a dose adjustment if amikacin is also being used systemically. Regional limb perfusion or a joint infusion pump is an alternative option for local delivery of antimicrobials.[22] NSAIDs should be used judiciously in foals due to the risk of gastrointestinal or renal injury.

Allogenic conditions[44] including neonatal isoerythrolysis (NI) and neonatal alloimmune thrombocytopenia (NAT) may cause severe anemia or thrombocytopenia. These conditions occur most commonly in foals born to a multiparous dam. These conditions occur at an increased frequency in mule foals. It is possible to prevent or manage these conditions in the field.[1] Prevention is focused on muzzling the postpartum foal and providing an alternative and tested replacement colostrum; this avoids a known carrier dam transferring antired blood cell (RBC) or antiplatelet antibodies in her colostrum. In cases of NI it is important to minimize stress and exercise. IV fluid support is indicated to promote diuresis in the face of hemolysis. Whole blood or RBC transfusion is recommended if the foal is weak and the PCV is less than 15%.[44] Cross-matching (major and minor) is recommended. If this is not possible, then a washed RBC transfusion from the dam is ideal.[44] Generally all foals with NI should be administered antibiotics to minimize sepsis. Therapy for foals affected by NAT includes administration of a whole-blood or cross-matched platelet-rich plasma transfusion. Thrombocytopenia secondary to sepsis should be a differential diagnosis to ensure appropriate therapy is initiated.

SUMMARY

Many conditions can be successfully managed with on-farm supportive care when referral to a hospital is not possible. There is a wide array of diagnostic and therapeutic possibilities in the field to support the appropriate diagnosis and treatment of foal emergencies.

CLINICS CARE POINTS

- Avoid alpha-2 agonist use in neonates or foals younger than 1 month. Benzodiazepines or butorphanol are safer alternatives.
- When the foal requires continuous monitoring and more intensive therapy, referral to a hospital is indicated. The foal can be stabilized in the field until referral is possible.
- Early initiation of supportive care in the field can be lifesaving in many emergent conditions of foals.

DISCLOSURE

The author declares no conflicts of interest.

REFERENCES

1. Carr EA. Field triage of the neonatal foal. Vet Clin North Am Equine Pract 2014; 30(2):283–300, vii.
2. McKenzie HC III. Disorders of Foals. Equine Intern Med 2018;1365–459.
3. Ramirez S, Gaunt SD, McClure JJ, et al. Detection and effects on platelet function of anti-platelet antibody in mule foals with experimentally induced neonatal alloimmune thrombocytopenia. J Vet Intern Med 1999;13(6):534–9.
4. Cummins C, Carrington S, Fitzpatrick E, et al. Ascending placentitis in the mare: a review. Ir Vet J 2008;61(5):307–13.
5. Macpherson ML. Diagnosis and treatment of equine placentitis. Vet Clin Equine Pract 2006;22(3):763–76.
6. Ericsson AC, Johnson PJ, Lopes MA, et al. A microbiological map of the healthy equine gastrointestinal tract. PLoS One 2016;11(11):e0166523.
7. Giguère S, Cohen ND, Chaffin MK, et al. Rhodococcus equi: clinical manifestations, virulence, and immunity. J Vet Intern Med 2011;25(6):1221–30.
8. Costa MC, Stämpfli HR, Arroyo LG, et al. Changes in the equine fecal microbiota associated with the use of systemic antimicrobial drugs. BMC Vet Res 2015; 11:19.
9. Streeter RM, Divers TJ, Mittel L, et al. Selenium deficiency associations with gender, breed, serum vitamin E and creatine kinase, clinical signs and diagnoses in horses of different age groups: a retrospective examination 1996-2011. Equine Vet J Suppl 2012;(43):31–5.
10. Robertson SA. Sedation and general anaesthesia of the foal. Equine Vet Educ 2005;15(S7):94–101.
11. Thomas WP, Madigan JE, Backus KQ, et al. Systemic and pulmonary haemodynamics in normal neonatal foals. J Reprod Fertil Suppl 1987;35:623–8.
12. Toth B, Aleman M, Brosnan RJ, et al. Evaluation of squeeze-induced somnolence in neonatal foals. Am J Vet Res 2012;73(12):1881–9.
13. Jones T, Bracamonte JL, Ambros B, et al. Total intravenous anesthesia with alfaxalone, dexmedetomidine and remifentanil in healthy foals undergoing abdominal surgery. Vet Anaesth Analg 2019;46(3):315–24.
14. Bidwell LA. Anesthesia for dystocia and anesthesia of the equine neonate. Vet Clin Equine Pract 2013;29(1):215–22.
15. Bidwell Lori. How to Anesthetize Foals on the Farm for Minor Surgical Procedures. Am Assoc Equine Pract Proc 2009;55:48–9.
16. Equine Emergencies. In: Magdesian KG, Neonatology, Orsini JA, Divers TJ, editors 2014;. p. 528–64.

17. Freeman DE, Orsini JA, Harrison IW, et al. Complications of umbilical hernias in horses: 13 cases (1972-1986). J Am Vet Med Assoc 1988;192(6): 804–7.

18. Borchers A, Wilkins PA, Marsh PM, et al. Sequential L-lactate concentration in hospitalised equine neonates: a prospective multicentre study. Equine Vet J Suppl 2013;(45):2–7.

19. Hultén C, Demmers S. Serum amyloid A (SAA) as an aid in the management of infectious disease in the foal: comparison with total leucocyte count, neutrophil count and fibrinogen. Equine Vet J 2002;34(7):693–8.

20. Sprayberry KA. Ultrasonographic examination of the equine neonate: thorax and abdomen. Vet Clin North Am Equine Pract 2015;31(3):515–43.

21. Porter MB, Ramirez S. Equine neonatal thoracic and abdominal ultrasonography. Vet Clin North Am Equine Pract 2005;21(2):407–29, vii.

22. Glass K, Watts AE. Septic arthritis, physitis, and osteomyelitis in foals. Vet Clin Equine Pract 2017;33(2):299–314.

23. Camacho-Luna P, Buchanan B, Andrews FM. Advances in diagnostics and treatments in horses and foals with gastric and duodenal ulcers. Vet Clin North Am Equine Pract 2018;34(1):97–111.

24. Wotman K, Wilkins PA, Palmer JE, et al. Association of blood lactate concentration and outcome in foals. J Vet Intern Med 2009;23(3):598–605.

25. Becht JL, Semrad SD. Hematology, blood typing, and immunology of the neonatal foal. Vet Clin North Am Equine Pract 1985;1(1):91–116.

26. Barton MH, Hart KA. Clinical pathology in the foal. Vet Clin North Am Equine Pract 2020;36(1):73–85.

27. Axon JE, Palmer JE. Clinical pathology of the foal. Vet Clin North Am Equine Pract 2008;24(2):357–85, vii.

28. Theelen MJP, Wilson WD, Byrne BA, et al. Initial antimicrobial treatment of foals with sepsis: Do our choices make a difference? Vet J 2019;243:74–6.

29. Hackett ES, Lunn DP, Ferris RA, et al. Detection of bacteraemia and host response in healthy neonatal foals. Equine Vet J 2015;47(4):405–9.

30. Corley KTT, Pearce G, Magdesian KG, et al. Bacteraemia in neonatal foals: clinicopathological differences between Gram-positive and Gram-negative infections, and single organism and mixed infections. Equine Vet J 2007;39(1):84–9.

31. Hollis AR, Wilkins PA, Palmer JE, et al. Bacteremia in equine neonatal diarrhea: a retrospective study (1990-2007). J Vet Intern Med 2008;22(5):1203–9.

32. Russell CM, Axon JE, Blishen A, et al. Blood culture isolates and antimicrobial sensitivities from 427 critically ill neonatal foals. Aust Vet J 2008;86(7):266–71.

33. Sanchez LC, Giguère S, Lester GD. Factors associated with survival of neonatal foals with bacteremia and racing performance of surviving Thoroughbreds: 423 cases (1982-2007). J Am Vet Med Assoc 2008;233(9):1446–52.

34. Theelen MJP, Wilson WD, Edman JM, et al. Temporal trends in in vitro antimicrobial susceptibility patterns of bacteria isolated from foals with sepsis: 1979-2010. Equine Vet J 2014;46(2):161–8.

35. Perkins GA, Miller WH, Divers TJ, et al. Ulcerative dermatitis, thrombocytopenia, and neutropenia in neonatal foals. J Vet Intern Med 2005;19(2):211–6.

36. Nunez R, Gomes-Keller MA, Schwarzwald C, et al. Assessment of Equine Autoimmune Thrombocytopenia (EAT) by flow cytometry. BMC Blood Disord 2001; 1(1):1.

37. Jokisalo JM, Corley KTT. CPR in the neonatal foal: has RECOVER changed our approach? Vet Clin Equine Pract 2014;30(2):301–16.

38. Magdesian KG. Antimicrobial pharmacology for the neonatal foal. Vet Clin Equine Pract 2017;33(1):47–65.
39. Drury PP, Bennet L, Gunn AJ. Mechanisms of hypothermic neuroprotection. Hypothermia Emerg Ther 2010;15(5):287–92.
40. Bentz BG. How to place a long-term over-the-wire catheter in a foal. Am Assoc Equine Pract Proc 2005.
41. McCue P, O'Fallon ES, Landolt G, et al. Foal formulary and field protocol guide. 2nd Edition. Colorado State University; 2020. Available at: https://books.google.com/books?id=c6WuyQEACAAJ.
42. Knottenbelt DC, Holdstock N, Madigan JE. Equine neonatology: medicine and surgery. Saunders; 2004. Available at: https://books.google.com/books?id=khRtQgAACAAJ.
43. Whiles BB, Deis AS, Simpson SQ. Increased time to initial antimicrobial administration is associated with progression to septic shock in severe sepsis patients. Crit Care Med 2017;45(4):623–9.
44. Giguère S, Polkes AC. Immunologic disorders in neonatal foals. Vet Clin North Am Equine Pract 2005;21(2):241–72.
45. Ryan CA, Sanchez LC. Nondiarrheal disorders of the gastrointestinal tract in neonatal foals. Vet Clin Equine Pract 2005;21(2):313–32.
46. Magdesian KG. Neonatal foal diarrhea. Vet Clin Equine Pract 2005;21(2):295–312.
47. Oliver-Espinosa O. Foal diarrhea: established and postulated causes, prevention, diagnostics, and treatments. Vet Clin North Am Equine Pract 2018;34(1):55–68.
48. Swain EA, Magdesian KG, Kass PH, et al. Pharmacokinetics of metronidazole in foals: influence of age within the neonatal period. J Vet Pharmacol Ther 2015;38(3):227–34.
49. Aleman M, Gray LC, Williams DC, et al. Juvenile idiopathic epilepsy in Egyptian Arabian foals: 22 cases (1985-2005). J Vet Intern Med 2006;20(6):1443–9.

Management of Colic in the Field

Diane M. Rhodes, DVM*, Rodolfo Madrigal, DVM

KEYWORDS

- Equine • Colic • Field • Treatment • Diagnosis • Fluids

KEY POINTS

- Recognition of critical colic cases is important for determining the need for aggressive management when referral is not an option.
- Fluid therapy is an integral part of field treatment and can be administered orally, intravenously, or rectally.
- Pain management should be initiated early for human and horse safety as well as animal welfare.
- Portable imaging and laboratory equipment have improved ambulatory diagnostic capabilities.

INTRODUCTION

Colic remains one of the most common reasons for equine practitioners to be called out on emergency, closely followed by wounds and lameness.[1] Studies investigating the incidence of colic estimate that there are 4.2 to 10.6 colic events per 100 horses per year and estimate the total economic impact at $115.3 million US dollars per year.[2,3] Approximately 76% of cases are considered mild, or noncritical; however, 24% of cases require surgery, intensive medical management, or humane euthanasia.[4] A United Kingdom study[5] found the mean cost for admitting a horse for treatment of colic to a referral hospital was £873.89 British pounds ($1141.00 US dollars). The mean cost for surgery and survival for greater than a 24-hour period was £6437.80 ($8411.00 US dollars).[5]

Quick and efficient identification of horses necessitating referral will reduce cardiovascular compromise, thereby improving survival. However, referral may not be an option because of several factors including transport, lack of referral facilities, financial constraints, patient behavior, or previous owner experience and/or lack of knowledge regarding treatment options and prognosis.[6,7]

Loomis Basin Equine Medical Center, 2973 Penryn Road, Penryn, CA 95603, USA
* Corresponding author.
E-mail address: drhodes@lbemc.com

Vet Clin Equine 37 (2021) 421–439
https://doi.org/10.1016/j.cveq.2021.04.010
0749-0739/21/© 2021 Elsevier Inc. All rights reserved.

Advances in portable imaging modalities and stall-side point-of-care (POC) equipment has improved the scope of diagnostics, monitoring capabilities, and treatment options in an ambulatory setting. This article aims to discuss management of colic in the field:

1. Diagnostic approach
2. Pain management
3. Fluid therapy

Performing diagnostics and intensive treatments in the field may be expensive; therefore, it is important to manage client expectations, particularly as many cases may require multiple visits.

DISCUSSION
Diagnostic Approach

Colic is abdominal pain commonly attributed to the gastrointestinal tract (GIT) or other abdominal viscera. Colic may be classified based on the segment of affected bowel and/or type of lesion (**Table 1**). The most common causes of colic include gas/spasmodic colic, large colon (LC) impactions, and LC displacements, with a significant number of cases remaining undiagnosed.[4,8,9]

Using a combination of history, physical examination (PE) findings, nasogastric intubation (NGT), rectal examination, as well as diagnostics including imaging and clinicopathologic data, the practitioner should be well equipped to differentiate the type of colic and determine the cardiovascular status of the patient. This is important when communicating the likelihood of successful field management.

Clinical Evaluation

History
Patient signalment, management, and environmental factors have been associated with an increased risk of colic and lesion type (**Table 2**). A middle-aged Arabian

Table 1 Classification of types of colic lesions and examples	
Type of Lesion	**Examples**
Strangulating obstruction	Strangulating lipoma Mesenteric rent Epiploic foramen entrapment Diaphragmatic hernia Volvulus or torsion
Physical nonstrangulating obstruction	Impaction (ingesta) Displacement Enterolithiasis Sand enteropathy
Functional nonstrangulating obstruction	Spasmodic colic Ileus Flatulent/gas colic
Inflammatory nonstrangulating	Enteritis/colitis Peritonitis Infarction Inflammatory bowel disease
Other	Proliferative enteropathy Neoplasia

Table 2		
Risk factors associated with colic		
Variable	**Risk Factor**	**Lesion**
Age	<2 y	Foreign body, ascarid impaction
	0–5 y	IFEE
	Geriatric	Strangulating lipoma, large colon impaction
Gender	Maiden mares[a]	LCV
	Mares[a] if ≥ 1 foal	LCV
	Stallion	Inguinal hernia
Breed	Arabian, Morgan and Miniature horses	Enterolithiasis
	Miniature horses	Fecalith, sand enteropathy
Behavior	Cribbing/windsucking	EFE
Housing/Turnout	Increased/change in hours of stabling	LCV, EFE
	Pasture grazing	DPJ (compared to other colics)
Feed	>2.5 kg/d concentrate diet	Duodenal proximal jejunitis
	Alfalfa (>50-70%)	Enterolithiasis
	Coastal Bermuda grass	Ileal impaction

Abbreviations: DPJ, duodenitis-proximal jejunitis; EFE, epiploic foramen entrapment; IFEE, idiopathic focal eosinophilic enteritis; LCV, large colon volvulus.

[a] Mares compared to geldings.

Adapted from: Curtis L, Burford JH, England GCW, Freeman SL. Risk factors for acute abdominal pain (colic) in the adult horse: A scoping review of risk factors, and a systematic review of the effect of management-related changes. Loor JJ, ed. *PLOS ONE.* 2019;14(7):e0219307. https://doi.org/10.1371/journal.pone.0219307.

with a history of recurrent colic on predominantly alfalfa forage, for example, should increase the level of suspicion for enterolithiasis, which may prompt referral for radiographic examination versus repeated field management.[10] The duration of an acute colic episode is another important factor to consider and has been associated with survival as it is likely related to cardiovascular status.[6] Additional information including fluid intake or losses, that is, via diarrhea, sweat, or reflux, is important to consider when formulating a fluid therapy plan.[11]

Physical examination

A thorough PE should be performed on all colic cases with special attention paid to pain level, presence or absence of gastrointestinal motility, and cardiovascular system parameters. Several pain scales, described elsewhere, have been developed with the goal of identifying critical cases and monitoring response to treatment.[12,13] Cardiovascular parameters associated with a critical outcome are listed in **Table 3**.[4,6,14]

Cardiovascular assessment should be focused on the following parameters associated with volume depletion and decreased perfusion[11]:

1. Mentation
2. Heart rate
3. Pulse quality
4. Jugular refill
5. Mucous membrane color
6. Capillary refill time
7. Urine output

Table 3
Physical examination parameters associated with a critical outcome

Variable	Change in Variable
Heart rate	Increased/tachycardia
Pulse character	Weak
Capillary refill time	$\geq$2.5 s
Pain	Moderate to severe (persistent)
Intestinal borborygmi	Absent
Mucous membrane color	Brick red or purple color

8. Extremity temperature

There is a common misconception that volume depletion is interchangeable with dehydration.[15] While dehydration and hypovolemia may co-exist, dehydration may be present without significant volume depletion; therefore, clinical markers of dehydration, including reduced skin turgor, dry mucous membranes, or sunken eyes, are less sensitive for assessing cardiovascular status.[15]

Nasogastric intubation
NGT may be therapeutic and diagnostic in the colicky horse. NGT allows for the determination and quantification of gastric reflux and facilitates enteral administration of fluids. Restraint using physical (twitch, lip chain) or chemical means is recommended (**Table 4**). Which combination of restraint is used depends on patient temperament, amount of technical help, cardiovascular status, and practitioner preference.

When to prioritize NGT:

1. Tachycardia (>60 bpm)
2. Spontaneous reflux
3. Palpation of small intestine on rectal examination
4. Significant abdominal pain

Rectal examination
A thorough PE combined with rectal palpation was considered sufficient to make a working diagnosis for most practitioners involved in a study evaluating horses for abdominal pain.[4] Considerations when performing a rectal examination include age,

Table 4
Commonly used drugs for sedation and safe rectal examination

Drug	Dose/Route	Average Dose for a 500-kg Horse
Alpha-2		
Xylazine	0.2-1 mg/kg IV	150–200 mg (1.5-2 mL)
Detomidine	0.005–0.01 mg/kg IV	3–5 mg (0.3–0.5 mL)
Romifidine	0.04–0.12 mg/kg IV	20–25 mg (2–2.5 mL)
Opioid		
Butorphanol	0.01–0.1 mg/kg IV	3-5 mg (0.3–0.5 mL)
Buscopan	0.3 mg/kg IV	150 mg (7.5 mL)
Lidocaine[a]	Not applicable	50–60 cc per rectum

[a] Limited data to support use.

size, temperament of the horse, and facilities. The most common rectal examination diagnoses include LC impactions and LC displacements (right dorsal displacement > left dorsal displacement).[4,8,16] Small colon, rectal, and cecal impactions are less frequently diagnosed.[4,8,17,18] Palpation of distended small intestine should heighten concern for a possible strangulating obstruction of the small intestine, although rectal palpation alone cannot differentiate between strangulating and nonstrangulating obstructions.

Practically, the following two questions are the main ones to ask:

1. Is the rectal examination normal or abnormal?
2. Is the lesion most likely in the large or small bowel?

Rectal examinations should only be performed if both practitioner and patient can be safe. Alpha-2 agonist combined with butorphanol provide an adequate level of sedation for most horses. N-butylscopolammonium bromide (Buscopan 0.3 mg/kg IV) is recommended to reduce straining and rectal pressure, which may allow for a more diagnostic evaluation.[19] Infusion of 50 to 60 mL of 2% lidocaine intrarectally using an extension set is also common practice. While this does not significantly reduce rectal pressure, lidocaine preparations may provide analgesia for perirectal palpation.[20]

Additional Diagnostics

Imaging and POC testing have become more widely available in ambulatory practice and may aid in the identification of a critical case requiring intensive management, referral, or euthanasia.

Imaging

Ultrasound
Several approaches to ultrasound of the acute abdomen have been described.[21,22] Typically, a low-frequency (2.5–5 MHz) curvilinear transducer will produce a diagnostic quality image while providing sufficient penetration to identify deeper structures. The fast, localized abdominal sonography of the horse is a rapid method requiring little previous experience in ultrasonographic examination. The method divides the abdomen into 7 sections (**Figs. 1** and **2**). The technique is most sensitive and specific for identifying small intestinal strangulating obstructions.[22] Interpretation of ultrasound of the large intestine is arguably more challenging as increased colon wall thickness may be seen with a variety of conditions. Significant thickening ($\geq$ 9 mm) often warrants intensive care and should be interpreted in light of clinical signs.[23]

Radiography
Digital radiography can be beneficial for diagnosis of sand enteropathy as well as to support the diagnosis of nonstrangulating obstructions in miniature horses and foals. Positioning the plate on an adult horse along the ventral abdomen a few centimeters caudal to the elbow allows visualization of sand, and occasionally enteroliths, in an average 450-kg horse (**Fig. 3**). In geographic locations where sand enteropathy is common, this may be helpful as the condition is frequently treated successfully with medical management.[24]

Clinical Pathology

There are POC hand-held devices that allow for the measurement of electrolytes, blood gases, creatinine, lactate, glucose, and serum amyloid A (SAA). POC devices for lactate, glucose, and SAA are fast; easy to use, store, and transport; relatively inexpensive; and can be used on plasma and/or abdominal fluid.

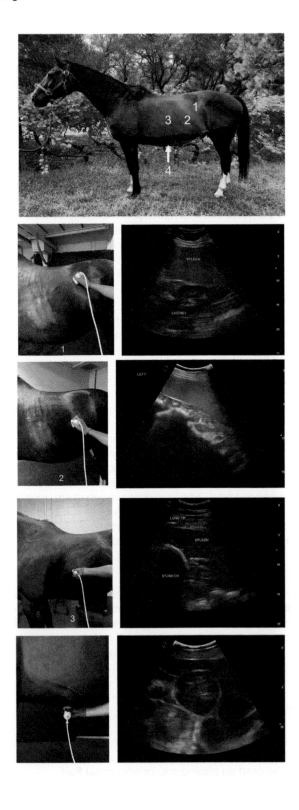

Blood work
Several clinicopathologic variables have been evaluated in acute colic to determine the need for medical versus surgical management. While not all the variables are practical for field use, measurement of lactate concentration has become an increasingly useful tool in colic diagnostic workups.

Plasma lactate
Lactate can be measured in the field using small portable lactate meters, with results being obtained within 10 to 60 seconds. Several models are available (Lactate Scout [SensLab GmbH, Leipzig, Germany], Accusport analyzer [Boehringer Mannheim, Germany], Lactate Pro 2 [Arkray Global Business, Kyoto, Japan]), and all have been shown to accurately measure lactate in equine blood.[25,26] Plasma lactate concentration helps determine the need for fluid therapy, monitor response to treatment, and predict survival. Typically, plasma lactate is <2 mmol/L in healthy horses. Increasing plasma lactate concentrations have long been associated with a poor prognosis for colic. In one study,[27] plasma lactate at hospital admission in horses with a LC volvulus was compared to survival. If plasma lactate was less than 6 mmol/L, 90% of horses survived compared with only 30% survival if lactate concentration was greater than 7 mmol/L. In addition, for horses with a suspected small intestinal strangulating lesion, comparison of blood and peritoneal fluid lactate concentrations can help identify the presence of ischemic injury in the intestine (see below).

Peritoneal fluid
Reasons for performing abdominocentesis are to determine the need for surgery or support a diagnosis (ie, septic peritonitis), monitor response to treatment, or determine the need for euthanasia, for example, in the case of ruptured bowel or the presence of a strangulating lesion with no referral option.[28] Cell counts often require submission to a reference laboratory; however, it is possible to visually assess color and turbidity. Normal peritoneal fluid should be clear and pale yellow. Total protein (TP) can be easily measured using refractometry, and normal values should be <2.0 g/dL. An increase in protein concentration indicates an increase in the permeability of the viscera, which allows plasma protein to leak out of the circulation into the peritoneal fluid. While sensitive for the presence of inflammation an increased protein concentration is not specific for the detection of a strangulating lesion. L-lactate and glucose can also be measured using hand-held devices. Peritoneal lactate should always be interpreted in conjunction with plasma lactate. An ischemic segment of intestine will leak lactate into the peritoneal fluid resulting in a rapid elevation in peritoneal fluid lactate. Plasma lactate does not rise so rapidly while the horse is systemically stable. Therefore, an elevated peritoneal fluid lactate compared with plasma lactate is a very sensitive indicator for the presence of ischemic intestine and the need for emergency surgery.[29] An abnormal color (serosanguinous) and peritoneal lactate greater than 8.45 mmol/L was associated with intestinal ischemia in one study.[29]

Fig. 1. Left-sided fast, localized abdominal sonography of the horse (FLASH) ultrasound in the order preferred by the author; left image shows the probe in the corresponding area, and right image shows sonographic image of the region. 1. Normal nephrosplenic space with the left kidney and spleen imaged. 2. Left middle one-third of the abdomen showing abnormal thickened left dorsal colon (LDC) wall deep to the spleen. 3. Normal gastric window with the stomach, spleen, and left lung tip visible. 4. Cranioventral abdomen showing multiple distended loops of small intestine; this image may also be taken from the inguinal region.

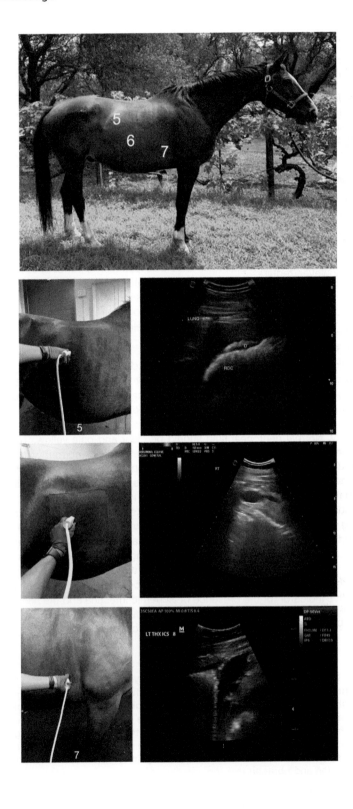

Pain Management

A summary of advantages and disadvantages of the options for pain management is listed in **Table 5**.

Nonsteroidal anti-inflammatories

Nonsteroidal anti-inflammatory drugs (NSAIDs) are frequently administered for alleviation of visceral pain, pyrexia, and inflammation.

Two NSAIDs frequently recommended for GIT pain include[30]

1. Flunixin meglumine (1.1 mg/kg IV, q12 hours)
2. Firocoxib (0.3 mg/kg IV loading dose; 0.1 mg/kg, IV q24 hours)

Flunixin meglumine and firocoxib provide superior analgesia compared with phenylbutazone and meloxicam for visceral pain.[30] Less data are available regarding the equipotency of ketoprofen and carprofen. The purported benefits of firocoxib, a selective COX-2 inhibitor, include decreased mucosal healing time and reduced biomarkers of endotoxemia in experimental models when compared with flunixin meglumine.[31,32] Firocoxib, however, requires a loading dose, and the IV formulation cannot be flushed with heparinized saline which can make its use more cumbersome than the traditionally used flunixin meglumine. Evidence does not suggest that combining NSAIDs, or using doses above the labeled dose, provides additional analgesia and may increase the risk of adverse side effects.[30]

Most horses will tolerate a full labeled dose; however, there are circumstances when a lower dose or delaying administration until after fluid therapy may be warranted:

1. Significant hypovolemia
2. History of renal disease
3. Endurance horses pulled from a ride for colic/metabolic reasons
4. Young animals (<6 months)

Dipyrone (metamizole)

Dipyrone, a nonclassical NSAID (30 mg/kg IV q12–24 hours for up to 3 days) belongs to the pyrazolone class of NSAIDs. Dipyrone has minimal anti-inflammatory effects and is labeled for the treatment of pyrexia but provides mild to moderate analgesia and has spasmolytic properties.[33] Analgesic properties are thought to be mediated by binding of metabolites to cannabinoid receptors. Minimal adverse effects have been reported in horses; however, there is a paucity of data regarding its use in cases of colic.

Acetaminophen

Acetaminophen (20 mg/kg by mouth q12–24 hours) is a nontraditional NSAID that has analgesic and antipyretic properties but few anti-inflammatory properties. In humans, acetaminophen is used for abdominal pain; however, little data are available in the horse.

Fig. 2. Right-sided fast, localized abdominal sonography of the horse (FLASH) ultrasound; left image shows the probe in the corresponding area, and right image shows sonographic image of the region. 5. Gastric outflow at the level of the right dorsal colon (RDC) and right liver lobe with the duodenum (D) imaged between these and the lung tip within the image (LUNG); this can also be imaged at the cranial pole of the right kidney. 6. Right middle one-third of the abdomen showing distended mesenteric vessels. 7. Right ventral thorax showing effusion and fibrin on the right pleural cavity.

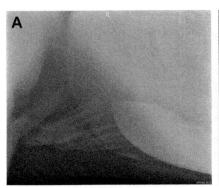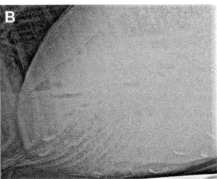

Fig. 3. (*A*) Abdominal radiograph taken with portable radiography until of a 450-kg QH for signs of colic. Radiographs confirmed the presence of sand along the ventral abdomen. (*B*) Radiograph of a miniature horse that presented for colic due to a suspect fecalith. Note a large amount of ingesta within the cranial abdomen. QH, Quarter horse.

Alpha-2 adrenoceptor agonists

Alpha-2 adrenergic agonists are routinely administered for their sedative and analgesic properties. The most commonly used alpha-2 agonists in equine practice are listed in **Table 4**. Alpha-2 agonists may be administered as a sole agent, or combined with an opioid. They may be administered as a bolus injection IV or IM as well as a continuous rate infusion (CRI). Alpha-2 agonists are not controlled substances; therefore, they provide an attractive option for field use as they can be dispensed to the client. The potency and duration of action vary with each drug (xylazine < romifidine < detomidine).

For colic pain control, it is common practice to start with administration of 1 to 3 doses of xylazine. Pain that is refractory to this protocol should alert the clinician of a more serious lesion. In these cases, the use of detomidine may improve the level and duration of analgesia. The concern for using detomidine at the onset stems from the conception that it may mask a surgical lesion.

When referral is not an option, the author has educated owners about the human risks of alpha-2 agonists and has dispensed detomidine to administer either by IV through a catheter or IM. Alternatively, these medications (typically detomidine) can be administered as a CRI by adding alpha-2s to fluid bags or via an infusion pump. A CRI may provide a smoother plane of sedation.[34] The author reserves infusion pumps for clients who are local and experienced in using medical equipment.

Detomidine can be added to a 5-L fluid bag and administered via a large bore fluid administration set, or diluted in a 1-L or 250-mL bag and piggybacked into the line using a drip set and needle. The separate bag allows for adjustment of the patient's fluid rate without changing the rate of alpha-2 administration.[11,34]

Calculation for a 5-L bag[11]

1. (Size of the IV fluid bag) ÷ (Liters per hour) = # hours per bag
   - Example: 5-L fluid bag ÷ 1 L/h = 5 hours per bag
2. (Dose of drug in mg/h) × (# of hours per bag) = # of mg of drug to add per bag
   - Example: 0.005 mg/kg/h → 2.5 mg/h for a 500-kg horse
   - 2.5 mg/h detomidine × 5 h/bag = 12.5 mg of detomidine to add to a 5-L bag

Detomidine in a 250-mL bag of 0.9% saline using a 60-drop/ml drip set[34]

Table 5
Summary of advantages and disadvantages of medications used to alleviate pain in horses

Drug or Class	Advantages	Disadvantages
Classical Nonsteroidal anti-inflammatories	• Oral and IV formulations • Rapid onset of action (IV) • Long dosing interval • Anti-inflammatory • Noncontrolled substances • Reasonable cost	• Increased risk of RDC • Increased risk of gastric ulcers • Nephrotoxic
Nonclassical, nonsteroidal anti-inflammatories		
Dipyrone	• Rapid onset of action • Moderate dosing interval (every 12–24 h) • Antipyretic • Some analgesic properties • Some antispasmodic properties	• Labeled for treatment of pyrexia • Increased risk of gastric ulcers • Increased risk of coagulopathy • As an NSAID, carries risk of GIT, renal and some liver toxicity
Acetaminophen	• Antipyretic • Analgesia • Low cost	• Minimally anti-inflammatory • Possible hepatotoxic effects • Limited safety data available
Alpha-2 adrenergic agonist	• Administer IV or IM • Rapid onset of action • Short duration of action • Noncontrolled drugs	• Reduce GI motility • Human safety concerns with inadvertent needle stick • Short duration of action • Hypertension followed by hypotension • May mask surgical lesion
Opioids	• Administer IV or IM • Rapid onset of action • Synergy with α-2 agonists	• Reduce GI motility • Excitation at high doses • Controlled substances • Level of analgesia has been questioned
Lidocaine	• Analgesia • Anti-inflammatory • +/− Prokinetic • Reasonable cost	• CRI administration • Ataxia, recumbency, anxiety seen with rapid administration • Loading dose required for faster onset of action

Abbreviations: CRI, continuous rate infusion; GIT, gastrointestinal tract; NSAID, nonsteroidal anti-inflammatory; RDC, right dorsal colitis.

1. Add 10 mg of detomidine to a 250-mL bag of saline
   • 10 mg detomidine ÷ 250 mL saline = 0.04 mg/mL solution
2. Rate of 1 drop/second = 60 mL/h
3. 60 mL/h × 0.04 mg/mL = 2.4 mg/h detomidine

One 250-mL saline bag will provide approximately 4 hours of sedation at this rate.

Opioids
Opioids are often combined with alpha-2 agonists to provide neuroleptanalgesia and a smoother plane of sedation. The most commonly used opioid in equine ambulatory practice is butorphanol, a synthetic mixed opioid agonist-antagonist. Butorphanol may be administered as a bolus (0.01–0.1 mg/kg IV or IM) or as a continuous infusion. The analgesic potency has been questioned, and in recent guidelines published by the

British Equine Veterinary Association (BEVA), the panel concluded that it provided inadequate analgesia for visceral pain.[30] Given this evidence, and that butorphanol is a scheduled IV substance, it is not recommended leaving this medication with clients.

Lidocaine
Lidocaine, a class 1B sodium channel blocker, is used for its anti-arrhythmic, anti-inflammatory, analgesic, and prokinetic properties.[35] Lidocaine is typically administered as a CRI using an infusion pump, although it can be added to fluid bags, similar to alpha-2 adrenoreceptor agonists. For visceral pain, a loading dose of 1.3 mg/kg is given as a slow bolus over 10 to 15 minutes, followed by 0.05-mg/kg/min infusion. Omitting the loading dose results in longer time to reach steady-state concentrations. Given the possible ataxia and recumbency, the author does not frequently use this in the field. In addition, in recent studies, its effects as a prokinetic on postoperative ileus and improved outcomes in surgery have been questioned.[36]

Adjunctive Treatments

N-butylscopolammonium bromide (Buscopan)
Buscopan (0.3 mg/kg IV or IM) is an anticholinergic drug that is routinely administered for colic to reduce smooth muscle spasm and facilitate rectal examination.[19,37] Owing to its anticholinergic effects, it will cause a transient increase in heart rate for approximately 20 to 30 minutes. Contraindications are predominantly impactions related to ileus, although one dose during evaluation and rectal examination is unlikely to have any detrimental effects and may help with intestinal spasm during medical treatment.[38] Owing to its rapid onset of action for cases of gas colic, a dose can be left with owners to administer IM.

Trocarization
Abdominal visceral distension is considered one of the causes of pain in horses with colic. Trocarization may be performed transabdominally or transrectally. The goal is to alleviate gas distension associated with the LC or cecum and possibly improve ventilation. The appropriate site for trocarizaton may be determined by auscultation of a dorsal ping, ultrasound, or via rectal palpation. Local cellulitis and peritonitis have been listed as complications in approximately 20% of cases.[39] Nonsurvival has been associated with the need for multiple procedures.[39] While not difficult to perform, it can be time-consuming, and the benefits may be short lived. If clinically indicated, and surgery is an option, prompt referral should be prioritized over trocarization, unless there is significant respiratory compromise.

Supplies needed for trocarization:

1. Sterile preparation supplies
2. 3 mL 2% lidocaine to block the skin
3. 15-blade
4. 14-g 5.25-cm angiocatheter for transabdominal or 18-g 40-mm needle
5. Extension set
6. Cup of water (to visualize gas)

Fluid therapy. Routes for administration of fluids include

1. Oral (enteral)
2. Intravenous
3. Rectal

Which routes are selected will largely depend on the clinical condition of the horse, type of lesion, owner preference, available facilities, and the field practitioner's time.

Enteral Fluids

A single oral bolus administration of fluids is the most common method and route of fluid administration in the field. Most horses can tolerate a 10 to 15 mL/kg bolus (5-8 L for a 500-kg horse) without difficulty.[40] Oral fluids have been shown to be relatively safe and effective at correcting fluid deficits and electrolyte imbalances and hydrating colonic ingesta.[41,42] The composition of fluids for a single administration may consist of water, electrolytes, and laxatives such as magnesium sulfate (MgSO4) or mineral oil. Horses with functional kidneys are unlikely to suffer ill effects from a single dose of a hypotonic or hypertonic solution; however, using a more balanced solution containing 5.27 g/L of NaCl, 0.37 g/L KCl, and 3.78 g/L of NaCHO3 has been recommended.[40]

The use of mineral oil as an effective laxative has been debated and is generally thought to be a good marker of gastrointestinal transit rather than effective at penetrating and hydrating colonic ingesta. MgSO4 (1 g/kg by mouth once daily) is considered more effective at penetrating ingesta when than mineral oil; however, systemic effects may be seen with repeated administration.[42]

Oral fluids may be repeated every 1 to 2 hours; however, this is impractical in the field setting. For complicated LC impactions and displacements, several visits to the farm may be necessary; therefore, time and cost must be factored into management.

Contraindications to enteral fluids include presence of gastric reflux (>2 L for a 500-kg horse) or ileus or lateral recumbency. Poor patient compliance may preclude administration via this route. Despite appropriate volumes and frequency of administration, some horses may experience more acute pain after the administration of oral fluids and develop intolerance to repeated administration. In these cases, reducing the volume and/or frequency of fluid administration may be beneficial.

Intravenous Fluid Therapy

Intravenous fluid therapy is an effective method to restore fluid volume, particularly when oral fluids are contraindicated. Commonly used resuscitation fluids are isotonic crystalloids, meaning they have the same osmolarity or solute concentration as plasma; however, they differ in their electrolyte composition. Examples include Normosol-R, lactated Ringer's solution, and 0.9% saline. Fluids with an electrolyte composition similar to plasma may be preferred over those with higher chloride, given the possible association of hyperchloremia and increased risk of acute kidney injury.[43] For rapid resuscitation and volume expansion, 7.2% hypertonic saline may be used (3-5 mL/kg as a bolus or 2 L per 500-kg horse). Owing to its short duration of effect, hypertonic saline administration must be followed with isotonic volume replacement.

Intravenous fluids may be administered as a bolus or as a CRI. Most horses will tolerate a bolus of 10 to 20 mL/kg over 30 minutes to 1 hour. The benefit of bolus administration is time; however, horses that are demonstrating marked hypovolemia may require anywhere from 1 to 3 boluses. After each bolus, the patient's cardiovascular parameters should be reassessed to determine the need for additional doses. From a practical standpoint, improvements in heart rate, mentation, and urine production are important indicators of effective volume support.

If a client is comfortable managing an IV catheter, continuous infusions of fluids is an option in the field. The maintenance rate for adult horses is 2-4 mL/kg/h. The rate may need to be adjusted depending on on-going losses (ie, gastric reflux or diarrhea). The benefit of a CRI is that it reduces the risk of volume overload and potentially allows for pain medications to be administered concurrently in the fluids. The client should be educated about the risk associated with IV catheters, chiefly, air emboli and thrombophlebitis.

Rectal Fluids

Anecdotal reports exist in humans and horses regarding the use of rectal fluids.[44,45] The benefits of rectal administration of fluids are that it is inexpensive, does not require sterility, and is associated with few risks. They can be administered as a fluid bolus or as a CRI (**Fig. 4**). A 500-kg horse will tolerate approximately 2 L of warmed fluids via rectal administration using gravity flow.[45] For bolus administration, the only equipment needed is a stallion catheter, lubrication, funnel, and warmed tap water. A recent study suggested that plain tap water at a CRI dose of 5 mL/kg/h was well tolerated and resulted in hemodilution. Interestingly, plain tap water was better tolerated than an isotonic electrolyte solution.[46] The author has used rectal fluids in a clinical setting as well as in field situations, particularly in miniature horses presenting with suspected fecaliths and/or financial constraints. In both these situations, the rectal fluids were combined with a bolus of oral and/or intravenous fluids. The only additional equipment needed for a CRI is a fluid bag, large bore fluid administration set, and a method to secure the stallion catheter to the tail.

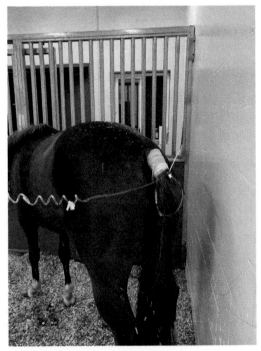

Fig. 4. Equine receiving rectal fluids as a CRI using fluid bags, large bore fluid administration set, transfer set, and foal enema catheter. The end of the fluid administration set has been cut, and a transfer set is being used to attach it to the enema tube. The ends have been secured with tape. (*Courtesy of* Madeline Courville, DVM, San Francisco Bay Area.)

Treatment of specific conditions

Sand enteropathy. Sand enteropathy results from the accumulation of sand or gravel in the large intestine. Clinical signs associated with sand accumulation include intermittent colic, abdominal distension, weight loss, ill-thrift, diarrhea, and pyrexia.[24,47] Horses of any age, including foals younger than 1 year, may be affected.[47] Blood work may be inflammatory and reveal a neutrophilia or neutropenia and hyperfibrinogenemia.[24] Diagnosis is supported by clinical signs, auscultation, and fecal sedimentation. However, radiography is by far the most objective diagnostic modality to definitively determine the presence of sand and the quantity. Ventral abdominal radiographs can be diagnostic in the field with current portable radiographic units.

Treatment consists of pain management and a combination of enteral and/or IV fluids. Nasogastric administration of psyllium with MgSO4 and/or mineral oil has been advocated for treatment, although few prospective, blinded studies exist comparing the efficacy of these treatments. Approximately 20% of nontreated horses in one study resolved sand with management changes alone; however, the control group was small.[48] There is evidence to suggest that feeding psyllium as a 10-day course (1 g/kg body weight) at home was less effective than daily administration via nasogastric tubing for 3 to 7 days.[49] The overall prognosis for medical management is good; however, owners should be warned that multiple treatments may be necessary.[24]

Septic peritonitis. Septic peritonitis may be idiopathic or secondary to abdominal surgery, gastrointestinal rupture, penetrating metallic foreign bodies, or internal abscesses.[50] Diagnostic testing includes peritoneal fluid evaluation and culture and/or PCR of abdominal fluid. In the field, the appearance of the abdominal fluid (cloudy, dark yellow/orange, turbid) along with a history of fever and colic is supportive. With portable hand-held devices, it is possible to assess TP, lactate, and glucose. A peritoneal fluid glucose concentration of less than 30 mg/dL has moderate sensitivity and specificity for diagnosing septic peritonitis.[51] Peritoneal glucose concentrations greater than 30 mg/dL should be compared with blood glucose concentration. If the blood glucose concentration is 50 mg/dL higher than peritoneal glucose concentration, it indicates the presence of septic peritonitis. While these results are used to guide initial diagnosis and therapy in the field, peritoneal fluid cytology and culture should always be performed to confirm the diagnosis.

In addition to supportive care, broad-spectrum antimicrobials should be administered. Ideally, antimicrobials are selected based on culture and antimicrobial sensitivity testing of the peritoneal fluid. Frequently administered antimicrobials include combinations of beta-lactams and aminoglycosides, trimethoprim sulfonamide combinations, and fluoroquinolones, possibly in combination with nitroimidazoles (metronidazole) if an anerobic component is suspected.[52-54]

SUMMARY

Many colic cases respond favorably to conservative medical management. Managing complicated cases can be daunting as they require significantly more professional time and financial commitment from the owner. When referral is recommended, but not an option, it is imperative to manage client expectations. Occasionally this may mean recommending euthanasia on humane grounds. Advances in portable imaging modalities and POC devices have expanded on-farm diagnostic and prognostic capabilities. Field management of colic should encompass a strategy to control pain, treat the primary lesion, and provide cardiovascular support, when indicated.

CLINICS CARE POINTS

- Pay close attention to pain severity and cardiovascular parameters to rapidly identify critical cases.
- Educate clients and manage expectations regarding finances, risks, and cost of management of critical cases.
- Fluid therapy is an integral part of cardiovascular support. Fluids may be administered enterally, intravenously, or rectally.
- Analgesia should be incorporated into the treatment of colic and will depend on pain severity, cardiovascular status, human safety, and cost.

DISCLOSURE

The authors declare no conflicts of interest.

Left Side FLASH.jpg	
FLASH 1.jpg	FLASH 1 US.jpg
FLASH 2.jpg	FLASH 2 US.jpg
FLASH 3.jpg	FLASH 3 US.jpg
FLASH 4.jpg	FLASH 4 US.jpg

Right Side FLASH.jpg	
FLASH 5.jpg	FLASH 5 US.jpg
FLASH 6.jpg	FLASH 6 US.jpg
FLASH 7.jpg	FLASH 7 US.jpg

REFERENCES

1. Bowden A, Boynova P, Brennan ML, et al. Retrospective case series to identify the most common conditions seen 'out-of-hours' by first-opinion equine veterinary practitioners. Vet Rec 2020;187(10):404.
2. Tinker MK, White NA, Lessard P, et al. Prospective study of equine colic incidence and mortality. Equine Vet J 1997;29(6):448–53.
3. Traub-Dargatz JL, Kopral CA, Seitzinger AH, et al. Estimate of the national incidence of and operation-level risk factors for colic among horses in the United States, spring 1998 to spring 1999. J Am Vet Med Assoc 2001;219(1):67–71.
4. Curtis L, Burford JH, Thomas JSM, et al. Prospective study of the primary evaluation of 1016 horses with clinical signs of abdominal pain by veterinary practitioners, and the differentiation of critical and non-critical cases. Acta Vet Scand 2015;57(1):69.
5. Barker I, Freeman SL. Assessment of costs and insurance policies for referral treatment of equine colic. Vet Rec 2019;185(16):508.
6. van der Linden MA, Laffont CM, Sloet van Oldruitenborgh-Oosterbann MM. Prognosis in equine medical and surgical colic. J Vet Intern Med 2003;17:343–8.

7. Mair TS, Smith LJ. Survival and complication rates in 300 horses undergoing surgical treatment of colic. Part 1: short-term survival following a single laparotomy. Equine Vet J 2010;37(4):296–302.
8. Jennings K, Curtis L, Burford J, et al. Prospective survey of veterinary practitioners' primary assessment of equine colic: clinical features, diagnoses, and treatment of 120 cases of large colon impaction. BMC Vet Res 2014;10(Suppl 1):S2.
9. Proudman CJ. A two year, prospective survey of equine colic in general practice. Equine Vet J 1992;24(2):90–3.
10. Cohen ND, Vontur CA, Rakestraw PC. Risk factors for enterolithiasis among horses in Texas. J Am Vet Med Assoc 2000;216(11):1787–94.
11. Fielding CL. Practical fluid therapy and treatment modalities for field conditions for horses and foals with gastrointestinal problems. Vet Clin North Am Equine Pract 2018;34(1):155–68.
12. Sutton GA, Dahan R, Turner D, et al. A behaviour-based pain scale for horses with acute colic: Scale construction. Vet J 2013;196(3):394–401.
13. van Loon JPAM, Van Dierendonck MC. Monitoring acute equine visceral pain with the Equine Utrecht University Scale for Composite Pain Assessment (EQUUS-COMPASS) and the Equine Utrecht University Scale for Facial Assessment of Pain (EQUUS-FAP): a scale-construction study. Vet J 2015;206(3):356–64.
14. Bowden A, England GCW, Brennan ML, et al. Indicators of 'critical' outcomes in 941 horses seen 'out-of-hours' for colic. Vet Rec 2020;187(12):492.
15. Asim M, Alkadi MM, Asim H, et al. Dehydration and volume depletion: How to handle the misconceptions. World J Nephrol 2019;8(1):23–32.
16. Abutarbush SM, Carmalt JL, Shoemaker RW. Causes of gastrointestinal colic in horses in western Canada: 604 cases (1992 to 2002). Can Vet J 2005;46:6.
17. Gillen A, Kottwitz J, Munsterman A. Meta-analysis of the effect of treatment strategies for nephrosplenic entrapment of the large colon. J Equine Vet Sci 2020;92: 103169.
18. Velloso Alvarez A, Reid Hanson R, Schumacher J. Caecal impactions: Diagnosis, management and prognosis. Equine Vet Educ 2020. https://doi.org/10.1111/eve. 13317.
19. Luo T, Bertone J, Greene H, et al. A comparison of N-butylscopolammonium and lidocaine for control of rectal pressure in horses. Vet Ther Res Appl Vet Med 2006; 7:243–8.
20. Verne GN, Sen A, Price DD. Intrarectal lidocaine is an effective treatment for abdominal pain associated with diarrhea-predominant irritable bowel syndrome. J Pain 2005;6(8):493–6.
21. Klohnen A. Abdominal ultrasonography in the equine patient with acute signs of colic. Lexington, Kentucky: American Association of Equine Practitioners; p. 8.
22. Busoni V, Busscher VD, Lopez D, et al. Evaluation of a protocol for fast localised abdominal sonography of horses (FLASH) admitted for colic. Vet J 2011;188(1): 77–82.
23. Biscoe EW, Whitcomb MB, Vaughan B, et al. Clinical features and outcome in horses with severe large intestinal thickening diagnosed with transabdominal ultrasonography: 25 cases (2003–2010). J Am Vet Med Assoc 2018;253(1):108–16.
24. Hart KA, Linnenkohl W, Mayer JR, et al. Medical management of sand enteropathy in 62 horses: sand colic. Equine Vet J 2013;45(4):465–9.
25. Nieto JE, Dechant JE, le Jeune SS, et al. Evaluation of 3 handheld portable analyzers for measurement of L-lactate concentrations in blood and peritoneal fluid of horses with colic. Vet Surg 2015;44(3):366–72.

26. Delesalle C, Dewulf J, Lefebvre RA, et al. Determination of lactate concentrations in blood plasma and peritoneal fluid in horses with colic by an accusport analyzer. J Vet Intern Med 2007;21(2):293–301.
27. Johnston K, Holcombe SJ, Hauptman JG. Plasma lactate as a predictor of colonic viability and survival after 360 degrees volvulus of the ascending colon in horses. Vet Surg 2007;36:563–7.
28. Curtis L, Trewin I, England GCW, et al. Veterinary practitioners' selection of diagnostic tests for the primary evaluation of colic in the horse. Vet Rec Open 2015; 2(2):e000145.
29. Latson KM, Nieto JE, Beldomenico PM, et al. Evaluation of peritoneal fluid lactate as a marker of intestinal ischaemia in equine colic. Equine Vet J 2005;37(4): 342–6.
30. Bowen IM, Redpath A, Dugdale A, et al. BEVA primary care clinical guidelines: analgesia. Equine Vet J 2020;52(1):13–27.
31. Ziegler AL, Freeman CK, Fogle CA, et al. Multicentre, blinded, randomised clinical trial comparing the use of flunixin meglumine with firocoxib in horses with small intestinal strangulating obstruction. Equine Vet J 2019;51(3):329–35.
32. Cook VL, Meyer CT, Campbell NB, et al. Effect of firocoxib or flunixin meglumine on recovery of ischemic-injured equine jejunum. Am J Vet Res 2009;70(8):9.
33. Jasiecka A, Maślanka T, Jaroszewski JJ. Pharmacological characteristics of metamizole. Pol J Vet Sci 2014;17(1):207–14.
34. Guedes A. How to maximize standing chemical restraint. In: AAEP proceedings. Lexington, Kentucky: American Association of Equine Practitioners; vol. 59. 2013. p. 461–3.
35. Torfs S, Delesalle C, Dewulf J, et al. Risk factors for equine postoperative ileus and effectiveness of prophylactic lidocaine. J Vet Intern Med 2009;23(3):606–11.
36. Salem SE, Proudman CJ, Archer DC. Has intravenous lidocaine improved the outcome in horses following surgical management of small intestinal lesions in a UK hospital population? BMC Vet Res 2016;12(1):157.
37. Boatwright CE, Fubini SLF, Grohn YT, et al. A comparison of N-butylscopolammonium bromide and butorphanol Tartrate for analgesia using a balloon model of abdominal pain in ponies. 4.
38. Hart KA, Sherlock CE, Davern AJ, et al. Effect of N-butylscopolammonium bromide on equine ileal smooth muscle activity in an ex vivo model: effects of N-butylscopolammonium bromide on equine ileum. Equine Vet J 2015;47(4):450–5.
39. Schoster A, Altermatt N, Torgerson PR, et al. Outcome and complications following transrectal and transabdominal large intestinal trocarization in equids with colic: 228 cases (2004-2015). J Am Vet Med Assoc 2020;257(2):189–95.
40. Lopes MAF. Enteral fluid therapy. In: Fielding CL, Magdesian KG, editors. Equine fluid therapy. Ames, Iowa: John Wiley & Sons, Inc; 2014. p. 261–78.
41. Lopes MAF, Walker BL, Ii NAW, et al. Treatments to promote colonic hydration: enteral fluid therapy versus intravenous fluid therapy and magnesium sulphate. Equine Vet J 2010;34(5):505–9.
42. Lopes MAF, White NA II, Donaldson L, et al. Effects of enteral and intravenous fluid therapy, magnesium sulfate, and sodium sulfate on colonic contents and feces in horses. Am J Vet Res 2004;65(5):695–704.
43. Oh TK, Song I-A, Kim SJ, et al. Hyperchloremia and postoperative acute kidney injury: a retrospective analysis of data from the surgical intensive care unit. Crit Care 2018;22(1):277.
44. Tremayne V. Proctoclysis: emergency rectal fluid infusion. Nurs Stand R Coll Nurs 2009;24:46–8.

45. Gardiner M. Administration of fluids per rectum in horses. Vet Rec 2013; 172(16):430.
46. Khan A, Hallowell GD, Underwood C, et al. Continuous fluid infusion per rectum compared with intravenous and nasogastric fluid administration in horses. Equine Vet J 2019;51(6):767–73.
47. Granot N, Milgram J, Bdolah-Abram T, et al. Surgical management of sand colic impactions in horses: a retrospective study of 41 cases. Aust Vet J 2008;86(10): 404–7.
48. Niinistö KE, Ruohoniemi MO, Freccero F, et al. Investigation of the treatment of sand accumulations in the equine large colon with psyllium and magnesium sulphate. Vet J 2018;238:22–6.
49. Kaikkonen R, Niinistö K, Lindholm T, et al. Comparison of psyllium feeding at home and nasogastric intubation of psyllium and magnesium sulfate in the hospital as a treatment for naturally occurring colonic sand (geosediment) accumulations in horses: a retrospective study. Acta Vet Scand 2016;58(1):73.
50. Odelros E, Kendall A, Hedberg-Alm Y, et al. Idiopathic peritonitis in horses: a retrospective study of 130 cases in Sweden (2002–2017). Acta Vet Scand 2019;61(1):18.
51. Alonso JM, Esper CS, Pantoja JCF, et al. Accuracy of differences in blood and peritoneal glucose to differentiate between septic and non-septic peritonitis in horses. Res Vet Sci 2020;132:237–42.
52. Browning A. Diagnosis and management of peritonitis in horses. In Pract 2005; 27(2):70–5.
53. Nógrádi N, Tóth B, Macgillivray K. Peritonitis in horses: 55 cases (2004–2007). Acta Vet Hung 2011;59(2):181–93.
54. Curtis L, Burford JH, England GCW, et al. Risk factors for acute abdominal pain (colic) in the adult horse: a scoping review of risk factors, and a systematic review of the effect of management-related changes. PLoS One 2019;14(7):e0219307.

Ophthalmic Emergencies in the Field

Ann E. Dwyer, DVM*

KEYWORDS

- Ophthalmic emergency • Corneal ulcer • Ocular desensitization • Eyelid laceration
- Uveitis

KEY POINTS

- Corneal ulcers and eyelid trauma or swelling are the most common ophthalmic emergencies, but a variety of other conditions prompt urgent evaluation.
- Thorough inspection of all regions inside and around both eyes with a bright light source is essential.
- Successful therapy relies on appropriate diagnostic tests and prompt initiation of targeted treatment.
- Key clinical skills include tonometry, ultrasound imaging, and acquisition/interpretation of corneal cytology.
- Field therapy may involve standing surgery of the eyelid or instillation of a subpalpebral lavage system. Topical treatment may involve frequent application of multiple medications.

INTRODUCTION

Ophthalmic emergencies are common in equine ambulatory practice. Of 615 emergencies seen during 2019 in a 5-veterinarian equine practice in the northeast United States, 98, or 16%, were ophthalmic emergencies (Dwyer AE. Unpublished data from practice records, 2019). Cases were most common between July and October, when 21% of emergencies (49 of 229 calls) involved the eye or periocular region (Dwyer AE. Unpublished data from practice records, 2019). A review of 6 years of records from the same practice documented 380 acute corneal ulcers, 120 urgent visits for unilateral eyelid swelling, and 57 surgical repairs of torn eyelids.[1]

EDUCATION OF OWNERS AND PRACTICE TEAM

Web sites and social media posts are effective vehicles for educating owners about the serious nature of ophthalmic emergencies. Images of horses with torn eyelids,

Genesee Valley Equine Clinic, 925 Chili Scottsville Road, Scottsville, NY 14546, USA
* Corresponding author.
E-mail address: adwyer7579@gmail.com

Vet Clin Equine 37 (2021) 441–460
https://doi.org/10.1016/j.cveq.2021.04.011
0749-0739/21/© 2021 Elsevier Inc. All rights reserved.

melting corneal ulcers, or uveitis motivate owners to call promptly for any sign of ocular discomfort or trauma. The practice staff should be coached on problems mandating "same day scheduling" including:

- Torn eyelid
- Trauma to the region around the eyes
- Acute swelling of an eyelid
- An eye that is partly shut, with/without profuse tearing, aversion to handling
- Portion of the globe that has suddenly turned white, red, or blue
- Sudden blindness

Ophthalmic emergencies threaten sight, but the outcome can be excellent if appropriate treatment is instituted after prompt, thorough examination and diagnostic testing.

EQUIPPING THE AMBULATORY VEHICLE

The author carries supplies and medications in a tote box dedicated for ophthalmic items (**Fig. 1**). Diagnostic supplies include microscope slides, scalpel blades, cytobrushes, culture swabs, ocular surface stains, Schirmer tear test strips, and topical tropicamide and anesthetic eye drops. Treatment items include subpalpebral lavage kits, adhesive tape, nasolacrimal flushing catheters, extra tuberculin syringes, and a box of 25-gauge 5/8″ needles. Surgical instruments include Bishop Harmon forceps, small Adson tissue forceps, small mosquito hemostats, curved Stevens tenotomy scissors, and short (5½″) Olsen-Hegar needle holders. Instruments reserved for ophthalmic work are sterilized and carried in the tote in individual packs along with several small-gauge (4–0) suture packs of a soft, absorbable polymer like vicryl or polygalactic acid. Stocked medications include ophthalmic ointments and solutions that have antibiotic, antifungal, mydriatic, hyperosmotic, nonsteroidal anti-inflammatory drug (NSAID), and corticosteroid activity as well as eye drops that support tear film function and treat glaucoma. Having all supplies readily at hand increases the efficiency of examination and treatment.

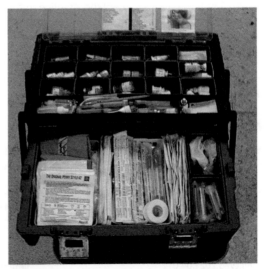

Fig. 1. Supplies and medications for ophthalmic emergencies are carried in a tote box.

EXAMINATION EQUIPMENT

A battery-powered 3.5-V coaxial direct ophthalmoscope kit is carried in the practice vehicle (Welch Allyn Co, Skaneateles, NY, USA, head part #11720, handle part #71000-C). The kit includes a halogen transilluminator (part #41100) with a removable cobalt blue filter (part #41102). A panoptic ophthalmoscope head (part #11820) is a useful accessory, as it provides a 5 times wider field of view of the fundus than the coaxial head.

Accurate ophthalmic examination requires a bright light source. Modern ophthalmoscope handles house rechargeable nickel-cadmium (NiCad) batteries and also can run on a pair of standard C batteries (Welch Allyn, part #71000-C). Powering the handle with C batteries minimizes field challenges; a spare set of batteries assures uninterrupted illumination when working in various temperatures away from reliable power sources. Some older power handles run solely on NiCad battery power, but one base (part #71000-A) can be retrofitted to run on C batteries by insertion of an inexpensive "converter ring" (part #71068-501).

Additional focal light sources aid management of ophthalmic problems. Military-grade tactical penlights provide bright focal light, facilitating dazzle, and pupillary reflex testing (Pelican LED 120 penlight [Pelican products, Torrance, CA, USA] or Maglite XL 50 penlight [MAG Instrument, Inc, Ontario, CA, USA]). A battery-powered headlamp aids diagnostic testing and field surgery. An inexpensive binocular headband provides a hands-free magnified view for close-up work and can be fitted with lenses that provide 1.5 to 3.5 times magnification (OptiVISOR, Donegan Optical Company, Inc, Lenexa, KS, USA).

A portable tonometer (TONOVET/TONOVET Plus, Icare, Helsinki, Finland, or Tono-Pen, Reichert, Inc, Depew, NY, USA) is used to measure the intraocular pressure (IOP) in horses. The TONOVET/TONOVET Plus, which records rebound motion parameters of a probe that bounces off the cornea, is a rugged choice for field conditions. Additional field examination equipment includes a handheld converging lens (+20 D or +28 D strength, Volk Optical, Inc, Mentor, OH, USA) for monocular indirect ophthalmoscopy and a battery-powered handheld slit lamp (SL-17, Kowa Co, Nagoya, Japan) for advanced inspection of the globe; use of a slit lamp and/or converging lens requires advanced training and practice.

PREPARATION AT THE FARM

Equine ophthalmic emergencies are examined in a darkened indoor area such as a stall or stable aisle. Four or five bales of hay, straw, or shavings are stacked to build a "table" to support the horse's head slightly above chest level, with edible components covered by a blanket (**Fig. 2**). A wheeled recycling bin or dental head stand provides head support if bales are unavailable. The field examination room is optimized by darkening outside light sources and minimizing disruptions from farm personnel, loose animals, or wind. Two or three lightweight folding aluminum tables placed nearby provide useful space for equipment and supplies (Ozark Trail aluminum camping tables, Walmart, Inc, Bentonville, AR, USA).

SEDATION AND REGIONAL ANESTHESIA

Examination and therapy for most ocular emergencies requires patient sedation. Intravenous xylazine (0.5–1.0 mg/kg) is effective if the horse has a calm temperament and is not in severe pain. Intravenous detomidine hydrochloride (0.02–0.04 mg/kg) is required if the horse is fractious, painful, or if standing surgery or installation of a sub-palpebral lavage system (SPL) is indicated. Butorphanol tartrate is rarely used

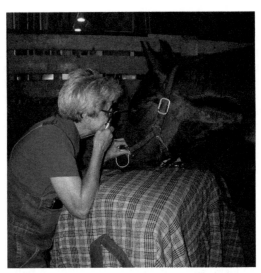

Fig. 2. Stacked bales of hay, covered by a blanket, provide a stable surface for examination and treatment.

because it produces troublesome head tremors. Sedative efficacy is optimized if the practitioner proceeds directly from examination to diagnostic testing to therapy so that procedures that require profound sedation occur promptly.

Motor and/or sensory denervation of the eyelid is required for handling many ocular emergencies.[2] The auriculopalpebral block produces temporary paralysis of the orbicularis oculi muscle of the upper eyelid. This branch of the facial nerve originates near the base of the ear and can be palpated through the skin over the zygomatic arch. Eyelid akinesia is induced by injecting 2 to 3 mL of 2% lidocaine or mepivacaine through a 25-gauge, 5/8″ needle along the nerve in one of 3 sites: (1) at the depression just in front of the base of the ear, (2) at the highest point of the caudal zygomatic arch, or (3) in the center of the dip of the arch just caudal to the rim of the orbit. The supraorbital (frontal) block desensitizes the nasal and central regions of the upper eyelid. This block involves subcutaneous injection of 1 mL lidocaine or mepivacaine through a 25-gauge, 5/8″ needle where the frontal nerve emerges from the supraorbital foramen. The foramen can be felt through the skin as a depression within the frontal bone in the superionasal quadrant above the orbital rim (**Fig. 3**).

Desensitization of the cornea is needed for debridement and acquisition of culture or cytology samples. Some horses tolerate procedures on the cornea after the surface is sprayed with 0.3 mL topical 0.5% proparacaine or tetracaine hydrochloride ophthalmic drops. If the horse remains uncooperative, subconjunctival injection of 0.25 to 0.50 mL 2% mepivacaine induces corneal desensitization. Injection of the bulbar conjunctiva is done with the horse sedated and the mandible supported on the head rest. The handler tips the poll away from the examiner, who then numbs the target conjunctival surface with a cotton bud soaked with topical anesthetic. The injection is delivered through a 25- or 27-gauge needle (**Fig. 4**).

CLEANING THE PERIOCULAR AND OCULAR REGION

The periocular region is cleaned with 4″×4″-gauze squares soaked with 2% povidone iodine solution (1 part povidone iodine/50 parts sterile saline). If needed, the

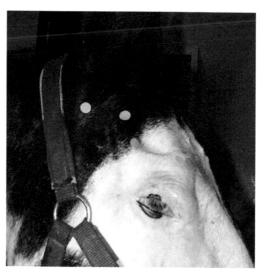

Fig. 3. Infiltration of local anesthetic over one of the 3 pink dotted sites induces eyelid aki-nesia (auriculopalpebral block). Infiltration over the foramen palpable in the green dotted area provides partial denervation of the eyelid (supraorbital block).

conjunctival sac is swabbed with cotton buds soaked in the same solution after any culture samples are obtained. Repeated applications of antiseptic will adequately cleanse the skin for nerve blocks or standing surgery; use of antiseptic "scrub" solutions containing soap near the eye is contraindicated.

EXAMINATION

A brief examination of the whole animal checks for concurrent or associated problems. A neuro-ophthalmic examination follows, using bright light to check the dazzle

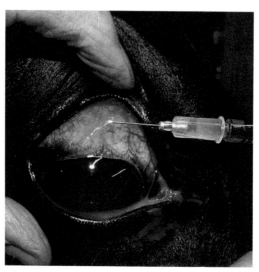

Fig. 4. A subconjunctival injection of local anesthetic provides corneal denervation if topical anesthetic drops are ineffective.

reflex and assess pupillary light reflexes. Hand motion around the globe and lid then checks for the menace and the palpebral (blink) response. Observation of cranial nerve function paired with reflex and response tests determines whether an intact visual and neural pathway is present. An absent dazzle reflex or fixed dilated pupil presents a grave prognosis for vision.

Many ophthalmic emergencies involve abnormalities of more than one region of the head or globe; a habitual "checklist" approach to ophthalmic examination guarantees consistent inspection of all anatomic parts of the globe. **Table 1** details the main questions to consider during assessment of the regions around and inside the eye.

The Finoff transilluminator (Welch Allyn Inc, Skaneatelas, NY, USA) is used to evaluate the periocular region, adnexa, and globe. The adnexa and anterior segment are examined with this bright halogen light, which easily illuminates this hemispherical area from all angles. The equine fundus can also be inspected with a transilluminator if the pupil is midrange or larger in size and the ocular media are transparent. A magnified image of the optic nerve and tapetal and nontapetal regions is visible if the transilluminator is held next to the examiner's cheek between 5″ and 8″ away from the globe and the light beam is aimed toward the tapetal-nontapetal border (**Fig. 5**). Examination with a direct ophthalmoscope follows, as well as tonometry, indirect ophthalmoscopy, and/or slit lamp examination if available. Study of references describing the finer points of examination and operation of ophthalmoscopes is advised for recognition of the pathologic condition.[3]

Table 1
Checklist for ophthalmic examination

Region	Questions to Consider During Examination
Whole horse	Body condition? Signs of other disease: PPID, laminitis, dermatitis, heaves, other?
Periorbit, head	Contour and symmetry of sinuses, orbit? Pain or skin abnormalities? Lymph node enlargement? Facial nerve dysfunction?
Globe function	Gaze: symmetric? Pupils: equal in size and shape? Dazzle and pupillary light reflexes? Menace response? Blink?
Adnexa	Tarsal margin: intact? Do eyelids meet when closed? Is eyelash position symmetric? Are both third eyelids present? Masses?
Sclera and conjunctiva	Abnormal color? Congestion, hyperemia? Masses? Swelling?
Cornea	Transparency? Color, size, shape, location of any focal opacities? Surface defects or foreign bodies? Vascularization? Pigmentation? Regions of stain uptake? Anatomy of drainage angle?
Anterior Chamber	Depth when viewed from side? Presence of flare, fibrin, hyphema or hypopyon?
Iris	Mobility? Color? Pupils: equal and reactive? Corpora nigrans: atrophy or cyst? Iris: synechia, atrophy, color change?
Lens	Lens clarity: focal or diffuse? Lens position: any luxation? Lens capsule: pigment rests or synechia?
Posterior chamber	Vitreous: any loss of clarity, color change? Any masses? Is the vitreous liquefied?
Fundus	Focal or diffuse depigmentation or scarring? Are optic nerve vessels normal? Is the image of the optic disc crisp? Any masses?

Abbreviations: PPID, pars pituitary intermedia dysfunction.

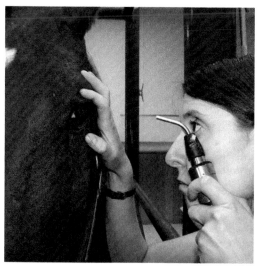

Fig. 5. A Finoff transilluminator is used to inspect the anterior and posterior segments of the globe, including the fundus.

The orbit, eyelid aperture, cornea, iris, lens, and optic nerve region are all round to oval, so the location of findings can be mapped in the medical record by noting the "clock hour" position and distance of the finding from a stable landmark like the orbital rim, limbus, pupil margin, or optic nerve head.

DIAGNOSTIC TESTS

The fluorescein dye test checks for corneal ulcers and assesses corneal integrity and patency of the nasolacrimal duct. Sterile paper strips impregnated with sodium fluorescein are applied directly to the tear film or mixed with 0.5 to 1 mL saline, which is then sprayed onto the cornea. Ulcers with exposed stroma stain bright green. Detection of stain uptake is enhanced by viewing with a cobalt blue light. Corneal perforations leak a tiny amount of aqueous humor; they are identified by a thin river of fluid (aqueous) flowing through the green staining tear film (Seidel test).

Corneal culture is performed to identify pathogens in corneal ulcers and determine sensitivity to available ophthalmic anti-infectives. Corneal cytology is indicated for any serious corneal ulcer to look for pathogens, inflammation, and microscopic foreign bodies. The blunt end of a scalpel blade or a cytology brush is used to place the specimen on a few slides, which are then stained with Diff-Quik solutions ± Gram stain.

Tonometry is used to obtain IOP readings on horses that present with any puzzling condition of the globe, particularly those suspected to have glaucoma or uveitis. References with detail on obtaining and interpreting cytology samples[4] and performing tonometry[5] are available to expand field expertise.

SUBPALPEBRAL LAVAGE SYSTEMS

Some ophthalmic emergencies cause severe pain that persists for days or weeks. Treatment of these conditions involves frequent topical application of multiple medications. Many horses resent handling around the eye and may not tolerate manual application of medication. Installation of an SPL is required for successful treatment of severe problems like mycotic keratitis, deep bacterial ulcers, and stromal abscesses. Practitioners must be prepared to place and manage SPLs on the farm when treating these emergencies.[6]

IMAGING

Ophthalmic emergencies that present with corneal opacity, cataracts, orbital trauma, or a prominent globe can be assessed with transpalpebral ultrasound as long as the globe is tectonically stable. Linear or microconvex probes used at frequencies of 7.5 to 10.0 MHz for orthopedic imaging produce images that evaluate globe size and echogenicity of intraocular structures.[7] Use of a homemade flexible standoff, created by filling a latex examination glove with water, is advised to aid image quality and preserve the conformation of the anterior chamber.

Ultrasonic gel is applied to the standoff and periocular skin taking care to avoid gel contact with the cornea. The standoff (inflated glove palm or finger) and probe are passed over the orbital margin: discontinuity of the bright white signal of the bony rim suggests fracture. The globe is then imaged through the standoff and eyelid over the most prominent curve of the axial cornea. Globe cross-sectional depth is measured and compared with the fellow eye; the average axial length of the globe is about 4 cm in a full-sized horse. The structures of the globe generate distinct echolucent or echodense signals that are summarized in **Table 2**. Alterations in echogenicity or position of any ocular structure suggests pathologic condition, displacement, or both: cataracts produce an echodense signal in the center of the spindle-shaped lens capsule, a luxated lens rests in the posterior chamber distant from the iris, and a complete retinal detachment appears as a V-shaped membrane emanating from the optic nerve region (**Fig. 6**A and **B**).

Many ophthalmic emergencies warrant photographic documentation of the periocular region and/or anterior segment.[8] Images downloaded to the medical record are invaluable for assessing progress and useful for owner education. The tiny lenses of cell phone cameras are suitable for recording images of fundic abnormalities; online tutorials are available for skill enhancement.[9]

Table 2
Ultrasonic signals generated by axial cross-sectional imaging of the globe

Echodense Signals	Dimensions	Echolucent Signals	Dimensions
Cornea: curved linear white signal	@1 mm thick	Anterior chamber: crescent-shaped black signal, fluid consistency	@ 4 mm deep
Iris: straight linear white signal. Corpora nigrans: cystic white projections	@2 mm thick (iris) @3–5 mm (Corpora nigrans)	Pupil: black linear "gap" in the center of iris signal	@ 12 mm wide
Lens capsule: spindle shaped white border signal; surrounds echolucent contents	< 1 mm thick both anterior and posterior borders	Lens contents (cortex/nucleus): elliptical black signal, solid consistency	@ 11–13 mm thick × @ 20 mm wide
Retina/choroid/sclera: hemispheric white signal	@ 2 mm thick	Vitreous contents: hemispheric black signal, gel consistency	@ 15–19 mm deep

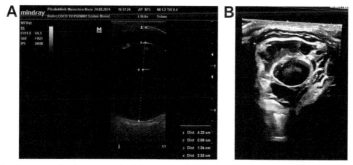

Fig. 6. (A) Ultrasound of a normal globe. Echodense structures include cornea (2) and lens capsule (3, 4). Anterior chamber, lens cortex, and vitreous are echolucent. (B) Ultrasound of an abnormal globe showing lens luxation, retinal detachment, and intraocular inflammatory debris. (*Courtesy of* Dr. Richard McMullen, Dr. med. vet., Dipl ACVO, Dipl ECVO, Alabama)

EMERGENCIES OF THE PERIOCULAR REGION

Periocular skin lacerations not involving the eyelid are straightforward; closure using standard wound repair techniques has an excellent outcome due to the abundant blood supply (**Fig. 7**). If a wound presents with loss of skin or margins that are difficult to close, the underlying planes of subcutaneous fascia are easily dissected off the surface of the skull bones, freeing skin flaps that are rotated for effective closure. Penrose drains are incorporated into the repair for drainage of any fluid that might accumulate in dead space.

Blunt trauma to the periocular region is commonly caused by kicks or collision with solid objects (**Fig. 8**). The force of the trauma is often associated with fracture of the roof of a sinus cavity near the orbit. Fractures are most often noted in the maxillary sinus, followed by the frontal sinus. Signs of an acute sinus fracture include unilateral

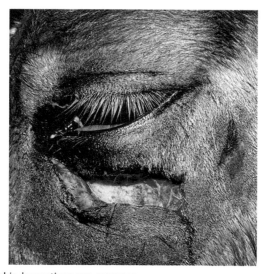

Fig. 7. Periocular skin lacerations are common.

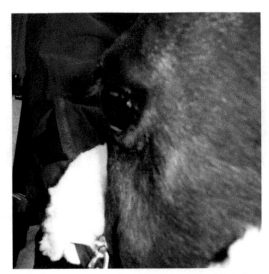

Fig. 8. Blunt trauma can fracture periocular sinuses or the orbital rim.

epistaxis and tenderness and swelling over the site. Occasionally these fractures are accompanied by subtle subcutaneous emphysema. Such injuries are treated as "open" fractures even if the skin is intact, as the sinus opening into the nasal passage can admit pathogens. Sinus fractures risk progression to orbital cellulitis; systemic treatment with broad-spectrum antibiotics for a minimum of 2 weeks is advised.

Orbital fractures are occasionally seen after trauma and cause pain and swelling of the orbital rim. Radiography of the orbit usually fails to document the extent of anatomic disruption, but ultrasound of the orbital rim is a useful procedure for the identification of bony fragments or fissures. The orientation and gaze of the affected globe is compared with the uninjured eye; strabismus, asymmetric pupil orientation, or restricted globe movement suggest compression of the orbital space secondary to injury. If orbital compression is present, referral to a tertiary center is advised, as advanced imaging and surgical manipulation or fixation is required to preserve globe integrity and function.

A torn eyelid is a common ophthalmic emergency that must be repaired promptly. These injuries are common in warm months because insect irritation induces horses to rub the periocular region, and the slim metal handles of ubiquitous stable buckets present convenient "rubbing posts." A gap in the J-shaped base that attaches the handle to the bucket rim will trap the tarsal margin. The eyelid will then rip if the horse pulls back (**Fig. 9**A–D). These dramatic injuries can have an excellent outcome if repaired on the day of occurrence and simple guidelines are followed:

- Support the head on a bale table or other stationary support. Use a strap on headlight for focal illumination.
- Administer detomidine for intravenous sedation. Clean the skin with an antiseptic solution of 2% povidone iodine solution/saline.
- Perform auriculopalpebral and supraorbital nerve blocks to achieve eyelid akinesia and partial desensitization of the upper eyelid (see earlier discussion)
- Administer a small volume of local anesthesia around the torn skin margins using a 25-gauge, 5/8″ needle. Test the efficacy of the local block with needle pricks before attempting closure.

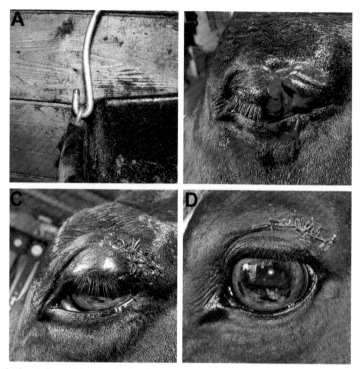

Fig. 9. (*A*) The J-shaped base of a bucket handle often traps eyelids. (*B*) A bucket handle caused a severe tear of this upper eyelid. (*C*) Immediate postoperative appearance after two-layer closure. (*D*) Appearance of eye at suture removal.

- Debride the torn tissue margins minimally, preserving as much eyelid skin as possible.
- Important: Perform a meticulous 2-layer closure, first apposing the subconjunctival tissues with 4–0 absorbable suture (see comment later in the article). All knots must be buried to avoid corneal irritation.
- Next, appose the skin (second layer) using 4–0 suture in a simple interrupted pattern. Particular attention should be paid to the tarsal margin, which must be closed exactly, using a figure-of-8 pattern so there is no "step." The suture tag ends of the tarsal margin suture can be left a little long and folded under adjacent interrupted suture knots to keep the ends away from the cornea.
- Prescribe systemic nonsteroidal anti-inflammatory medication and systemic antibiotics for 5 to 7 days.

Some eyelid tears are challenging due to multiplanar damage and/or substantial chemosis. The repair of such injuries can be cosmetic and functional if great care is taken with the closure of the conjunctiva and tarsal margin. Many texts describe closure of the conjunctiva with a simple continuous pattern, but judicious use of a small number of simple interrupted sutures may be more effective in complex multiplanar injuries. Simple plastic surgery techniques like V-Y plasty are used to bring the lid pieces into exact alignment without excess tension.[10,11] Poor repair, no repair, or amputation of any portion of the tarsal margin must be avoided, as resultant complications of trichiasis, entropion, ectropion or lagophthalmos cause lifelong suffering.

Most eyelid tears are preventable if stable managers cover the handle hooks on all farm buckets with duct or electrical tape.

Concurrent corneal damage with periocular trauma is surprisingly rare, but fluorescein dye is always applied to the cornea on the injured side to screen for ulceration. Both globes are inspected for miosis or other signs of uveitis; administration of systemic nonsteroidal anti-inflammatory medication is usually appropriate. Owners are warned that blunt periocular trauma can be followed by cataract development weeks to months later in the instance that the lens capsule was disrupted by the force of the accident.

Emergency calls reporting unilateral eyelid swelling are frequent in warm months, and the most common cause is allergic chemosis involving the eyelid and conjunctiva. The conjunctival sac can swell to 4 times the normal size: resultant lid turgidity that blocks full inspection of the globe presents a diagnostic challenge, as eyelid swelling is often seen accompanying corneal ulceration or uveitis. Corneal or intraocular problems are accompanied by miosis; if the pupil diameter of the affected eye is comparable to that of the normal eye (not miotic), the eyelid swelling is likely due to allergy (**Fig. 10**A and **B**). Such cases respond quickly to systemic and topical anti-inflammatory therapy.

EMERGENCIES OF THE CORNEA

Horses are often discovered with unilateral epiphora, blepharospasm, and ocular discharge. This cluster of signs may indicate ulcerative keratitis, the most common equine ophthalmic emergency.[12] If application of sodium fluorescein shows a small area on the corneal surface that stains weakly green, a minor corneal erosion, or loss of a few superficial layers of epithelial cells, is present. These lesions often respond well to empirical therapy with a broad-spectrum antibiotic ointment applied 3 to 4 times per day, plus a few applications of atropine sulfate ointment to induce mydriasis. Intense uptake of bright green stain is a more serious concern as this indicates a corneal ulcer, a focal region where the epithelium is absent and underlying stroma is exposed. All corneal ulcers, particularly those that present with infiltrate, vascularization, and/or severe pain, warrant cytologic evaluation, followed by focal debridement (**Fig. 11**A and **B**). These procedures require perineural and topical anesthesia, as well as sedation, done in the following order:

- Obtain a culture sample by swabbing material from the lesion edge.
- Use the blunt end of a sterile scalpel blade or a cytology brush to dislodge cellular material from the lesion, preparing 2 or 3 microscope slides for cytologic analysis.

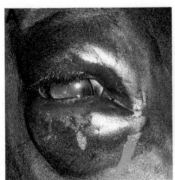 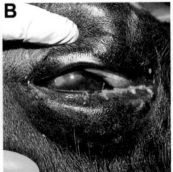

Fig. 10. (*A*) Severe eyelid swelling due to allergy; normal pupil size. (*B*) Severe eyelid swelling accompanying corneal ulcer; miotic pupil.

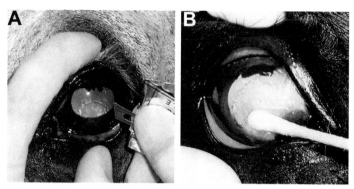

Fig. 11. (A) Corneal cytology sampling. (B) Corneal debridement.

- Debride the ulcer with the blunt end of a scalpel blade followed by swabbing the defect with a series of dry sterile cotton buds. Remove all surface debris and loose the epithelium.
- After treating the patient and returning to the practice, stain one cytology slide with Diff-Quik stain and evaluate using 100× microscopic magnification. If bacteria are seen, Gram stain a second slide and evaluate the staining characteristics of the organisms.
- Modify treatment plan that was started at the farm visit as needed to address the cause.

The importance of diagnostic sampling at the emergency visit, coupled with prompt analysis of cytology, cannot be overemphasized. Corneal ulcers have multiple causes; gross appearance does not distinguish between the various causes (**Fig. 12**A–F). Prompt evaluation of ulcer cytology assures prescription of appropriate evidence-based therapy, optimizes outcome, and ultimately saves expense and ineffective treatment effort. Failure to collect and analyze samples at the initial visit can result in progressive, painful keratitis requiring weeks to months of therapy, or even lead to sight loss or enucleation.

Many corneal ulcers are infected. Abundant, uniform numbers of extracellular or intracellular rods or cocci on cytology indicate bacterial keratitis and the need for topical antibiotics specific to the class of pathogen. Presence of fungal hyphae with or without spores confirms *mycotic keratitis*, a serious condition requiring weeks to months of antifungal therapy administered through an SPL. Heavy neutrophilic infiltrate coupled with tangles of cytokeratin debris in a cytology sample is evidence of stromal malacia and collagenolysis. Such cases risk progression to a melting ulcer, a serious condition that threatens globe integrity. Frequent application of anticollagenase agents, in addition to mydriatic and anti-infective therapy, is mandatory to counter stromal malacia.

On the other hand, some corneal ulcers have a noninfectious cause; anti-infectives, although appropriate as a component of the treatment plan, will not resolve these conditions.[13,14] Findings like small pieces of plant material or calcium crystals embedded in corneal epithelium indicate a role of foreign bodies in ulcer development. The presence of abundant eosinophils interspersed among corneal epithelial cells is consistent with eosinophilic keratitis, an immune-mediated condition requiring aggressive debridement and systemic immune suppression in addition to broad-spectrum topicals. Absence of pathogens, foreign bodies, and inflammatory cells suggests that the lesion may be an indolent ulcer that will require surgical debridement for healing.

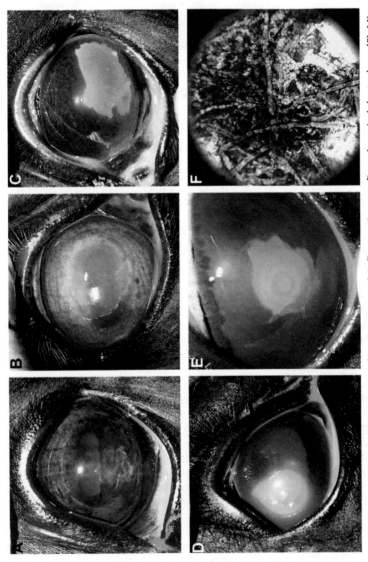

Fig. 12. Cytologic evaluation is essential: (*A*) Absence of pathogens and inflammation confirmed an indolent ulcer. (*B*) Microscopic plant parts confirmed a foreign body ulcer. (*C*) Abundant eosinophils confirmed eosinophilic keratitis. (*D*) Abundant extracellular Gram and cocci confirmed bacterial keratitis. (*E*) Abundant fungal hyphae confirmed mycotic keratitis. (*F*) 100× magnification showing fungal hyphae in previous figure.

Failure to institute appropriate treatment of ulcers with noninfectious causes may result in a nonhealing ulcer that will persist for months.

Treatment choice for corneal ulcers depends on the severity of signs, horse temperament, and farm resources as well as cause.[14] Initial selection of treatment on the farm, summarized in **Table 3**, follows basic principles of reducing pathogen presence and debris, controlling pain and secondary uveitis, minimizing collagenolytic activity, and providing broad-spectrum anti-infectives to sterilize the ocular surface. Topical therapy with ointments is effective for many cases of ulcerative keratitis, but installation of an SPL system at the emergency call is appropriate for severe cases and therapy may need to shift to an SPL later if the case is refractory.

Treatment prescribed at the emergency may need modification once cytology results are known. At that point either the owner is contacted to change the spectrum of topicals or another visit is scheduled to address the ulcer cause. Treatment may need further modification when culture results are available. The reader is directed to current references reviewing therapeutic details of the spectrum of agents in use for ulcerative keratitis treatment.[15,16] Follow-up will involve additional visits to assess progress.

A descemetocele is a deep ulcer where stroma is absent; these serious ulcers do not stain with fluorescein and appear black. Referral of these rare cases may be indicated because they are at risk for perforation and will require intense medical or possibly surgical treatment.

A stromal abscess is another painful corneal condition that presents with blepharospasm and epiphora. However, in contrast to ulcerative keratitis, surface staining with fluorescein is negative because the epithelium is intact. Stromal abscesses present as focal, usually singular, round yellow, tan, or white opacities buried within the deeper layers of the cornea (**Fig. 13**B). The lesion is often surrounded by a halo of edema and/or infiltrate; vascularization may be present or absent. Secondary uveitis, manifesting as miosis ± flare, hypopyon, or hyphema, is severe. Recognition of stromal abscesses is critical; if the focal opacity is not noted and negative surface staining causes a case to be misdiagnosed as equine recurrent uveitis (ERU) and consequently

Table 3		
Clinical guidelines for treatment of infectious keratitis		
Therapy	**Reason**	**Agents Prescribed**
Mydriatic	Dilate pupil, treat secondary uveitis	Topical atropine ointment or eye drops, 1–2×/day
Anticollagenase	Protect corneal integrity	Topical autologous serum, dilute EDTA, or 5%–10% acetylcysteine, 4–6×/day
Antibacterial	Treat bacterial keratitis, prevent secondary infection	Topical triple antibiotic or chloramphenicol ointment, or tobramycin, ciprofloxacin, ofloxacin, gatifloxacin, or moxifloxacin eye drops, 4–6×/day
+/− Antifungal	Treat mycotic keratitis	Topical voriconazole or miconazole solution, or itraconazole/DMSO ointment, 4–6×/day
Systemic NSAIDs	Treat ocular pain and secondary uveitis	Oral flunixin meglumine, phenylbutazone, firocoxib 1–2×/day

Abbreviation: DMSO, dimethyl sulfoxide.
Noninfectious causes may require additional interventions.

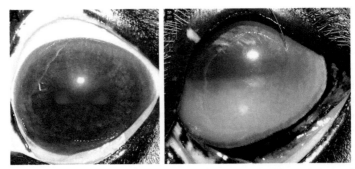

Fig. 13. (*A*) Equine recurrent uveitis (ERU). Cardinal signs are miosis and lack of stain uptake, +/− circumlimbal edema, and vascularization. (*B*) Stromal abscess. Focal opacity, +/− asymmetric infiltrate, or edema are distinguishing features.

treated with topical corticosteroids, the eye will worsen rapidly and vision may be lost. Stromal abscesses are often caused by fungal infections buried deep in the cornea; prognosis is guarded and management must be intense so referral may be needed for optimal treatment.[17]

Horses occasionally present with a foreign body embedded in the cornea. The material is usually vegetative material. Treatment must not risk driving the foreign body deeper into the cornea. The corneal surface around the object is flushed using a 12-mL syringe to force a stream of sterile saline through the broken off hub of a 25-gauge needle. The pressure generated is often sufficient to dislodge the body[18] (**Fig. 14A–14C**). If that approach is unsuccessful, an attempt is made to "scoop" the body out with a 2-mm biopsy punch, an ophthalmic foreign body spud, or careful direction of the bevel of a 20-gauge needle under the "piercing" end of the body. If such efforts do not dislodge the foreign material, referral is appropriate.

Corneal lacerations that penetrate the central stroma and/or result in a stromal flap are rare, but serious. Referral to a tertiary center is indicated if the laceration extends to 50% or more of the stromal depth, as the eye is at risk for rupture. Lacerations that are shallow may be amenable to management with installation of an SPL and frequent administration of mydriatic, anti-infective, and anticollagenase therapy. Some small flaps can be amputated with curved Stevens tenotomy scissors and the exposed ulcerated cornea managed with intense topical treatment, but deep or large flaps require referral for resolution.

INTRAOCULAR EMERGENCIES

Horses that present with eyes that are closed, red, and/or photophobic may have ERU. ERU can affect one or both eyes and can present acutely or as chronic, insidious inflammation of various anatomic regions of the globe. The cardinal signs of acute ERU are miosis, lack of fluorescein stain uptake on the ocular surface, and absence of focal opacity in the cornea that would indicate a stromal abscess (see **Fig. 13**A and **B**).[19] Signs of corneal inflammation may include deep circumlimbal neovascularization and symmetric edema or haze. The anterior chamber may harbor flare, fibrin, hypopyon, or hyphema. In addition to miosis, the iris may have a muddy appearance. If vitritis is present the fundus image will appear hazy with an orange or green tint. Hypotension of the globe is common; an IOP of less than 12 mm Hg is suspicious for uveitis. Horses with chronic or persistent ERU may present with synechia, cataracts, lens luxation, vitritis, and/or focal chorioretinitis or retinal detachment.

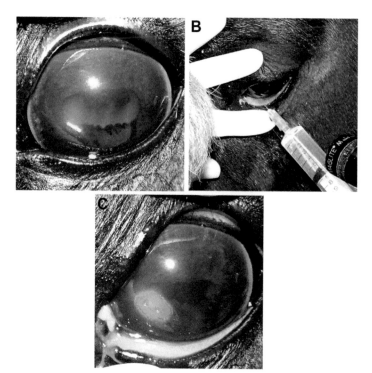

Fig. 14. (*A*) Wood sliver embedded in cornea. (*B*) A stream of saline successfully removed the sliver. (*C*) Entry and egress tract are seen.

ERU is suspected if the horse presents with any combination of the aforementioned signs, especially if it is an at-risk breed (Appaloosa, other spotted breed, Warmblood, or draft horse). Diagnosis includes staining the corneal surface with fluorescein and careful examination to rule out an ulcer or stromal abscess. Treatment of ERU focuses on controlling pain, quelling inflammation, and opening up the pupil. Topical atropine sulfate ointment or eye drops are prescribed, initially 2 to 4 times per day, tapered to once daily administration once dilation is confirmed, and combined with a topical corticosteroid, usually dexamethasone ointment, which is started 4 times daily and then tapered over several weeks. A systemic NSAID (flunixin meglumine or phenylbutazone) is administered intravenously and continued in an oral format. In some instances, oral corticosteroids are prescribed. ERU is by definition a chronic disease that progresses to vision loss in at least 50% of cases; owners should be counseled to plan frequent monitoring.

Horses that present with a cornea showing complete or regional bluish white opacity may have glaucoma (**Fig. 15**). Loss of transparency is due to stromal edema from endothelial dysfunction; tonometry is indicated as part of the ocular examination. An IOP greater than 30 mm Hg is suspicious for glaucoma; horses with eyes that are "big and blue" often present with IOP between 40 and 80 mm Hg. Most cases of glaucoma are secondary to chronic, persistent ERU; medication to reduce uveitis is appropriate in addition to topical treatment that reduces production of aqueous humor.[20] Eye drops containing a β-blocker (timolol maleate) +/− a carbonic anhydrase inhibitor (dorzolamide) are prescribed to reduce ciliary body production of aqueous; signs may improve with concurrent administration of topical and/or systemic corticosteroids.

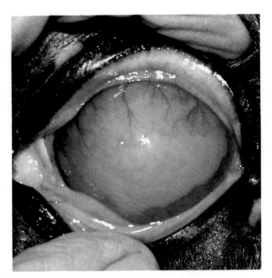

Fig. 15. Chronic glaucoma.

Prognosis for retention of vision in horses with ERU that progress to glaucoma is poor. Diffuse stromal edema signals a loss of endothelial function that may be complicated by a rupture of Descemet's membrane. A condition called bullous keratopathy may result wherein the opaque cornea develops small blister-like bullae on the surface as well as limbal vascularization (**Fig. 16**). Options for treatment of these cases are limited; once vision is lost enucleation may be required to control pain.

Occasionally horses suffer severe trauma that causes globe rupture or irreversible blinding intraocular damage. The weakest region of globe anatomy is the limboscleral junction; severe trauma mandates close inspection of this region. The presence of

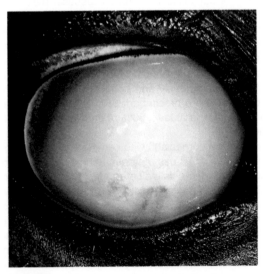

Fig. 16. Bullous keratopathy.

hyphema that occupies more than 50% of the anterior chamber is a grave prognostic sign. Treatment of severe trauma should center on immediate control of pain and uveitis. Re-evaluation of the neural and visual pathway a few days after the trauma will determine if vision is salvageable. Eyes that suffer blinding damage often require enucleation.

CLINICS CARE POINTS

- Patient head support, sedation and regional anesthesia are required for examination and treatment of serious ophthalmic emergencies.

- Subconjunctival injection of a small amount of local anesthetic provides good corneal desensitization if topical anesthetic is ineffective.

- Corneal cytology is indicated for all corneal ulcers; results will dictate targeted therapy.

- Transpalpebral ultrasound aids in diagnosis of orbital rim fractures, lens luxation and retinal detachment.

- Eyelid tears should be repaired in two layers, using small gauge (4-0) suture.

- Miosis is a cardinal sign of ERU as well as stromal abscesses. Careful examination is required to distinguish the two conditions.

- While many eyes with ERU initially present with low IOP, most cases of glaucoma (high IOP) are secondary to chronic ERU. Glaucoma is difficult to control in horses and usually results in blindness.

DISCLOSURE

I have no commercial or financial conflicts of interest, and I have no funding sources to disclose.

REFERENCES

1. Dwyer AE. Practical Field Ophthalmology. In: Equine Ophthalmology. 3rd ed. Ames, IA: BC Gilger; 2017. p. 91.
2. Labelle AL, Clark-Price SC. Anesthesia for ophthalmic procedures in the standing horse. Vet Clin North Am Equine Pract 2013;29(1):179–91.
3. Allbaugh RA. How to perform a thorough equine eye exam in the field. Am Assoc Equine Pract Proc 2013;59:145–8.
4. Dwyer AE. How to obtain and interpret corneal cytology samples. Am Assoc Equine Pract Proc 2017;63:154–66.
5. Stoppini R, Gilger BC. Equine ocular examination basic techniques. In: Equine Ophthalmology. 3rd ed. Ames, IA: BC Gilger; 2017. p. 21–2.
6. Dwyer AE. How to insert and manage a subpalpebral lavage system. Am Assoc Equine Pract Proc 2013;59:164–73.
7. Hallowell GD, Bowen IM. Practical ultrasonography of the equine eye. Equine Vet Educ 2007;12:600–4.
8. Dwyer AE. How to take digital photographs of equine eyes in practice. Am Assoc Equine Pract Proc 2010;56:1–10.
9. Available at: http://www.theeyephone.com/. Tutorials on cell phone ocular photography, Accessed August 1, 2020.
10. Hendrix DV. How to repair eyelid lacerations. AAEP Proc 2013;59:149–54.

11. Henriksen MD. Standing ophthalmic surgery-how to perform standing surgery of the periocular region in the field. Am Assoc Equine Pract Proc 2017;63:139–53.

12. Brooks DE, Mathews A, Clode AB. Diseases of the cornea. In: Equine Ophthalmology. 3rd ed. Ames, IA: BC Gilger; 2017. p. 252–368.

13. Monk C. How to diagnose the cloudy eye. Am Assoc Equine Pract Proc 2013;59: 181–6.

14. Brooks DE. How to use the clinical examination to determine the significance of abnormalities of the horse cornea and adnexa. Am Assoc Equine Pract Proc 2014;60:19–25.

15. Clode AB. Therapy of infectious keratitis: a review. Equine Vet J Suppl 2010;37: 19–23.

16. Nunnery C. How to select appropriate treatment for corneal ulcers. Am Assoc Equine Pract Proc 2017;63:167–78.

17. Brooks DE. How to recognize and treat corneal stromal abscesses. Am Assoc Equine Pract Proc 2017;63:179–85.

18. LaBelle AL. Use of hydropulsion for the treatment of superficial corneal foreign bodies: 15 cases (1999-2013). J Am Vet Med Assoc 2014;244(4):476–9.

19. Gilger BC, Hollingsworth SR. Diseases of the uvea, uveitis and recurrent uveitis. In: Equine Ophthalmology. 3rd ed. Ames, IA: BC Gilger; 2017. p. 369–415.

20. Wilkie DA, Gemensky-Metzler AJ, Lassaline M, et al. Glaucoma. In: Equine Ophthalmology. 3rd ed. Ames, IA: BC Gilger; 2017. p. 453–68.

Antimicrobial Selection for the Equine Practitioner

W. David Wilson, BVMS, MS*, K. Gary Magdesian, DVM, CVA

KEYWORDS

- Horses • Infection • Antimicrobial • Stewardship • Resistance • Susceptibility
- Treatment • Extralabel

KEY POINTS

- Antimicrobial drugs frequently play a central role in the therapeutic management of mature horses and foals with a variety of bacterial illnesses, including those requiring critical care.
- The rapidly progressive course of infection often necessitates implementation of empirical antimicrobial treatment before culture and susceptibility test results are available. Empirical initial treatment should take into account the likely identity of the infecting organisms, the likely antimicrobial susceptibility of those organisms, and several other factors.
- The emergence of antimicrobial resistance in human and animal pathogens has led the World Health Organization (WHO) to categorize antimicrobials based on their importance to human health and to the concept of antimicrobial stewardship, which promotes judicious use to preserve the utility of antimicrobials in the future.
- Of the seven available antimicrobial drugs or combinations approved by the Food and Drug Administration (FDA) for use in horses, four are designated as being of critical importance to human health.
- The paucity of FDA-approved antimicrobials marketed for use in horses frequently necessitates extralabel drug use and places increased responsibility on the prescribing veterinarian.
- The inconsistent and often poor absorption of orally administered drugs in adult horses limits the serum concentrations that are attained and often necessitates use of more conservative interpretive breakpoints for susceptibility than are used for humans.

INTRODUCTION

Diseases caused by primary or secondary bacterial infection are commonly encountered in horses and may contribute to malfunction or failure of single or multiple organs. Consequently, antimicrobial drugs play an important, and often central, role in the therapeutic management of mature horses and foals with a variety of illnesses, including those requiring critical care. Antimicrobial use must be based on rational

Department of Medicine (VM: VME), School of Veterinary Medicine, University of California-Davis, Davis, CA 95616, USA
* Corresponding author.
E-mail address: wdwilson@ucdavis.edu

Vet Clin Equine 37 (2021) 461–494
https://doi.org/10.1016/j.cveq.2021.04.012
0749-0739/21/© 2021 Elsevier Inc. All rights reserved.

principles involving thorough patient evaluation and sound clinical judgment that indicate a high likelihood that the patient has a bacterial infection and that antimicrobials are indicated to promote recovery. Thereafter, actual or predicted information regarding the identity of bacterial species involved in the particular disease syndrome, measured or predicted susceptibility profiles of likely bacterial isolates, and the antimicrobial spectrum, mode of action, indications, dose, ease of administration, cost, and potential adverse effects of selected antimicrobials are important considerations.[1] These considerations become the basis for formulation of a dosage regimen appropriate to the infectious agent, the disease process, the patient, and the caretaker, after assessment of the benefits and risks of the chosen treatment.[1] The ultimate aim of antimicrobial treatment is to inflict an insult on infecting bacteria sufficient to kill the organism or render it susceptible to inactivation by natural host defenses or the local microenvironment without adversely affecting the patient.[1]

ANTIMICROBIAL STEWARDSHIP, CRITICALLY IMPORTANT ANTIMICROBIALS, AND EXTRALABEL DRUG USE

Equine practitioners have many issues to consider when deciding whether antimicrobials are indicated for treatment of a particular patient and which antimicrobial regimen to choose. Such antimicrobial use is implemented on the backdrop of concern for ever-increasing acquired resistance of bacteria isolated from humans and animals (including horses) to existing antimicrobial drugs and the paucity of new drugs coming to market.[2] These and other concerns have led the World Health Organization (WHO) to designate drugs of critical importance to human health and to the concept of antimicrobial stewardship (AMS).[2,3] This concept places responsibility on practicing clinicians (human and veterinary) to be judicious in their use of antimicrobials so as to minimize the emergence and spread of antimicrobial resistance (AMR) and preserve the future utility of antimicrobials that are important to human and animal health.[2,3]

Although AMR in equine bacterial pathogens seems to be less widespread and to be developing less rapidly than AMR in human pathogens, several notable examples have emerged over the past few decades and now pose real challenges, particularly in referral hospitals.[2] These include methicillin-resistant *Staphylococcus aureus*; extended-spectrum ß-lactamase-producing *Escherichia coli*; and multidrug resistance (ie, resistance to drugs from three or more antimicrobial classes) in *E coli* and in opportunists, including those often referred to as ESKAPE pathogens (*Enterococcus faecium*, methicillin-resistant *S aureus*, *Klebsiella pneumoniae*, *Acinetobacter baumanii*, *Pseudomonas aeruginosa*, and *Enterobacter* spp).[2,4–6] Additionally, increasing resistance of *Clostridium difficile* to metronidazole and of *Rhodococcus equi* to rifampin and macrolides are disturbing recent trends.[7–10] AMR has been associated with poorer treatment outcomes for infections in several body systems of horses.[11,12]

An in-depth discussion of AMS is beyond the scope of this article; therefore, the reader is referred to several excellent recent reviews on the subject.[2,13–17] The general approach is multifaceted and is aimed at continuous improvement embodied in the "5R" approach: responsibility, review, refinement, reduction, and replacement.[2,17,18] Important elements of AMS programs include development, use, and review of practice guidelines for antimicrobial use; prevention and control of infection; use of clinical microbiology; surveillance of antimicrobial use and AMR; dosage, pharmacokinetics, and pharmacodynamics of antimicrobials; regulation; education; owner compliance; leadership; coordination; and measurement.[2,19] A model AMS approach, the "Protect ME" program developed by the British Equine Veterinary Association in 2012, has gained increasing traction in Britain in recent years and, in those practices in which it has become an integral component of the practice culture, has resulted in substantial reduction in use of critically important antimicrobials (CIAs).[20,21] Implementation has been greatly facilitated by development of a useful multimedia Protect ME toolkit, an important component of which is peer review of antimicrobial prescribing practices by individual veterinarians and practices as a whole.[20] Whereas equine veterinarians in the United Kingdom and Europe seem to be several years ahead of practitioners here in North America with regard to AMS, we are in the fortunate position of being able to avail ourselves of excellent educational materials that already exist.

Decision-making by the practitioner regarding choice of antimicrobial treatment regimens is further complicated by the paucity of antimicrobials that are Food and Drug Administration (FDA)-approved for parenteral or oral use in horses; therefore, extralabel drug use is frequently necessary and the prescribing clinician must shoulder an increased responsibility for adverse events. Extralabel use of antimicrobials in horses in the United States is permitted under the provisions of the Animal Medicinal Drug Use Clarification Act of 1994.[22] This act includes the provision that there is no approved new animal drug that is labeled for the proposed use (eg, treatment of systemic sepsis in a foal) or that contains the same active ingredient that is in the required dosage form and concentration, except where a veterinarian finds, within the context of a valid veterinarian-client-patient relationship, that the approved new animal drug is clinically ineffective for its intended use. This latter statement implies that the patient has failed to respond to an appropriate course of treatment with an FDA-approved drug at an approved dose, dosing interval, and route of administration before another drug can be used on that patient in an extralabel manner.[22] Extralabel drug use is defined not only by whether the drug in question is approved by the FDA for use in horses, but also whether the treatment indication (eg, strangles), dose, dosing interval, route of administration, and treatment duration comply with approved label directions for use (**Table 1**). In several instances, the FDA-approved dose is suboptimal (eg, procaine penicillin G and ampicillin sodium), the approved dosing interval is longer than optimal (eg, procaine penicillin G and one of the available trimethoprim-sulfadiazine products), or the commonly used route of administration is not approved (eg, amikacin, gentamicin, and ceftiofur sodium are not approved for intravenous [IV] use).

The information presented in **Table 1** may surprise some veterinarians, because extralabel use of antimicrobials is necessary and so routine in equine practice in North America that little thought is typically given to this issue. The following are but a few of the many examples of treatment protocols that are used regularly in equine practice in North America but may not intuitively be considered by practitioners as representing extralabel drug use:

1. IV injection of amikacin (20 mg/kg every 24 hours) or gentamicin (6.6 mg/kg every 24 hours) to treat systemic sepsis (reason for extralabel designation: nonapproved route, dose, and disease indication).
2. IV use of ceftiofur sodium to treat peritonitis (nonapproved route and disease indication).
3. Intramuscular (IM) administration of procaine penicillin G at a dose of 22,000 IU/kg every 12 hours to treat upper respiratory tract infection (nonapproved dose and dosing interval).
4. Oral administration of trimethoprim-sulfamethoxazole at a dose of 30 mg/kg every 12 hours to treat upper respiratory tract infection (use of a nonapproved potentiated sulfonamide product when several approved products containing trimethoprim-sulfadiazine are available for the stated disease indication).

Table 1
Details of active FDA approvals and WHO designations of antimicrobial drugs approved for use in horses in the United States[3]

Antimicrobial Drugs	Preparation	Approved Route	Approved Dose	Approved Indication	WHO Designation
Ceftiofur, Na	Aqueous solution (50 mg/mL after reconstitution of dry powder)	IM	2.2–4.4 mg/kg q 24 h for up to 10 d	Respiratory infection associated with *Streptococcus equi* subsp. *zooepidemicus*	CIA-HP1
Ceftiofur, crystalline free acid	Aqueous suspension (200 mg/mL)	IM	6.6 mg/kg on Day 1, repeated on Day 4 (no more than 20 mL per injection site)	Respiratory disease caused by *S equi* subsp. *zooepidemicus*	CIA-HP1
Ampicillin, Na	Aqueous solution (300 mg/mL) after reconstitution of dry powder	IV, IM	6.6 mg/kg q 12 h[a]	Respiratory, soft tissue, and skin infections (wounds, abscesses)	CIA-HP2
Amikacin sulfate	Aqueous solution (250 mg/mL)	IU	Infuse 2.0 g mixed in 200 mL saline q 24 h for 3 d	Treatment of uterine infection in mares caused by susceptible organisms	CIA-HP2
Gentamicin sulfate	Aqueous solution (100 mg/mL)	IU	Infuse 2.0–2.5 g diluted with 200–500 mL saline IU q 24 h for 3–5 d	Control of uterine infection in mares and as an aid to improved conception	CIA-HP2
Penicillin G, procaine	Aqueous suspension (300,000 IU/mL)	IM	6600 IU/kg q 24 h[a] for up to 4 d (no more than 10 mL per injection site)	Strangles caused by *S equi* subsp. *equi*	HIA
TMP-SDZ	Aqueous suspension (333 mg SDZ + 67 mg TMP = 400 mg/mL)	PO	24 mg/kg of combination PO q 12 h for 10 d	Lower respiratory tract infection caused by susceptible strains of *S equi* subsp. *zooepidemicus*	HIA
TMP-SDZ	Powder	PO	30 mg/kg of combination PO q 24 h[b] for 5–7 d	Acute strangles, respiratory tract infection, acute urogenital infection, wound infection, abscess	HIA

| PYR-SDZ | Suspension of 250 mg SDZ + 12.5 mg PYR/mL | PO | 20 mg/kg of SDZ + 1 mg/kg PYR (4 mL/50 kg) PO q 24 h for 90–270 d | Equine protozoal myeloencephalopathy | HIA |

Abbreviations: CIA-HP1, critically important highest priority antimicrobial; CIA-HP2, critically important high priority antimicrobial; HIA, highly important antimicrobial; IU, intrauterine; PYR, pyrimethamine; SDZ, sulfadiazine; TMP, trimethoprim.
[a] Approved dose is lower than recommended dose.
[b] Approved dosing frequency is lower than recommended dosing frequency.

The WHO has classified antimicrobials into three categories according to their level of importance to human health: (1) critically important (CIA), (2) highly important (HIA), and (3) important (IA).[3] The CIA category is further divided into highest priority (CIA-HP1) and high priority (CIA-HP2). Two classification criteria (C1 and C2) and three prioritization factors (P1, P2, P3) are used to assign the level of importance to human health, taking into account that all antimicrobials used in human medicine are designated as IA or higher. Classification C1 is assigned to an antimicrobial class that is the sole, or one of limited number of therapies available, to treat serious bacterial infections in people. Antimicrobials of C2 are used to treat infections in people caused by bacteria that may be transmitted to humans from nonhuman sources, or may acquire resistance genes from nonhuman sources.[3] Prioritization factor P1 is assigned when a large number of people in the community or in certain high-risk populations are affected by diseases for which there are limited antimicrobial choices. Factor P2 is assigned when there is a high frequency of use of the antimicrobial class for any indication in human medicine or in certain high-risk groups and such use may favor selection of resistance. An antimicrobial class designated P3 is used to treat infections in people for which there is already extensive evidence of transmission of resistant bacteria (eg, nontyphoidal *Salmonella* spp and *Campylobacter* spp) or resistance genes (high for *E coli* and *Enterococcus* spp) from nonhuman sources. Criteria and prioritization factors applied for categorization of antimicrobial classes are as follows[3]:

- CIA-HP1: Meet C1 and C2, and all prioritization factors (P1+P2+P3).
- CIA-HP2: Meet C1 and C2, and one or more prioritization factors.
- HIA: Meet either C1 or C2 but not both.
- IA: Used in humans but meet neither C1 or C2.

Of the seven antimicrobial agents licensed for parenteral or oral administration to horses in North America, one (ceftiofur) is assigned CIA-HP1, three (amikacin, gentamicin, and ampicillin) are CIA-HP2, and three (penicillin G, trimethoprim-sulfadiazine, pyrimethamine-sulfadiazine) are HIA (see **Table 1**). Please note that the drug doses detailed in **Table 1** shows the FDA-approved doses and may differ from doses in common use based on results of pharmacokinetic, bacterial susceptibility, and other studies.

PRINCIPLES OF RESPONSIBLE ANTIMICROBIAL USE

Adherence to the following principles contributes to responsible AMS and serves as a guide for antimicrobial use in horses. However, the authors recognize that not all principles can be followed, particularly in the critical care patient because progression of the disease process is frequently rapid and delay in initiating antimicrobial treatment would adversely impact survival.[1,23–26] In particular, the identity and susceptibility profile of the etiologic agent is rarely known when therapy is initiated, extralabel drug use is frequently necessary, and combination therapy with more than one antibiotic is often indicated in critical care patients because a mixed infection is likely or the suspected infecting organism has an unpredictable antimicrobial susceptibility profile. Although the term "antimicrobial stewardship" is a recent addition to the vocabulary of veterinarians, the principles on which it is based have been in existence for many decades and are summarized in the following questions or issues that the clinician should consciously consider before prescribing an antimicrobial drug:

1. Is an infectious bacterial agent involved in the disease process?
    a. Antimicrobials are not indicated for treatment of noninfectious inflammatory disease (eg, inflammatory airway disease) or viral respiratory tract infection unless secondary bacterial infection is present.

2. Is antimicrobial treatment necessary to rid the host of the infectious agent?
3. Is the identity of the infecting agent known or at least reasonably suspected based on clinical findings and/or results of tests that can be obtained quickly (eg, cytologic examination with Gram stain)?
4. What are the most appropriate samples for collection and submission to the laboratory for pathogen identification tests cytologic examination and culture of appropriately collected samples, or through use of pathogen identification techniques, such as polymerase chain reaction or matrix-assisted laser desorption ionization time-of-flight mass spectrometry (MALDI-TOF MS)?
5. Are the infecting organisms likely to be susceptible to the available antimicrobial drugs under consideration? Confirm by susceptibility testing of bacteria isolated above.
6. Are host defense mechanisms sufficiently active to contribute to the patient's recovery?
7. Are ancillary treatments (eg, drainage, debridement, lavage) available and appropriate to remove infected debris and reduce the bacterial load?
8. Will therapeutic concentrations of the drug be achieved at the site of infection and will the microenvironment at this site support activity of the drug?
9. Can I use a narrow-spectrum drug rather than a broad-spectrum drug?
   a. Unless a mixed infection is likely or the suspected infecting organism likely has an unpredictable susceptibility pattern, narrower spectrum drugs are preferred.
10. Can I avoid concurrent use of more than one antimicrobial drug?
    a. Concurrent use of more than one antimicrobial drug is discouraged except under the following circumstances:
       i. Life-threatening conditions: insufficient time to wait for culture and susceptibility results.
       ii. Mixed infections: more than one drug is needed to provide the appropriate antimicrobial spectrum.
       iii. Need for synergistic activity (eg, penicillin G and an aminoglycoside).
11. Is there a drug available that is FDA-approved for use in horses and is likely to be effective for the intended indication when used via the approved route, at the approved dose, and for the intended duration?
12. If not, is there a drug available that is FDA-approved for use in horses and is likely to be effective for the intended indication when used via a nonapproved route or at a nonapproved dose?
13. If not, is there a drug available that is FDA-approved for use in animals or people, is likely to be safe and effective for the intended indication, and is available in a suitable dosage form without the need for other than "horse side" compounding (eg, grinding tablets and mixing with water to prepare a suspension for oral administration)?
14. If not, is there a drug available that is FDA-approved for use in animals or people, is likely to be safe and effective for the intended indication, and can be compounded into a suitable dosage form?
15. Can I avoid using an antimicrobial that is critically important to human health (CIA)? The goal should be to use the drug or drugs with the lowest WHO classification (IA<HIA<CIA-HP2<CIA-HP1) that will likely be effective for the intended indication without compromising the outcome for the patient. It is often difficult to comply with this latter stipulation because there are few published controlled studies comparing the efficacy of different antimicrobial regimens for treating specific infections in horses.

16. Be aware that supportive therapy often plays a role at least as important as antimicrobials in promoting a positive outcome, and adverse effects of antimicrobial drugs used individually or in combination may actually lead to negative consequences.
17. Adverse reactions should be recognized, investigated, and reported to the manufacturer of the drug and, in the United States, to the FDA/Center for Veterinary Medicine (1–888–332–8387 or 1–888-FDA-VETS; www.fda.gov/cvm/), or to the Veterinary Practitioners' Reporting Network (USPPRN) of the US Pharmacopeia (1–800–487–7776 or 1–800-4-USPPRN; www.usp.org/).

UTILITY AND INTERPRETATION OF CULTURE AND SUSCEPTIBILITY TESTING RESULTS

Culture of appropriately collected samples from sites of infection and susceptibility testing of bacterial isolates obtained should be pursued whenever possible before starting antimicrobial treatment and is a requirement for use of CIAs in many countries.[2] By helping guide selection of the appropriate antimicrobial drug and dosing regimen, culture and susceptibility testing aids in maximizing the potential for therapeutic success of an antimicrobial on an individual horse level, and in reducing acquisition of resistance among bacterial isolates affecting horses at the population level. Antimicrobial susceptibility tests are typically performed by either the disk diffusion (Kirby Bauer) or the broth or plate microdilution. The microdilution test is the preferred susceptibility test because it provides quantitative information (minimum inhibitory concentration [MIC]) that is helpful for selecting dose and route of administration, whereas the disk diffusion test provides only qualitative information (susceptible [S] or resistant [R]).

Interpreting susceptibility test results from the microbiology laboratory is more complex than simply looking for the "S" versus "R" interpretation on the report. It is important to evaluate the actual MIC value reported or, if not reported, it should warrant a call to the diagnostic laboratory. The MIC is defined as the lowest concentration of an antimicrobial that prevents visible growth of bacteria in the diffusion susceptibility test. The susceptibility breakpoint is an antimicrobial drug concentration, usually determined by the Clinical Laboratory Standards Institute, that defines whether a species of bacteria is considered to be susceptible to the antimicrobial tested in the context of the drug concentrations that can be achieved in a particular patient using commonly accepted dosing regimens.[27] This latter statement is particularly important to consider for orally administered drugs because, with the exception of foals in some instances, absorption of orally administered drugs in horses is generally poor and is often further compromised by administration after feeding. Concentrations that can be achieved in blood and tissues are generally substantially lower than those achieved in humans, the species for which breakpoints were initially established by Clinical Laboratory Standards Institute, making interpretive breakpoints established in people inapplicable to horses. Use of the human breakpoints could lead to a false sense of security that the chosen antibiotics will be effective, when in actuality horses cannot achieve the high plasma or tissue concentrations necessary to be effective. Fortunately, the Clinical Laboratory Standards Institute has increased the number of recommended equine-specific susceptibility breakpoints for antimicrobials as new research and results of pharmacokinetic studies have become available.[27] **Tables 2** and **3** list antimicrobial drugs that are used parenterally or orally in horses, together with recommended doses, equine-specific breakpoints for susceptibility, the WHO classification of level of importance to human or animal health, and whether the stated use is on-label or extralabel. The recommended dosing regimen for a particular antimicrobial may be different from that approved by the FDA.

Table 2
Recommended doses, equine-specific breakpoints, WHO classification, and extralabel status of antimicrobials administered parenterally to horses

Antimicrobial	Recommended Dose	Route	Extralabel Use?	Breakpoint (μg/mL)			WHO Class
				S	I	R	
Penicillin G, procaine	22,000 IU/kg q 12–24 h	IM	Yes	≤0.5	1.0	≥2	HIA
Penicillin G, Na or K	22,000–44,000 IU/kg q 6 h	IV	Yes	≤0.5	1.0	≥2	HIA
Ampicillin, Na	25–40 mg/kg q 6 h	IV, IM	Yes	≤0.25		≥0.5	CIA-HP2
Amoxicillin, Na	20–40 mg/kg q 6–12 h	IV, IM	Yes	≤0.25		≥0.5	CIA-HP2
Amikacin[a] (adult)	10–20 mg/kg q 24 h	IV, IM	Yes	≤4.0[a]	8.0	≥16.0	CIA-HP2
Amikacin[a] (foal)	20–25 mg/kg q 24 h	IV, IM	Yes	≤2.0[a]	4.0	≥8.0	CIA-HP2
Gentamicin[a] (adult)	6.6 mg/kg q 24 h	IV, IM	Yes	≤2.0[a]	4.0	≥8.0	CIA-HP2
Gentamicin[a] (foal)	8.8 mg/kg q 24 h	IV, IM	Yes	≤2.0[a]	4.0	≥8.0	CIA-HP2
Cefazolin[a] (1st-generation)	20–25 mg/kg q 6–8 h	IV	Yes	≤2.0[a]	4.0	≥8.0	HIA
Ceftiofur[a,b], Na (3rd-generation)	2.2–5.0 mg/kg q 12–24 h	IV, IM, SQ	Yes/no[c]	≤2.0[a,b]	4.0	≥8.0	CIA-HP1
Ceftiofur[a,b], crystalline free acid (3rd-generation)	6.6 mg/kg q 72 h	SQ	Yes	≤2.0[a,b]	4.0	≥8.0	CIA-HP1
Cefotaxime[a] (3rd-generation)	25–40 mg/kg q 6 h	IV	Yes	≤1.0[a]	2.0	≥4.0	CIA-HP1
Ceftazidime[a] (3rd-generation)	40 mg/kg q 6–8 h	IV	Yes	≤4.0[a]	8.0	≥16.0	CIA-HP1
Ceftizoxime[a] (3rd-generation)	10–40 mg/kg q 8–12 h	IV, IM	Yes	≤8.0[a]		≥16.0	CIA-HP1
Ceftriaxone[a] (3rd-generation)	25–50 mg/kg q 12 h	IV, IM	Yes	≤1.0[a]	2.0	≥4.0	CIA-HP1
Cefepime[a] (4th-generation)	11 mg/kg q 8 h	IV	Yes	≤2.0[a]		≥4.0	CIA-HP1
Cefquinome[a] (4th-generation)	1–4.5 mg/kg q 6–12 h	IV, IM	Yes	≤2.0[a]		≥4.0	CIA-HP1
Oxacillin	20–40 mg/kg q 6–8 h	IV, IM	Yes	≤4.0		≥8.0	HIA
Oxytetracycline	5–10 mg/kg q 12–24 h	IV	Yes	≤2.0	4.0	≥8.0	HIA
Enrofloxacin[a]	5 mg/kg q 24 h	IV	Yes	≤0.12[a]	0.25	≥0.5	CIA-HP1
Chloramphenicol	25–50 mg/kg q 6–8 h	IV	Yes	≤8.0	16	≥32	HIA
Gamithromycin (foals-only)	6 mg/kg q 7 d	IM	Yes	≤4.0	8.0	≥16.0	CIA-HP1
Ticarcillin-clavulanate	50 mg/kg q 6 h	IV	Yes	≤16.0		≥32.0	CIA-HP2

(continued on next page)

Table 2
(continued)

Antimicrobial	Recommended Dose	Route	Extralabel Use?	Breakpoint (µg/mL)			WHO Class
				S	I	R	
Imipenem-cilastatin	10–15 mg/kg q 8–12 h	IV, IM	Yes	≤1.0	2.0	≥4.0	CIA-HP2
Vancomycin	4.5–7.5 mg/kg q 8 h	IV	Yes	≤1.0		≥2.0	CIA-HP1

[a] Aminoglycosides, cephalosporins, fluoroquinolones, and potentiated sulfonamides are ineffective against *Enterococcus* spp infection in the clinical setting, regardless of measured MIC.
[b] *Streptococcus* spp susceptibility breakpoint for ceftiofur is 0.25 µg/mL.
[c] Depends on whether approved dose and dosing frequency are used.

Table 3
Recommended doses, equine-specific breakpoints, WHO classification, and extralabel status of antimicrobials administered orally to horses

Antimicrobial	Recommended Oral Dose	Extralabel Use?	Breakpoint (μg/mL) S	I	R	WHO Classification
TMP-SDZ	24–30 mg/kg q 12–24 h	Y/Nᵃ	≤0.5/9.5ᵇ	1/18ᵇ	≥2/38ᵇ	HIA
TMP-SMZ	24–30 mg/kg q 12 h	Y	≤0.5/9.5	1/18	≥2/38	HIA
PYR-SDZ	21 mg/kg q 24 h	N	NA	NA	NA	HIA
Doxycycline	10–20 mg/kg q 12 h	Y	≤0.12	0.25	≥0.5	HIA
Minocycline	4 mg/kg q 12 h	Y	≤0.12	0.25	≥0.5	HIA
Enrofloxacin	7.5 mg/kg q 12 h	Y	≤0.12	0.25	≥0.5	CIA-HP1
Rifampin	5 mg/kg q 12 h	Y	≤1.0	2.00	≥4.0	CIA-HP1
Erythromycinᶜ	20–25 mg/kg q 6–8 h	Y	≤0.5	1–4	≥8.0	CIA-HP1
Azithromycinᶜ	10 mg/kg q 24 h, then q 48 h	Y	≤2.0	4	≥8.0	CIA-HP1
Clarithromycinᶜ	7.5 mg/kg q 12 h	Y	≤2.0	4	≥8.0	CIA-HP1
Chloramphenicol	50 mg/kg q 6–8 h	Y	≤1.0		≥2.0	HIA
Cefpodoximeᶜ	10 q 6–12 h	Y	≤2.0	4	≥8.0	CIA-HP1
Metronidazole	15 mg/kg q 8 h oral or 20 mg/kg q 8 h per rectum	Y	≤8.0	16	≥32	IA

Abbreviations: PYR, pyrimethamine; SDZ, sulfadiazine; SMZ, sulfamethoxazole; TMP, trimethoprim.
ᵃ Optimal dosing interval is every 12 hours.
ᵇ MIC results for the trimethoprim and sulfonamide components of the combination are reported. Comments in footnote to **Table 2** regarding interpretation of *Enterococcus* spp susceptibility test also apply to **Table 3**.
ᶜ For use only in foals age 4 months or younger; unsafe for adult horses.

BACTERIA ASSOCIATED WITH DISEASE SYNDROMES IN HORSES

In critical care situations, there is insufficient time to wait for results of culture and susceptibility testing of samples before initiating antimicrobial therapy.[26,28] The appropriate approach is therefore to:

a. Collect and submit appropriate samples for culture and susceptibility testing.
b. Begin treatment based on knowledge of bacteria most likely to be involved in particular syndromes/clinical presentations and their most likely susceptibility patterns.
c. Adjust therapy (antimicrobial, dose, route, frequency) based on response to initial treatment, results of initial culture and susceptibility tests, physiologic status of patient, ability to administer antimicrobials by the preferred route (eg, continued IV access), adverse effects, and feasibility (including cost) of treatment.

This approach is predicated on veterinarians having a sound working knowledge of the major bacterial pathogens of horses by body system, age, use, geographic location, and the type of facility on which the horses reside. In referral centers, nosocomial infection with resistant bacteria including *Salmonella* spp, other enteric species, *Staphylococcus* spp, and *C difficile* influence the situation and antibiotic-associated colitis involving *Clostridium* spp or *Salmonella* spp is an ever-present concern. In general, the following are the most commonly encountered bacterial pathogens of horses:

- β-Hemolytic *Streptococcus* spp (*Streptococcus equi* subsp. *zooepidemicus* and *S equi* subsp. *equi*)
- Nonenteric gram-negative bacteria
  Actinobacillus equuli
  Actinobacillus spp
  Pasteurella spp
- Enteric gram-negative bacteria (Enterobacteriales)
  E coli
  K pneumoniae
  Enterobacter spp
  Salmonella spp
- *Corynebacterium pseudotuberculosis* (United States)
- *R equi* (in foals and weanlings)
- *P aeruginosa*
- *Bordetella bronchiseptica*
- Coagulase-positive *Staphylococcus* spp including *S aureus*
- Coagulase-negative *Staphylococcus* spp
- *Enterococcus* spp
- Nonhemolytic *Streptococcus* spp
- Anaerobic gram-negative bacteria
  Bacteroides fragilis
  Bacteroides spp
  Fusobacterium spp
- Anaerobic gram-positive bacteria
  Clostridium spp
  Peptostreptococcus spp

EMPIRICAL SELECTION OF ANTIMICROBIALS TO INITIATE TREATMENT OF INFECTIONS IN HORSES BASED ON LIKELY SUSCEPTIBILITY OF BACTERIAL ISOLATES

Antibacterial susceptibility profiles of bacteria, such as β-hemolytic *Streptococcus* spp, *Actinobacillus* spp, *Pasteurella* spp, and anaerobes, with the exception of *Bacteroides* spp, are somewhat predictable and do not show great variation between different geographic locations. In contrast, Enterobacteriales, *Pseudomonas* spp, *Bordetella* spp, *Enterococcus* spp, coagulase-positive *Staphylococcus* spp, α-hemolytic *Streptococcus* spp, *B fragilis*, and, more recently, *R equi*, have either unpredictable susceptibility or are predictably resistant to particular antibiotics or classes of antibiotics.[28] It is thus particularly important to perform susceptibility tests on these isolates. Clinicians should become familiar with antimicrobial susceptibility patterns of isolates in their practice area, and work with their microbiology laboratories to update information every few years. Although it is acknowledged that there may be substantial variation in susceptibility patterns of bacteria between different geographic locations, and organisms isolated from patients in hospitals or on farms where antibiotics are used frequently are likely to show more resistance than bacteria isolated from horses on premises on which antimicrobial use is not prevalent, the following overall guidelines apply to most situations (**Table 4**). Although these guidelines take into account the desire to limit extralabel drug use, and minimize use of high priority CIAs, the extent to which these goals can be accomplished is limited by the paucity of antimicrobials licensed for use in horses and that four of the seven antimicrobials approved for use in horses are CIAs.

Table 4
Initial choice of antimicrobials for use in horses based on likely susceptibility of bacterial isolates, consideration of WHO classification of antimicrobials, prioritization of "on-label" use, and other factors

Bacterial Species	First Choices Antimicrobials	Alternate Parenterally Administered Options	Other Orally Administered Options
β-Hemolytic Streptococcus spp	Penicillin G	Ampicillin; ceftiofur; cefazolin	TMS; doxycycline; minocycline; chloramphenicol; azithromycin (foals only); rifampin
Coagulase-positive Staphylococcus spp	Amikacin; cefazolin; rifampin (oral); enrofloxacin (IV or oral)	Oxacillin; ceftiofur	Chloramphenicol; azithromycin (foals only)
Coagulase-negative Staphylococcus spp	Amikacin; cefazolin; rifampin (oral)	Enrofloxacin (IV); ceftiofur; gentamicin; oxytetracycline; oxacillin	Enrofloxacin; chloramphenicol; doxycycline; minocycline
Enterococcus spp	Ampicillin	Oxytetracycline	Chloramphenicol; doxycycline; minocycline
Rhodococcus equi (foals)	Clarithromycin + rifampin (both oral); azithromycin + rifampin (both oral)	Gentamicin (IV) + rifampin (oral)	Doxycycline; minocycline
Corynebacterium pseudotuberculosis	TMS (oral); TMS + rifampin (both oral); doxycycline (oral); minocycline (oral); penicillin G (IV or IM)	Enrofloxacin (IV)	Enrofloxacin
Actinobacillus spp Pasteurella spp	TMS (oral); gentamicin; ceftiofur; ampicillin	Penicillin G oxytetracycline	Doxycycline; minocycline; chloramphenicol
Escherichia coli	Amikacin	Gentamicin; ceftiofur; enrofloxacin; ticarcillin/clavulanate	TMS; chloramphenicol; enrofloxacin
Salmonella spp	Amikacin; ceftiofur	Gentamicin; enrofloxacin; other 3rd-generation cephalosporin; oxytetracycline; ticarcillin/clavulanate	Enrofloxacin; chloramphenicol; TMS; doxycycline; minocycline

(continued on next page)

Table 4
(continued)

Bacterial Species	First Choices Antimicrobials	Alternate Parenterally Administered Options	Other Orally Administered Options
Bordetella bronchiseptica	TMS (oral)	Gentamicin; oxytetracycline	Doxycycline; minocycline
Klebsiella pneumoniae	Amikacin	Ceftiofur; enrofloxacin; gentamicin; ticarcillin/clavulanate	Enrofloxacin; chloramphenicol; TMS
Pseudomonas aeruginosa	Amikacin	Ticarcillin/clavulanate; gentamicin; ceftazidime; imipenem	
Bacteroides spp (except *Bacteroides fragilis*)	Metronidazole (oral or intrarectal)	Penicillin G; oxytetracycline	Chloramphenicol; doxycycline; minocycline
Bacteroides fragilis	Metronidazole (oral or intrarectal)	Oxytetracycline	Chloramphenicol; doxycycline; minocycline
Gram-positive (*Clostridium* spp, *Peptostreptococcus* spp) and gram-negative (*Fusobacterium* spp) anaerobic bacteria	Penicillin G; metronidazole (oral or intrarectal)	Oxytetracycline; ceftiofur	Chloramphenicol; doxycycline; minocycline

EMPIRIC SELECTION OF ANTIMICROBIALS FOR INITIATING TREATMENT OF DISEASE SYNDROMES IN HORSES WHILE AWAITING CULTURE AND SUSCEPTIBILITY TEST RESULTS

The following guidelines are based on the most likely etiologic agent; probability of susceptibility of the etiologic agents to antimicrobial drugs; prioritization of "on-label" use; consideration of WHO classification of antimicrobials; and other factors, such as feasibility and ease of administration, potential adverse effects, cost, and human health risks.

Neonatal Septicemia

Blood culture is an important component of the diagnostic work-up of neonatal foals with signs suggestive of systemic or localized sepsis (eg, joint infection).[29,30] Regional and temporal differences have been observed with regard to the distribution of bacterial species causing sepsis in neonatal foals; however, reports from all geographic regions document that a high proportion of septicemic foals are infected with gram-negative bacteria, including E coli (the most common isolate), A equuli, Actinobacillus suis–like spp, K pneumoniae, Enterobacter spp, Citrobacter spp, and Salmonella spp.[4,29–38] As many as 50% of septicemic foals have polymicrobic infection with more than one gram-negative species or with a gram-negative bacterium along with a gram-positive species, usually Streptococcus zooepidemicus, Enterococcus spp, Staphylococcus spp, or non–group D Streptococcus spp.[30,31,38] The prevalence of gram-positive infections is increasing, particularly in hospital-acquired infections,[30,38,39] which emphasizes the need to do repeat blood cultures in hospitalized foals that are not responding well to the initial antimicrobial regimen.[39] Staphylococcus spp, Enterococcus spp, and non–group D Streptococcus spp have unpredictable susceptibility patterns and frequently demonstrate multiple drug resistance (ie, resistance to three or more antimicrobial classes).[30] Anaerobic bacteria are uncommonly involved in neonatal septicemia, except secondary to enterocolitis caused by Clostridium perfringens or Clostridium septicum.[40]

Suggested antimicrobial protocols for treating neonatal septicemia

Treatment protocols for neonatal septicemia must include antimicrobials with a high level of activity against gram-negative enteric bacteria. Because a substantial number of septicemic foals are also infected with gram-positive bacteria and the activity of aminoglycosides against gram-positive organisms is generally poor, inclusion of a gram-positive spectrum antimicrobial drug in the treatment regimen is recommended. Use of bactericidal agents that do not require extensive hepatic metabolism is preferred, as is the parenteral, rather than oral, route of administration. The clinical condition of foals with sepsis declines rapidly if appropriate antimicrobial treatment is not started early in the disease course. Sound evidence was published recently documenting that use of an antimicrobial treatment regimen to which all bacterial isolates were susceptible ("correct choice") resulted in significantly better outcomes than regimens to which one or more isolates were resistant ("incorrect choice").[41]

> First choice: Amikacin + ampicillin. Serum creatinine should be monitored often, and therapeutic drug monitoring of amikacin is recommended during treatment.
> Alternate choices: Amikacin + penicillin G; amikacin + ceftiofur; amikacin + cefazolin; gentamicin + ampicillin, penicillin G, or cefazolin; ceftiofur; other third-generation cephalosporin (eg, cefotaxime, ceftazidime); amikacin or gentamicin + ceftiofur; imipenem (for resistant infections if supported by culture and susceptibility (C&S) results).
> Continued oral therapy: Trimethoprim-sulfonamide (TMS) may be appropriate for continued oral therapy for infections caused by susceptible organisms.

Pneumonia in Foals and Weanlings

Pneumonia in neonatal foals frequently occurs in association with septicemia; therefore, the predominant bacterial isolates and antimicrobials recommended for use are the same as those listed for septicemia in the preceding section.[38,41,42] Polymicrobial infection is common, as it is in older foals and weanlings, in which the most frequent bacterial isolate is S zooepidemicus, followed closely by gram-negative non-enteric bacteria (A equuli, Actinobacillus spp, and Pasteurella spp). E coli, K pneumoniae, other enteric bacteria, B bronchiseptica, P aeruginosa, Staphylococcus spp, and anaerobic bacteria are less commonly involved.[26,42–44] R equi, either alone or as part of a polymicrobic infection with any of the isolates listed previously, is typically the most likely etiologic agent on farms on which R equi infection is endemic and occurs year after year.[43–45]

Morbidity related to respiratory tract infection is high in foals on breeding farms in many geographic regions, approaching 100% on some farms, particularly those on which R equi is endemic.[46–50] The first foal to present with signs of lower respiratory tract infection, such as cough, nasal discharge, tachypnea, altered respiratory character, abnormal auscultation findings, and fever, often represents the tip of the iceberg and close inspection of the group frequently reveals other foals with respiratory tract disease.[47] Whereas early recognition and treatment of those foals with significant lower respiratory tract involvement (pneumonia) is considered to be important to minimize mortality and treatment costs, it should be recognized that spontaneous resolution of infectious respiratory disease occurs in many foals.[46,49,50] The decision whether or not to treat affected foals with antimicrobials and for how long is, therefore, difficult and opinions vary considerably. Although laboratory parameters, such as total white blood cell (WBC) count, neutrophil count, plasma fibrinogen concentration, and serum amyloid A, can provide useful information to inform decisions regarding treatment,[51,52] thoracic ultrasound is likely the most useful diagnostic tool. Ultrasound is a highly sensitive modality that is widely used in the field to screen foals for the presence of pulmonary consolidation, abscesses, and pyogranulomas.[48–50,53] The presence of such lesions raises the index of suspicion of R equi pneumonia, to the extent that many clinicians regard them as sufficient justification to start specific treatment directed at R equi on farms on which R equi is endemic.[53] Similarly, routine prophylactic administration of azithromycin every 48 hours during the first 2 weeks of life has been shown to effectively reduce the cumulative incidence of R equi pneumonia on endemic farms.[54]

Recent studies have concluded that these approaches result in treatment of many foals that would not otherwise develop pneumonia or would resolve their pneumonia without antimicrobial treatment.[49,50] Such approaches undoubtedly contribute to the development of resistance of R equi to macrolides or rifampin, both of which are WHO classified as CIA-HP1, as has been observed increasingly during the last decade.[9,49,55–59] An intermediate approach, whereby cumulative ultrasound lesion scores are calculated and only foals with lesion scores greater than a specific cutoff are treated with antibiotics, has gained favor in recent years.[49,50,58] Depending on the severity of clinical illness, foals with lesion scores lower than the cutoff are monitored clinically and by ultrasound but not treated with antimicrobial drugs.[49,50] This approach, particularly when coupled with culture and susceptibility testing of tracheobronchial aspirates, has not resulted in higher mortality but has substantially reduced use of CIAs, thereby representing sound AMS.[49] Gallium maltolate, a semi-metal compound with antimicrobial activity, was shown not to be inferior to clarithromycin + rifampin when administered orally to treat foals affected subclinically with presumptive R equi pneumonia based on ultrasonographically visible lung lesions.[60] This approach would be less likely to select for AMR to macrolides and rifampin and merits further investigation.[58]

Resistance of *R equi* to all macrolides, lincosamides, and streptogramins type B is conferred by the ribosomal RNA methylase gene designated *erm*(46), a gene that is transferred to susceptible isolates by conjugation and thereby spread rapidly.[61] Although resistance to rifampin is mediated through a different gene (the *rpoB* gene), many macrolide-resistant isolates are also resistant to rifampin,[59,62] thereby creating challenges for antimicrobial selection and resulting in increased mortality in affected foals.[9] Many macrolide- and rifampin-resistant isolates are susceptible in vitro to enro-floxacin, tetracycline, doxycycline, chloramphenicol, TMS, imipenem, linezolid, and lincomycin.[58,63] Unfortunately, no published information is available regarding the effi-cacy of these antimicrobials in treating *R equi* pneumonia caused by macrolide- and rifampin-resistant isolates. Lincomycin should not be used in horses.

Suggested antimicrobial protocols for treating pneumonia in foals and weanlings
When *R equi* is not the suspected pathogen:

First choice: Penicillin G; ceftiofur or TMS.
Alternate choices: Penicillin G or ampicillin + gentamicin.

When *R equi* is the suspected or confirmed pathogen:

First choices: Clarithromycin + rifampin. (Administration of these drugs should be
    staggered because coadministration reduces the bioavailability of rifampin. The
    combination of clarithromycin and rifampin has been shown to have superior ef-
    ficacy in treating *R equi* pneumonia than azithromycin and rifampin or erythro-
    mycin and rifampin.[64])
Alternate choices: Azithromycin + rifampin.
For macrolide-resistant *R equi*: Rifampin + gentamicin; doxycycline; minocycline.

Pneumonia and Pleuropneumonia in Adult Horses

The distribution of bacterial species isolated from adult horses with pneumonia is similar to that described for older foals, except that *R equi* is rarely involved, and anaerobic bacteria are much more commonly isolated from pneumonic adult horses than from pneumonic foals.[26] Unlike foals, adult horses frequently develop pleural effusion in association with bacterial pneumonia. This effusion quickly becomes septic and the condition is typically termed pleuropneumonia.[65,66] Polymicrobic infection is common in horses with pleuropneumonia and frequently involves combinations of gram-positive aerobes (*S zooepidemicus*), gram-negative aerobes (*Actinobacillus* spp, *Pasteurella* spp, *E coli*, or *K pneumoniae*), and anaerobes (*B fragilis*, *Bacteroides* spp, *Fusobacterium* spp, *Porphyromonas* spp, *Prevotella* spp, or *Peptostreptococcus* spp).[65–75] Consequently, antimicrobials used in treatment regimens should provide a broad spectrum of activity and take into account that anaerobic bacteria are involved in 30% to 50% of cases and the most important anaerobe, *B fragilis*, has a high likeli-hood of resistance to penicillins and cephalosporins, including ceftiofur.[70,75,76] *Myco-plasma* spp is the etiologic agent in sporadic cases, in which case the use of oxytetracycline, doxycycline, minocycline, enrofloxacin, or azithromycin (foals only) may be necessary.[77]

Suggested antimicrobial protocols for treating pneumonia and pleuropneumonia in adult horses
Administration of antimicrobials as early in the course of disease as possible is the most important part of the therapeutic plan for horses with bronchopneumonia or

pleuropneumonia.[75] Choice depends on stage and severity of disease; cost; ease of administration; and, when available, results of C&S testing of tracheobronchial aspirates.[75]

Early bronchopneumonia without pleural involvement or significant consolidation is often treated successfully with ceftiofur, or penicillin G + gentamicin or TMS.[75]

When pleural involvement is suspected or confirmed and marked pulmonary consolidation is present:

First choices: Penicillin G or ampicillin + gentamicin + metronidazole.
Alternate choices: Penicillin G or ampicillin + amikacin + metronidazole; ceftiofur ± metronidazole.
Special circumstances: Penicillin G or ampicillin + enrofloxacin (when azotemia precludes use of aminoglycosides); oxytetracycline.
Continued oral therapy: Chloramphenicol (pending susceptibility testing if documented or predicted MIC $\leq$1–2 µg/mL); TMS; doxycycline or minocycline.

Inhalation treatment, via a nebulizer or inhaler, with ceftiofur, gentamicin, enrofloxacin, or cefquinome, has been described and achieves higher intrabronchial concentrations of the respective antibiotics than those achieved after parenteral administration.[70,75] Further studies regarding efficacy are warranted.[70]

Septic Peritonitis

Peritonitis is classified as either primary (also called idiopathic), in which peritoneal infection and inflammation occurs without a predisposing cause, or secondary to a variety of insults to the bowel or body wall, including complications of abdominal surgery, bowel leakage, severe enteritis, migration of metallic foreign bodies from the gut, body wall trauma, uterine rupture, rupture of abdominal abscess, foaling, castration, or rectal examination.[78–80] The gram-negative nonenteric pleomorphic organism, A equuli, is the predominant isolate from horses with primary peritonitis in most geographic locations.[78,80–84] The route of infection with this organism and its predilection for the peritoneal lining remain to be determined, although translocation from the bowel seems to be the most plausible explanation.[78] Other Actinobacillus spp, ß-hemolytic Streptococcus spp, E coli, Bacteroides spp, and Fusobacterium spp are involved in a smaller percentage of primary peritonitis cases and, in endemic areas, C pseudotuberculosis may be involved, particularly in association with abdominal abscesses.[78,80]

Considering that the source of infection in secondary peritonitis is often the bowel or external environment through breaches in the body wall, it is not surprising that gram-negative enteric bacteria (especially E coli and K pneumoniae) are the predominant pathogens involved (about 50% of cases), that obligate anaerobic bacteria are also often isolated, and that polymicrobic infection is common.[28,80,85] C perfringens or other anaerobes may induce peritonitis in foals in association with acute necrotizing enterocolitis.[40,86] History, careful examination, and a diagnostic work-up that typically includes ultrasound examination of the abdomen, and gross and laboratory assessment of peritoneal fluid, help in establishing a diagnosis of primary or secondary peritonitis and in guiding antimicrobial therapy while awaiting culture results. Treatment of secondary peritonitis involves identification and correction of the primary cause, peritoneal lavage, treatment or prevention of adhesions, supportive (often intensive) care, and antimicrobial therapy. Treatment is often prolonged and prognosis is guarded. Peritoneal lavage is typically not necessary in primary peritonitis, the response to antimicrobial treatment and supportive care is often rapid, the course of treatment rarely needs to exceed 2 weeks, and abdominal adhesions rarely form.

Suggested antimicrobial protocols for treating primary peritonitis

First choices: Penicillin G alone[78]; penicillin or ampicillin + gentamicin; ceftiofur.
Alternate choices: Penicillin G or ampicillin + enrofloxacin; TMS.
Continued oral therapy: TMS; doxycycline; minocycline.

Suggested antimicrobial protocols for treating secondary peritonitis

First choices: Penicillin G or ampicillin + gentamicin or amikacin; ceftiofur.
Alternate choices: Penicillin G or ampicillin + enrofloxacin; add metronidazole if anaerobic bacteria suspected.
Continued oral therapy: Doxycycline; TMS; minocycline.

Primary Abdominal Abscess

Most abdominal abscesses seem to be primary in nature and result from hematogenous seeding or lymphatic spread of a single bacterial species from a primary site, such as the respiratory tract or infected lymph node.[87] *Streptococcus zooepidemicus* and *S equi* are the most likely etiologic agents in most geographic locations,[87–89] whereas *C pseudotuberculosis* may be the predominant isolate in the western United States, particularly California, where the organism is endemic.[88,90–92] In recent years, the area of endemicity for *C pseudotuberculosis* has expanded eastward and northward; therefore, cases are now encountered in areas where they had not previously been diagnosed.[90,91,93,94] In foals, *R equi* may also cause primary abdominal abscesses or pyogranulomas.[87]

Suggested antimicrobial protocols for treating primary abdominal abscess
Antimicrobials that are active against gram-positive aerobic bacteria should be selected to initiate treatment of primary internal abscess, as follows:

First choices: Penicillin G or ampicillin (preferably IV initially) + rifampin; ceftiofur + rifampin.[89,92]
Alternate choices: Penicillin G + gentamicin; penicillin G alone; penicillin G + TMS.
For continued oral therapy: Rifampin + TMS; TMS alone; chloramphenicol; doxycycline; minocycline.

Rifampin is recommended because of its high level of activity against causal gram-positive organisms, excellent ability to penetrate cells and tissues and remain active within the acid environment present in abscesses, and oral route of administration. Diarrhea and colitis are, however, a risk in adult horses. Because of the poor lipid solubility of penicillin and ampicillin, they penetrate abscesses poorly unless a high serum to tissue concentration gradient is achieved; therefore, IV administration of high doses is recommended to initiate treatment. A prolonged course of antimicrobial treatment is necessary for resolution; a range from 31 to 131 days (mean, 72 days) was reported for horses with *S equi* internal abscesses in a recent study.[89] As with secondary abdominal abscesses, surgical drainage and lavage may expedite recovery in those horses with accessible abscesses that are visualized with ultrasound.[95]

Secondary Abdominal Abscess

Abdominal abscesses may occur secondary to abdominal trauma, ulceration or perforation of the intestinal tract, abdominal surgery, or ascending infection after castration and often occur as a sequela to, or concomitant with, secondary peritonitis as the body deposits fibrin in an attempt to wall off infection in the peritoneal cavity.[87,96–98] Abdominal abscesses involving lymph nodes, mesentery, and parenchymal organs, such as the spleen or liver, may result from migration of metallic foreign bodies from the intestine resulting in seeding of bacteria.[87,97] Considering that the bowel is often the source of bacteria causing secondary abdominal abscess, a broad range of gram-positive and gram-negative aerobic and anaerobic bacteria may be involved, often as a polymicrobic infection.[99] Broad-spectrum antimicrobial treatment is therefore indicated, as outlined for the treatment of secondary peritonitis.[87] The prognosis for horses with secondary abdominal abscesses is guarded and surgical procedures, such as drainage or marsupialization of abscesses, removal of foreign bodies and adhesions, and bypass of portions of the bowel, followed by peritoneal lavage may be indicated, in addition to supportive care and prolonged broad-spectrum antimicrobial treatment.[87,95]

Suggested antimicrobial protocols for secondary treating abdominal abscess.[87]

Suppurative Cholangiohepatitis

Most cases of cholangiohepatitis are thought to result from ascending infection of the biliary tree with bacteria from the proximal small intestine, although seeding of infection from the gut via the portal circulation is also a possibility.[100–102] Gram-negative enteric organisms (E coli, Salmonella spp, Citrobacter spp, Enterobacter spp, or K pneumoniae) are therefore the predominant isolates, whereas gram-positive aerobes, enterococci, A equuli, and anaerobic bacteria are less commonly involved.[100–104] Affected horses often have choleliths or excessive biliary "sludge" at the time of presentation and some have a history of recent or ongoing proximal enteritis.[100–102,104] Confirmation of the bacterial species involved relies on results of culture of liver biopsies, which may be negative even in the presence of active suppurative cholangiohepatitis.[102] Antimicrobials with a broad gram-negative spectrum of activity that includes enteric organisms are indicated, and those that achieve therapeutic concentrations in the bile (either as parent drug or active metabolites) are preferred but not essential. A positive initial response to antimicrobials may take several days and treatment should be continued until serum concentrations of the hepatobiliary enzyme, γ-glutamyl transaminopeptidase, have returned to normal, which may take several weeks or months.[102]

Suggested antimicrobial protocols for treating septic cholangiohepatitis

First choices: Enrofloxacin; ceftiofur; TMS (add metronidazole if anaerobic infection is suspected or confirmed).
Alternate choices: Penicillin G + gentamicin; ampicillin + gentamicin.
Continued oral therapy: Enrofloxacin; TMS; doxycycline; minocycline; chloramphenicol.

Septic Arthritis and Osteomyelitis

Septic arthritis, polysynovitis, physitis, and osteomyelitis in neonatal foals most often occur by hematogenous spread in association with or as a sequel to septicemia; therefore, the bacterial species involved and recommended antimicrobials are the same as those listed previously for foal septicemia.[105–107] S zooepidemicus is more commonly isolated from older foals than from foals less than 3 weeks of age and may be the sole etiologic agent in these cases.[26] R equi should be considered in cases of septic arthritis, synovitis, or osteomyelitis in foals age 1 to 8 months on farms with endemic R equi infection, particularly when the individual foal has also shown signs of R equi pneumonia.[108] When R equi is the suspected or confirmed pathogen, systemic antimicrobial treatment with clarithromycin (or azithromycin) + rifampin is indicated as detailed in the foal pneumonia section discussed previously.

Septic arthritis or synovitis in adult horses most often occurs secondary to trauma, intrasynovial injection, or surgical intervention.[109,110] The mechanism by which infection was introduced influences the bacterial species isolated. *Staphylococcus* spp account for more than 50% of the isolates from synovial structures infected by injection or surgery, whereas gram-negative enteric bacteria and anaerobes predominate in synovial structures infected via a wound.[109–111] *Pseudomonas* spp, β-hemolytic *Streptococcus* spp, nonhemolytic *Streptococcus* spp, and *Actinobacillus* spp are also commonly isolated from infected synovial structures. Polymicrobial infection is common in joints that become infected via a wound.[109–111]

Suggested antimicrobial protocols for treating septic arthritis in adult horses
The high likelihood of involvement of penicillinase-producing *Staphylococcus* spp and Enterobacteriales should be considered when initiating treatment of septic arthritis or septic tenosynovitis in adult horses:

First choices: Penicillin G or ampicillin + gentamicin; penicillin G or ampicillin + amikacin.
Alternate choices: Cefazolin or cephalothin + gentamicin or amikacin; oxacillin + gentamicin or amikacin; rifampin + amikacin; enrofloxacin; ceftiofur.
Continued oral therapy: Enrofloxacin; doxycycline or minocycline; chloramphenicol.

In all cases of septic arthritis or synovitis, lavage with or without arthroscopic debridement is important to remove inflammatory debris from the synovial cavity. Thereafter, instillation of appropriate antimicrobials, usually amikacin, gentamicin, or a third-generation cephalosporin, is indicated.[112] More effective inactivation of bacteria in synovial cavities and bone may be accomplished using the technique of regional limb perfusion, which accomplishes high drug concentrations in infected tissue.[113,114] This technique involves application of a tourniquet proximal to the involved structure, followed by IV or intraosseus injection of the appropriate antimicrobial to create local concentrations of an antimicrobial that are much higher than those achieved through conventional parenteral or oral dosing. This approach is particularly appropriate for antimicrobials, such as aminoglycosides, that show concentration-dependent bacterial killing (an in-depth review on clinical applications of IV regional limb perfusion in the field is found elsewhere in this issue). Alternate approaches, particularly in horses with septic osteomyelitis or physitis lesions that have been debrided surgically, include local instillation of antibiotic-impregnated sponges or polymethyl methacrylate beads that release the antimicrobial into the local environment.[115,116]

Osteomyelitis and Orthopedic Infection

Selection of antimicrobials for treatment of osteomyelitis secondary to trauma or surgical intervention follows the same principles as outlined previously for septic arthritis/synovitis in adult horses because the distribution and species of bacteria isolated are similar in the two conditions. Enterobacteriales, *Streptococcus* spp, and *Staphylococcus* spp each account for 20% to 25% of bacterial isolates.[111] The overall treatment plan must include identification, curettage, and/or removal of sequestrate or devitalized bone. Long-term treatment is warranted.

Urinary Tract Infection

Clinical disease resulting from infection of the urinary tract is uncommon in horses compared with humans and dogs, most often manifesting as cystitis and generally occurring secondary to conditions that impede urine flow and thereby predispose to ascending infection of the urinary tract.[117] Consequently, gram-negative enteric bacteria, particularly *E coli* and *K pneumonia*, are involved in more than 50% of cases and *P aeruginosa* is isolated from approximately 10%.[26,117] Gram-positive bacteria, predominantly β-hemolytic *Streptococcus* spp and *Staphylococcus* spp, are isolated from approximately 20% of cases, often in association with gram-negative organisms.[26,117]

Resolution of urinary tract infection in horses depends on correcting the primary cause of impeded urinary flow, such as by removing or dissolving calculi; surgical correction of congenital anomalies, traumatic sequelae or masses; or treatment of the neurologic disease underlying detrusor muscle atony, supplemented by appropriate antimicrobial treatment.[117]

Suggested antimicrobial protocols for treating urinary tract infection

A high proportion of the administered dose of most ß-lactam and aminoglycoside antibiotics and TMS is eliminated in the active form in urine. Concentrations of these antibiotics in urine are therefore generally much higher than those achieved in serum, allowing them to kill bacteria that would otherwise be considered resistant by virtue of an MIC higher than the standard breakpoint for susceptibility. This concept, termed conditional susceptibility, is exploited in the treatment of infections of the urinary tract.

First choices: TMS; gentamicin + penicillin G or ampicillin; ceftiofur.

Alternate choices: Gentamicin alone; doxycycline; minocycline; enrofloxacin if indicated by susceptibility testing.

Limb Cellulitis/Lymphangitis

Cellulitis and lymphangitis involving the limbs of horses have each been reported as separate syndromes; however, both occur concurrently in many cases, resulting in extensive limb swelling, heat, pain, lameness, and often fever.[118–122] In one recent study, about 50% of cases were classified as primary (ie, no history of recent trauma or invasive procedure) and about 50% as secondary to recent trauma, puncture wound, surgical incision, or injection.[120] Unlike other causes of "big leg syndrome," such as purpura hemorrhagic and "stocking up," the condition typically involves only one limb.[118–120,122] Thoroughbreds are overrepresented,[119] the hind limbs are affected more commonly than the fore limbs, swelling often extends the entire length of the leg, and in primary cases there is often evidence of chronic dermatitis (eg, pastern dermatitis) or an old keloid-like scar that may diminish local defenses against infection.[118–120] The hock or pastern region are frequently the site for such keloid-type scars and in these cases limb cellulitis is often chronic and/or recurrent. It is frequently not possible to isolate bacteria from affected horses because a successful therapeutic outcome relies on aggressive antimicrobial therapy early in the disease course before development of abscesses or skin sloughs that provide material for culture. Ultrasound examination not only helps delineate involvement of deep structures and define the relative contributions of cellulitis, lymphangitis, and vasculitis, but also identifies pockets of fluid that can be aspirated for laboratory analysis and culture, or drained to facilitate recovery.[118–120] Coagulase-positive *Staphylococcus* spp are the most common isolates, especially in racehorses, whereas β-hemolytic *Streptococcus* spp, coagulase-negative *Staphylococcus* spp, gram-negative aerobic bacteria, and anaerobic bacteria are involved less often.[118–123] Polymicrobic infection is common.[119] In states where *C pseudotuberculosis* infection is endemic, this organism is an important cause of external abscesses and limb cellulitis, and sporadic cases of ulcerative lymphangitis.[90]

Suggested systemic antimicrobial protocols for treating limb cellulitis/lymphangitis

Treatment protocols for limb cellulitis should take into account the high likelihood that penicillinase-producing *Staphylococcus* spp are involved and that the condition can progress rapidly and lead to serious complications including laminitis, skin slough, and death.[121] Systemic antimicrobials are the cornerstone of treatment, along with administration of nonsteroidal anti-inflammatory drugs to control inflammation and pain, local hydrotherapy, bandaging and laminitis prevention, together with ultrasound-guided drainage, debridement, and wound care as appropriate.[119] Regional limb perfusion with amikacin or a β-lactam antimicrobial[124] has been used with success,[120] as have compression techniques and controlled exercise to enhance lymphatic and tissue drainage and promote reduction or resolution of limb swelling.[125] Antithrombotic medications may also be indicated.

> First choices: Penicillin G or ampicillin + amikacin or gentamicin; cephalothin or cefazolin + amikacin or gentamicin; cephalothin or cefazolin + enrofloxacin.
> Alternate choices: Enrofloxacin alone; rifampin + gentamicin; oxacillin + amikacin or gentamicin; rifampin + TMS; cephalothin or cefazolin alone.

Bacterial Myositis

Most cases of septic myositis and associated cellulitis in horses occur secondary to IM injection of a variety of nonantimicrobial drugs or, less commonly, deep puncture wounds.[126,127] Common injection sites in the neck and hind limb are the sites most often affected and the anaerobic histotoxic or tissue-destroying clostridia (*C perfringens*, *C septicum*, *C chauvoei*, *C novyi*, *C sordelli*, and *C fallax*) are the bacterial species most often involved.[126–129] A recent study demonstrated the presence of dormant clostridial spores in muscle tissue of normal horses, suggesting that inflammatory reactions in muscle secondary to injections may create an anaerobic environment favoring proliferation of clostridial organisms; release of toxins; and induction of profound muscle inflammation, necrosis, and gas production.[128] Alternatively, clostridial spores residing on the skin could be introduced during needle placement for injection, or spores could potentially persist in contaminated injectable solutions, particularly in multidose vials. The terms clostridial myositis, myonecrosis, malignant edema, and gas gangrene have been used to describe the condition when clostridia are involved.[126,127] Affected horses typically show fever, obtundation and severe swelling, and pain centered on the injection site, and may quickly develop systemic signs of toxemia and septic shock.[126,127] Subcutaneous crepitus from gas accumulation is often, although not invariably, present and is virtually pathognomonic for clostridial involvement.

Treatment protocols should include fasciotomy to improve tissue aeration and promote drainage; debridement of necrotic tissue; drainage of abscesses; and supportive care to reduce inflammation, improve comfort, maintain hydration, address systemic illness, and prevent laminitis.[126,127] Parenteral administration (preferably IV initially) of high doses of antimicrobials that are highly active against *Clostridium* spp is indicated. Suitable antimicrobials include penicillin G (potassium of sodium), ampicillin, or oxytetracycline, of which penicillin G is the treatment of choice and is associated with survival rates of almost 75% for a disease that would otherwise have a high mortality rate if left untreated.[126,127] Although aminoglycosides are not active against anaerobic bacteria, they are often included initially in empirical treatment regimens to increase gram-negative coverage. Metronidazole has excellent activity against clostridia and is used as a front-line treatment by some clinicians; however, the IV formulation is expensive and oral administration may cause horses to go off feed. In this author's opinion, metronidazole should be reserved for use in horses that do not respond to penicillin G or for continued oral treatment after discontinuing IV treatment. Metronidazole can also be administered per rectum, which has less profound effects on appetite suppression and has high bioavailability. This can be combined with parenteral penicillin treatment.

Suggested antimicrobial protocol for treating bacterial myositis

First choice: Penicillin G ($\pm$ gentamicin).
Alternate choices: Ampicillin ($\pm$ gentamicin); metronidazole (alone or in combination with combinations listed above); oxytetracycline.
Continued oral therapy: Metronidazole; doxycycline or chloramphenicol.

Mastitis

Mastitis occurs sporadically in lactating, nonlactating, and nulliparous mares, fillies, and even young foals.[130–133] *S zooepidemicus* is the most common etiologic agent, being involved in approximately 40% to 50% of cases, whereas gram-negative enteric bacteria (*E coli, K pneumoniae, Enterobacter* spp) are isolated from approximately 20% and gram-negative nonenteric bacteria (*Actinobacillus* spp or *Pasteurella* spp) from about 15%.[130–134] A wide range of other microbial isolates, including *Staphylococcus* spp, *Nocardia* spp, *S equi, Streptococcus agalactia, Streptococcus viridans, P aeruginosa, Arcanobacterium pyogenes,* and *Coccidioides immitis,* have also been reported.[130–133,135] In states where *C pseudotuberculosis* is endemic, it may cause mastitis and/or perimammary abscess or cellulitis.[90]

Treatment with parenteral or oral nonsteroidal anti-inflammatory drugs, frequent stripping of the affected mammary gland, and local application of warm compresses or hydrotherapy are useful adjuncts to systemic antimicrobial therapy. If tolerated, intramammary infusion of antimicrobials after stripping may be beneficial. Considering the range of gram-positive and gram-negative bacteria that may cause mastitis, broad-spectrum systemic antimicrobial treatment is indicated while awaiting culture and susceptibility test results.

Suggested antimicrobial protocols for treating mastitis

First choices: Ceftiofur; penicillin G + gentamicin.
Alternate choices: Ampicillin + gentamicin; penicillin G or ampicillin + amikacin.
Continued oral therapy: TMS.

Acute Colitis in Adult Horses

In many instances, the cause of acute colitis is not determined. *C difficile* and, to a lesser extent, *C perfringens* should be considered the likely cause of colitis in horses that have a history of antimicrobial administration, particularly if the resulting diarrhea has a foul "spoiled fish" odor.[86,136–139] *Salmonella* spp also cause diarrhea in stressed horses, particularly those that have undergone surgery or have experienced another stressful illness and have been treated with antimicrobials, but can also cause outbreaks of diarrhea in otherwise healthy horses.[140] *Neorickettsia risticii* should be suspected when signs of colitis occur in horses, particularly pastured horses or those kept near open water sources in endemic areas during the summer and fall.[141–143] Diarrhea and colic may also be manifestations of infection during coronavirus outbreaks.[144]

Suggested antimicrobial protocols for treating acute colitis

In general, administration of antimicrobials should be discontinued in horses that develop diarrhea during a course of antimicrobial treatment. Antimicrobials are generally not indicated for the treatment of undifferentiated colitis, except in horses with profound neutropenia, persistent high fever, or other evidence of severe compromise to the integrity of the bowel wall. In these instances, the antibiotic of choice is gentamicin (6.6–8.8 mg/kg every

24 hours) administered IV for a short (3–5 day) course, provided renal function is adequate and fluid deficits are addressed. When *C difficile* or *C perfringens* are the suspected or confirmed etiologic agents, oral administration of metronidazole (15 mg/kg orally every 8 hours) is the treatment of choice. Whereas a high proportion of *C difficile* isolates remain susceptible to metronidazole, an increasing number are resistant,[7,10] necessitating carefully controlled use of other CIAs, such as vancomycin. Resistance should be suspected in horses that develop colitis while being treated with metronidazole, by lack of response to metronidazole for cases not on metronidazole at the onset of signs, by identification of *C difficile* strain B, or by documentation of resistance through antimicrobial susceptibility testing.[7] Neonatal foals with enterocolitis should be treated with broad-spectrum antimicrobials to prevent bacterial translocation and dangerous sequelae, such as septic arthritis. In neonatal foals with clostridial enterocolitis IV metronidazole (10 mg/kg every 12 hours) is indicated and often effective, especially when gastric reflux is present. When *N risticii* is the suspected or confirmed cause of colitis, early administration of oxytetracycline (6.6 mg/kg IV every 12 hours for 5 days) seems to be the treatment of choice[141,145] and is preferred over oral administration of tetracycline drugs because of concern for poor absorption in horses with diarrhea. If twice daily IV injection is not feasible for the entire 5-day treatment period, oral administration of doxycycline (10 mg/kg orally every 12 hours) or minocycline (4 mg/kg orally every 12 hours) are reasonable alternatives, especially after initial treatment with one or more IV doses of oxytetracycline.

Equine Proliferative Enteropathy (Lawsonia intracellularis Infection)

In weanling foals and young horses up to 2 years of age, and rarely older, *Lawsonia intracellularis* causes equine proliferative enteropathy resulting in diarrhea (cow pie to loose stool), unthriftiness, weight loss, and edema associated with profound hypoproteinemia.[146–148] Although *L intracellularis* is susceptible to a wide range of antimicrobial agents in vitro, its obligate intracellular nature in vivo dictates that antimicrobials that penetrate cell membranes well are strongly preferred.[149] Rifampin and clarithromycin were shown to be the most highly active antimicrobials against intracellular *L intracellularis* in a recent study, and doxycycline, minocycline, erythromycin, chloramphenicol, and enrofloxacin were shown to be moderately to highly active.[149] Azithromycin and oxytetracycline were not tested in that study. The choice of antimicrobial regimen must consider the risks of inducing adverse effects, such as renal toxicity or colitis, because of further disturbances in gastrointestinal flora, the risk of which increases in older foals, particularly when macrolides are used.[146–148]

Suggested antimicrobial protocols for treating equine proliferative enteropathy

Oral rifampin with azithromycin or clarithromycin are often recommended for foals less than 500 lb, whereas IV oxytetracycline (3–7 days) followed by oral doxycycline or minocycline, or oral chloramphenicol are frequently used to treat older weanlings, yearlings, and mature horses.[146–148] The required course of treatment is typically 2 to 3 weeks in cases diagnosed early in the disease course but may be longer in more advanced cases.[148] Supportive care including IV fluids, colloids, plasma transfusion, appropriate enteral or parenteral nutrition, and antiulcer medications are also necessary in many cases.[148]

Meningitis and Meningoencephalitis

Bacterial infection of the central nervous system (CNS), although rare in horses, can occur via direct invasion through the calvarium from adjoining structures secondary to accidental or surgical trauma; from ascending infection from ocular, nasal, paranasal sinus, guttural pouch, lymph node, oral cavity, or regional bony structures; or from hematogenous spread.[150–153] Considering the diversity of sources and routes of infection, a wide range of aerobic and anaerobic gram-positive and gram-negative bacteria and fungi may be involved. Reported infectious agents include *Cryptococcus neoformans*, *S equi*, *S zooepidemicus*, *Streptococcus suis*, *S aureus*, *Actinomyces* spp, *K pneumoniae*, *E coli*, *A equuli*, *Pasteurella caballi*, *C pseudotuberculosis*, *Capnocytophaga canimorphus*, *Fusobacterium* spp, and *Bacteroides* spp[150–153]; however, antemortem culture of cerebral spinal fluid frequently yields negative results.[150] In neonatal foals, CNS infection is most often the result of hematogenous spread of bacteria in patients with systemic sepsis. Gram-negative enteric bacteria are, therefore, the most common etiologic agents in foals. The primary treatment regimen is typically directed at the underlying systemic sepsis and usually includes amikacin or an alternate aminoglycoside antimicrobial, together with a β-lactam antimicrobial (see neonatal sepsis).

Apart from inherent activity against the infecting organisms, factors that affect the potential effectiveness of drugs to treat CNS infection include ability to penetrate into meningeal and neural tissues, activity in a purulent environment, and the pharmacodynamic relationship between the CNS concentration of drugs and their bactericidal activity.[152] Antimicrobial agents with good CNS penetration include potentiated sulfonamides, chloramphenicol, rifampin, macrolides, doxycycline, fluoroquinolones, metronidazole, and some third- and fourth-generation cephalosporins.[152] Horses have a well-developed blood-brain barrier that impedes distribution to the brain of antimicrobials, particularly those that are polar and have low lipid solubility (eg, aminoglycosides and most β-lactams) or are highly protein bound (many β-lactams, including ceftiofur), under normal circumstances. When the meninges are inflamed, however, as is the case in bacterial meningitis, permeability to antimicrobials has been shown to increase, thereby extending the range of antimicrobials that are used in treatment regimens. Many third-generation cephalosporins (eg, cefotaxime and ceftriaxone) that have been shown to cross the "normal" blood-brain barrier and are highly active against gram-negative enteric bacteria have been used to treat meningitis in foals and are considered to be the antimicrobials of choice. They are administered IV at high doses every 4 to 6 hours to establish a high blood/CNS concentration gradient and thereby maximize diffusion into the CNS. Amikacin is typically also included in treatment regimens for the reasons stated previously.

Suggested antimicrobial protocols for treating meningitis in adult horses

Potassium or sodium penicillin G or ampicillin plus amikacin or gentamicin; TMS; chloramphenicol; minocycline; rifampin and enrofloxacin have all been used to treat CNS infection in adult horses.[150,152] If anaerobic involvement is suspected, as in cases secondary to dental or sinus disease, it is rational to add metronidazole to the treatment protocol. Third-generation cephalosporins can be used; however, ceftiofur does not penetrate the blood-brain barrier well and cefotaxime and ceftriaxone are expensive and carry a definite risk of inducing antimicrobial-associated colitis in adult horses. Despite intensive antimicrobial and supportive treatment, prognosis is poor. A mortality rate of more than 95% was reported for 22 horses age 2 days to 21 years with CNS infection treated at a referral hospital.[150]

DISCLOSURE

The authors have no affiliations or agreements that would constitute conflicts of interest.

REFERENCES

1. Brumbaugh GW, Langston VC. Principles of antimicrobial therapy. In: Smith BP, editor. Large animal internal medicine. 2nd edition. St. Louis: Mosby; 1996. p. 1587–613.
2. Prescott JF. Outpacing the resistance tsunami: antimicrobial stewardship in equine medicine, an overview. Equine Vet Educ 2020.
3. Organization WH. Critically important antimicrobials for human medicine: ranking of medically important antimicrobials for risk management of antimicrobial resistance due to non-human use. In: AGISAR, editor. WAGolSoAR. 6th Revision edition. Switzerland: World Health Organization; 2018. Available at: https://creativecommons.org/licenses/by-nc-sa/3.0/igo.
4. Theelen MJ, Wilson WD, Edman JM, et al. Temporal trends in in vitro antimicrobial susceptibility patterns of bacteria isolated from foals with sepsis: 1979-2010. Equine Vet J 2014;46:161–8.
5. Johns IC, Adams EL. Trends in antimicrobial resistance in equine bacterial isolates: 1999-2012. Vet Rec 2015;176:334.
6. Isgren CM, Edwards T, Pinchbeck GL, et al. Emergence of carriage of CTX-M-15 in faecal *Escherichia coli* in horses at an equine hospital in the UK; increasing prevalence over a decade (2008-2017). BMC Vet Res 2019;15:268.
7. Magdesian KG, Dujowich M, Madigan JE, et al. Molecular characterization of *Clostridium difficile* isolates from horses in an intensive care unit and association of disease severity with strain type. J Am Vet Med Assoc 2006;228:751–5.
8. Huber L, Giguère S, Slovis NM, et al. Emergence of resistance to macrolides and rifampin in clinical isolates of *Rhodococcus equi* from foals in Central Kentucky, 1995 to 2017. Antimicrob Agents Chemother 2019;63:e01714–8.
9. Giguère S, Berghaus LJ, Willingham-Lane JM. Antimicrobial resistance in *Rhodococcus equi*. In: Schwarz S, Cavaco L, Shen J, editors. Antimicrobial Resistance in Bacteria from Livestock and Companion Animals. Washington, DC: ASM Press; 2017. p. 229–36.
10. Baverud V, Gustafsson A, Franklin A, et al. *Clostridium difficile*: prevalence in horses and environment, and antimicrobial susceptibility. Equine Vet J 2003;35:465–71.
11. Gilbertie JM, Schnabel LV, Stefanovski D, et al. Gram-negative multi-drug resistant bacteria influence survival to discharge for horses with septic synovial structures: 206 cases (2010-2015). Vet Microbiol 2018;226:64–73.
12. Willis AT, Magdesian KG, Byrne BA, et al. Enterococcus infections in foals. Vet J 2019;248:42–7.
13. Bowen M. Antimicrobial stewardship: time for change. Equine Vet J 2013;45:127–9.
14. Slater JD. Antimicrobial resistance, equine practitioners and human health: a true one health issue or political interference? Equine Vet J 2015;47:750–2.
15. Raidal SL. Antimicrobial stewardship in equine practice. Aust Vet J 2019;97:238–42.
16. Rendle D, Gough S. Antimicrobial stewardship in equine practice. UK-Vet Equine 2019;3:200–5.
17. Weese JS. Antimicrobial use and antimicrobial resistance in horses. Equine Vet J 2015;47:747–9.
18. Page S, Prescott J, Weese S. The 5Rs approach to antimicrobial stewardship. Vet Rec 2014;175:207–8.
19. Hardefeldt LY. Implementing antimicrobial stewardship programmes in veterinary practices. Vet Rec 2018;182:688–90.

20. Bowen I, Slater J, Protect ME. The responsible antimicrobial toolkit for equine practitioners 2012. Available at: https://www.beva.org.uk/Portals/0/Documents/ResourcesForVets/1beva-antimicrobial-policy-template-distributed.pdf.

21. Directorate. VM. UK-VARSS. Veterinary antibiotic resistance and sales surveillance report (UK-VARSS 2019) 2020. New Haw, Addlestone, Surrey KT15 3LS, UK.

22. (FDA) FaDA. Animal Medicinal Drug Use Clarification Act of 1994 (AMDUCA). Administration FaD; 1994. Available at: http://www.ecfr.gov/cgi-bin/text-idx?SID=054808d261de27898e02fb175b7c9ff9&node=21:6.0.1.1.16&rgn=div5.

23. Baggot JD, Prescott JF. Antimicrobial selection and dosage in the treatment of equine bacterial infections. Equine Vet J 1987;19:92–6.

24. Hirsh DC, Ruehl WW. A rational approach to the selection of an antimicrobial agent. J Am Vet Med Assoc 1984;185:1058–61.

25. Prescott JF, Baggot JD, Walker RD. Antimicrobial therapy in veterinary medicine. 3 edition. Ames, Iowa: Iowa State University Press; 2000. p. 796.

26. Wilson WD. Rational selection of antibiotics for use in horses. Lexington: Proceedings of the 47th Annual Convention of the American Association of Equine Practitioners (AAEP); 2001. p. 75–93.

27. CLSI. Performance standards for antimicrobial disk and dilution susceptibility tests for bacteria isolated from animals. 4th edition. Wayne, PA: Clinical Laboratory Standards Institute; 2018.

28. Hirsh DC, Jang SS. Antimicrobic susceptibility of bacterial pathogens from horses. Vet Clin North Am Equine Pract 1987;3:181–90.

29. Carter GK, Martens RJ. Septicemia in the neonatal foal. Compend Contin Educ Pract Vet 1986;8:S256–71.

30. Russell CM, Axon JE, Blishen A, et al. Blood culture isolates and antimicrobial sensitivities from 427 critically ill neonatal foals. Aust Vet J 2008;86:266–71.

31. Wilson WD, Madigan JE. Comparison of bacteriologic culture of blood and necropsy specimens for determining the cause of foal septicemia: 47 cases (1978-1987) [published erratum appears in J Am Vet Med Assoc 1990 Feb 1;196(3):438]. J Am Vet Med Assoc 1989;195:1759–63.

32. Fouche N, Gerber V, Thomann A, et al. Antimicrobial susceptibility patterns of blood culture isolates from foals in Switzerland. Schweiz Arch Tierheilkd 2018; 160:665–71.

33. Toombs-Ruane LJ, Riley CB, Kendall AT, et al. Antimicrobial susceptibility of bacteria isolated from neonatal foal samples submitted to a New Zealand veterinary pathology laboratory (2004 to 2013). N Z Vet J 2016;64:107–11.

34. Hepworth-Warren KL, Wong DM, Fulkerson CV, et al. Bacterial isolates, antimicrobial susceptibility patterns, and factors associated with infection and outcome in foals with septic arthritis: 83 cases (1998-2013). J Am Vet Med Assoc 2015;246:785–93.

35. Brewer BD, Koterba AM. Bacterial isolates and susceptibility patterns in foals in a neonatal intensive care unit. Compend Contin Educ Pract Vet 1990;12:1773–9.

36. Koterba AM, Brewer BD, Tarplee FA. Clinical and clinicopathological characteristics of the septicaemic neonatal foal: review of 38 cases. Equine Vet J 1984;16:376–82.

37. Platt H. Septicaemia in the foal. A review of 61 cases. Br Vet J 1973;129:221–9.

38. Theelen MJ, Wilson WD, Edman JM, et al. Temporal trends in prevalence of bacteria isolated from foals with sepsis: 1979-2010. Equine Vet J 2014;46:169–73.

39. Theelen MJP, Wilson WD, Byrne BA, et al. Differences in isolation rate and antimicrobial susceptibility of bacteria isolated from foals with sepsis at admission and after >/=48 hours of hospitalization. J Vet Intern Med 2020;34:955–63.
40. Jones SL, Wilson WD. *Clostridium septicum* septicemia in a neonatal foal with hemorrhagic enteritis. Cornell Vet 1993;83:143–51.
41. Theelen MJP, Wilson WD, Byrne BA, et al. Initial antimicrobial treatment of foals with sepsis: do our choices make a difference? Vet J 2019;243:74–6.
42. Reuss SM, Cohen ND. Update on bacterial pneumonia in the foal and weanling. Vet Clin North Am Equine Pract 2015;31:121–35.
43. Giguère S, Jordan LMI, Glass K, et al. Relationship of mixed bacterial infection to prognosis in foals with pneumonia caused by *Rhodococcus equi*. J Vet Intern Med 2012;26:1443–8.
44. Leclere M, Magdesian KG, Kass PH, et al. Comparison of the clinical, microbiological, radiological and haematological features of foals with pneumonia caused by *Rhodococcus equi* and other bacteria. Vet J 2011;187:109–12.
45. Cohen ND. *Rhodococcus equi* foal pneumonia. Vet Clin North Am Equine Pract 2014;30:609–22.
46. Hoffman AM, Viel L, Juniper E, et al. Clinical and endoscopic study to estimate the incidence of distal respiratory tract infection in Thoroughbred foals on Ontario breeding farms. Am J Vet Res 1993;54:1602–7.
47. Wilson WD. Foal pneumonia: an overview. Lexington: Proceedings of the 38th Annual Convention of the American Association of Equine Practitioners (AAEP); 1993. p. 203–29.
48. Arnold-Lehna D, Venner M, Berghaus LJ, et al. Efficacy of treatment and survival rate of foals with pneumonia: retrospective comparison of rifampin/azithromycin and rifampin/tulathromycin. Pferdeheilkunde 2019;35:423–30.
49. Arnold-Lehna D, Venner M, Berghaus LJ, et al. Changing policy to treat foals with *Rhodococcus equi* pneumonia in the later course of disease decreases antimicrobial usage without increasing mortality rate. Equine Vet J 2020;52:531–7.
50. Chaffin MK, Cohen ND, Blodgett GP, et al. Evaluation of ultrasonographic screening parameters for predicting subsequent onset of clinically apparent *Rhodococcus equi* pneumonia in foals. Lexington: Proceedings of the 59th Annual Convention of the American Association of Equine Practitioners (AAEP); 2013. p. 268–9.
51. Thomé R, Rohn K, Venner M. Clinical and haematological parameters for the early diagnosis of pneumonia in foals. Pferdeheilkunde 2018;34:260–6.
52. Thomé R, Weber C, Rohn K, et al. Serum amyloid A concentration in foals: can it help when making a treatment decision in foals with pneumonia? Pferdeheilkunde 2018;34:61–7.
53. McCracken JL, Slovis NM. Use of thoracic ultrasound for the prevention of *Rhodococcus equi* pneumonia on endemic farms. Lexington: Proceedings of the 55th Annual Convention of the American Association of Equine Practitioners (AAEP); 2009. p. 38–44.
54. Chaffin MK, Cohen ND, Martens RJ. Chemoprophylactic effects of azithromycin against *Rhodococcus equi*-induced pneumonia among foals at equine breeding farms with endemic infections. J Am Vet Med Assoc 2008;232:1035–47.
55. Willingham-Lane JM, Berghaus LJ, Berghaus RD, et al. Effect of macrolide and rifampin resistance on fitness of *Rhodococcus equi* during intramacrophage replication and in vivo. Infect Immun 2019;87:e00281–9.

56. Huber L, Giguere S, Cohen ND, et al. Prevalence and risk factors associated with emergence of *Rhodococcus equi* resistance to macrolides and rifampicin in horse-breeding farms in Kentucky, USA. Vet Microbiol 2019;235:243–7.

57. Giguère S, Lee E, Williams E, et al. Determination of the prevalence of antimicrobial resistance to macrolide antimicrobials or rifampin in *Rhodococcus equi* isolates and treatment outcome in foals infected with antimicrobial-resistant isolates of *R equi*. J Am Vet Med Assoc 2010;237:74–81.

58. Giguère S. Treatment of infections caused by *Rhodococcus equi*. Vet Clin North Am Equine Pract 2017;33:67–85.

59. Burton AJ, Giguère S, Sturgill TL, et al. Macrolide- and rifampin-resistant *Rhodococcus equi* on a horse breeding farm, Kentucky, USA. Emerg Infect Dis 2013; 19:282–5.

60. Cohen ND, Slovis NM, Giguère S, et al. Gallium maltolate as an alternative to macrolides for treatment of presumed *Rhodococcus equi* pneumonia in foals. J Vet Intern Med 2015;29:932–9.

61. Anastasi E, Giguere S, Berghaus LJ, et al. Novel transferable erm(46) determinant responsible for emerging macrolide resistance in *Rhodococcus equi*. J Antimicrob Chemother 2016;71:1746.

62. Fines M, Pronost S, Maillard K, et al. Characterization of mutations in the rpoB gene associated with rifampin resistance in *Rhodococcus equi* isolated from foals. J Clin Microbiol 2001;39:2784–7.

63. Riesenberg A, Fessler AT, Erol E, et al. MICs of 32 antimicrobial agents for *Rhodococcus equi* isolates of animal origin. J Antimicrob Chemother 2014;69: 1045–9.

64. Giguère S, Jacks S, Roberts GD, et al. Retrospective comparison of azithromycin, clarithromycin, and erythromycin for the treatment of foals with *Rhodococcus equi* pneumonia. J Vet Intern Med 2004;18:568–73.

65. Sweeney CR, Divers TJ, Benson CE. Anaerobic bacteria in 21 horses with pleuropneumonia. J Am Vet Med Assoc 1985;187:721–4.

66. Sweeney CR, Holcombe SJ, Barningham SC, et al. Aerobic and anaerobic bacterial isolates from horses with pneumonia or pleuropneumonia and antimicrobial susceptibility patterns of the aerobes. J Am Vet Med Assoc 1991;198: 839–42.

67. Mair TS, Yeo SP. Equine pleuropneumonia: the importance of anaerobic bacteria and the potential value of metronidazole in treatment. Vet Rec 1987;121:109–10.

68. Raphel CF, Beech J. Pleuritis secondary to pneumonia or lung abscessation in 90 horses. J Am Vet Med Assoc 1982;181:808–10.

69. Tomlinson JE, Reef VB, Boston RC, et al. The association of fibrinous pleural effusion with survival and complications in horses with pleuropneumonia (2002-2012): 74 CASES. J Vet Intern Med 2015;29:1410–7.

70. Tallon R, McGovern K. Bacterial pneumonia in adult horses. UK-Vet Equine 2018;2:34–41.

71. Arroyo MG, Slovis NM, Moore GE, et al. Factors associated with survival in 97 horses with septic pleuropneumonia. J Vet Intern Med 2017;31:894–900.

72. Carvallo FR, Uzal FA, Diab SS, et al. Retrospective study of fatal pneumonia in racehorses. J Vet Diagn Invest 2017;29:450–6.

73. Estell KE, Young A, Kozikowski T, et al. Pneumonia caused by *Klebsiella* spp. in 46 horses. J Vet Intern Med 2016;30:314–21.

74. Ferrucci F, Zucca E, Croci C, et al. Bacterial pneumonia and pleuropneumonia in sport horses: 17 cases (2001-2003). Equine Vet Educ 2008;20:526–31.

75. Reuss SM, Giguère S. Update on bacterial pneumonia and pleuropneumonia in the adult horse. Vet Clin North Am Equine Pract 2015;31:105–20.
76. Samitz EM, Jang SS, Hirsh DC. In vitro susceptibilities of selected obligate anaerobic bacteria obtained from bovine and equine sources to ceftiofur. J Vet Diagn Invest 1996;8:121–3.
77. Hoffman AM, Baird JD, Kloeze HJ, et al. *Mycoplasma felis* pleuritis in two show-jumper horses. Cornell Vet 1992;82:155–62.
78. Odelros E, Kendall A, Hedberg-Alm Y, et al. Idiopathic peritonitis in horses: a retrospective study of 130 cases in Sweden (2002-2017). Acta Vet Scand 2019;61:18.
79. Elce YA. Infections in the equine abdomen and pelvis: perirectal abscesses, umbilical infections, and peritonitis. Vet Clin North Am Equine Pract 2006;22: 419–36.
80. Arndt S, Kilcoyne I, Vaughan B, et al. Clinical and diagnostic findings, treatment, and short- and long-term survival in horses with peritonitis: 72 cases (2007-2017). Vet Surg 2021;50:323–35.
81. Matthews S, Dart AJ, Dowling BA, et al. Peritonitis associated with *Actinobacillus equuli* in horses: 51 cases. Aust Vet J 2001;79:536–9.
82. Golland LC, Hodgson DR, Hodgson JL, et al. Peritonitis associated with *Actinobacillus equuli* in horses: 15 cases (1982-1992). J Am Vet Med Assoc 1994;205: 340–3.
83. Hawkins JF, Bowman KF, Roberts MC, et al. Peritonitis in horses: 67 cases (1985-1990). J Am Vet Med Assoc 1993;203:284–8.
84. Gay CC, Lording PM. Peritonitis in horses associated with *Actinobacillus equuli*. Aust Vet J 1980;56:296–300.
85. Nógrádi N, Tóth B, MacGillivray KC. Peritonitis in horses: 55 cases (2004-2007). Acta Vet Hung 2011;59:181–93.
86. Diab SS, Kinde H, Moore J, et al. Pathology of *Clostridium perfringens* type C enterotoxemia in horses. Vet Pathol 2012;49:255–63.
87. Arnold CE, Chaffin MK. Abdominal abscesses in adult horses: 61 cases (1993-2008). J Am Vet Med Assoc 2012;241:1659–65.
88. Rumbaugh GE, Smith BP, Carlson GP. Internal abdominal abscesses in the horse: a study of 25 cases. J Am Vet Med Assoc 1978;172:304–9.
89. Pusterla N, Whitcomb MB, Wilson WD. Internal abdominal abscesses caused by *Streptococcus equi* subspecies *equi* in 10 horses in California between 1989 and 2004. Vet Rec 2007;160:589–92.
90. Aleman M, Spier SJ, Wilson WD, et al. *Corynebacterium pseudotuberculosis* infection in horses: 538 cases (1982-1993). J Am Vet Med Assoc 1996;209: 804–9.
91. Miers KC, Ley WB. *Corynebacterium pseudotuberculosis* infection in the horse: study of 117 clinical cases and consideration of etiopathogenesis. J Am Vet Med Assoc 1980;177:250–3.
92. Pratt SM, Spier SJ, Carroll SP, et al. Evaluation of clinical characteristics, diagnostic test results, and outcome in horses with internal infection caused by *Corynebacterium pseudotuberculosis*: 30 cases (1995-2003). J Am Vet Med Assoc 2005;227:441–8.
93. Mayfield MA, Martin MT. *Corynebacterium pseudotuberculosis* in Texas horses. Southwest Vet 1979;32:133–6.
94. Corbeil LE, Morrissey JF, Léguillette R. Is *Corynebacterium pseudotuberculosis* infection (pigeon fever) in horses an emerging disease in western Canada? Can Vet J 2016;57:1062–6.

95. Mair TS, Sherlock CE. Surgical drainage and post operative lavage of large abdominal abscesses in six mature horses. Equine Vet J Suppl 2011;123–7.

96. Zicker SC, Wilson WD, Medearis I. Differentiation between intra-abdominal neoplasms and abscesses in horses, using clinical and laboratory data: 40 cases (1973-1988). J Am Vet Med Assoc 1990;196:1130–4.

97. Marley LK, Soffler C, Hackett ES. Clinical features, diagnostic methods, treatments, and outcomes associated with ingested wires in the abdomen of horses: 16 cases (2002-2013). J Am Vet Med Assoc 2018;253:781–7.

98. Carvalho A de M, Xavier ABdS, Santos JPVd, et al. Post-castration abdominal abscess in horses: case report. Rev Bras Ciência Vet 2017;24:125–7.

99. Coleman MC, Schmitz DG. Splenic abscessation in the horse: a retrospective study of 12 cases. Equine Vet Educ 2019;31:67–70.

100. Davis JL, Jones SL. Suppurative cholangiohepatitis and enteritis in adult horses. J Vet Intern Med 2003;17:583–7.

101. Johnston JK, Divers TJ, Reef VB, et al. Cholelithiasis in horses: ten cases (1982-1986). J Am Vet Med Assoc 1989;194:405–9.

102. Peek SF, Divers TJ. Medical treatment of cholangiohepatitis and cholelithiasis in mature horses: 9 cases (1991-1998). Equine Vet J 2000;32:301–6.

103. Durando MM, MacKay RJ, Staller GS, et al. Septic cholangiohepatitis and cholangiocarcinoma in a horse. J Am Vet Med Assoc 1995;206:1018–21.

104. Reef VB, Johnston JK, Divers TJ, et al. Ultrasonographic findings in horses with cholelithiasis: eight cases (1985-1987). J Am Vet Med Assoc 1990;196:1836–40.

105. Wright L, Ekstrøm CT, Kristoffersen M, et al. Haematogenous septic arthritis in foals: short- and long-term outcome and analysis of factors affecting prognosis. Equine Vet Educ 2017;29:328–36.

106. Annear MJ, Furr MO, White NA. Septic arthritis in foals. Equine Vet Educ 2011; 23:422–31.

107. Neil KM, Axon JE, Begg AP, et al. Retrospective study of 108 foals with septic osteomyelitis. Aust Vet J 2010;88:4–12.

108. Ruocco NA 3rd, Luedke LK, Fortier LA, et al. *Rhodococcus equi* joint sepsis and osteomyelitis is associated with a grave prognosis in foals. Front Vet Sci 2019; 6:503.

109. Schneider RK, Bramlage LR, Moore RM, et al. A retrospective study of 192 horses affected with septic arthritis/tenosynovitis. Equine Vet J 1992;24:436–42.

110. Moore RM, Schneider RK, Kowalski J, et al. Antimicrobial susceptibility of bacterial isolates from 233 horses with musculoskeletal infection during 1979-1989. Equine Vet J 1992;24:450–6.

111. Snyder JR, Pascoe JR, Hirsh DC. Antimicrobial susceptibility of microorganisms isolated from equine orthopedic patients. Vet Surg 1987;16:197–201.

112. Schneider RK, Bramlage LR, Mecklenburg LM, et al. Open drainage, intra-articular and systemic antibiotics in the treatment of septic arthritis/tenosynovitis in horses. Equine Vet J 1992;24:443–9.

113. Murphey ED, Santschi EM, Papich MG. Regional intravenous perfusion of the distal limb of horses with amikacin sulfate. J Vet Pharmacol Ther 1999;22:68–71.

114. Whitehair KJ, Blevins WE, Fessler JF, et al. Regional perfusion of the equine carpus for antibiotic delivery. Vet Surg 1992;21:279–85.

115. Butson RJ, Schramme MC, Garlick MH, et al. Treatment of intrasynovial infection with gentamicin-impregnated polymethylmethacrylate beads. Vet Rec 1996; 138:460–4.

116. Summerhays GES. Treatment of traumatically induced synovial sepsis in horses with gentamicin-impregnated collagen sponges. Vet Rec 2000;147:184–8.

117. Frye MA. Pathophysiology, diagnosis, and management of urinary tract infection in horses. Vet Clin North Am Equine Pract 2006;22:497–517.
118. Koskenranta E, Mykkänen A, Määttä M, et al. Cellulitis, lymphangitis or vasculitis? Retrospective study of 66 equine cases treated in the University of Helsinki Veterinary Teaching Hospital. Suomen Eläinlääkärilehti 2020;126:14–22.
119. Fjordbakk CT, Arroyo LG, Hewson J. Retrospective study of the clinical features of limb cellulitis in 63 horses. Vet Rec 2008;162:233–6.
120. Adam EN, Southwood LL. Primary and secondary limb cellulitis in horses: 44 cases (2000-2006). J Am Vet Med Assoc 2007;231:1696–703.
121. Markel MD, Wheat JD, Jang SS. Cellulitis associated with coagulase-positive staphylococci in racehorses: nine cases (1975-1984). J Am Vet Med Assoc 1986;189:1600–3.
122. Rendle D. Cellulitis and lymphangitis. UK-Vet Equine 2017;1:16–20.
123. Vyetrogon T, Dubois MS. Perisuspensory abscessation in eight horses with hindlimb cellulitis. Equine Vet Educ 2019;31:e66–70.
124. Dietz O, Kehnscherper G, Neubauer J. Further observations on retrograde intravenous antibiotic therapy for pyogenic infections of the lower limb of horses. Monatshefte für Vet 1991;46:605–7.
125. Rötting A, von Rautenfeld DB, Schubert T, et al. Manual lymphatic drainage in the horse for treatment of the hindlimb. Part 2: findings and treatment in horses affected with "chronic cellulitis. Pferdeheilkunde 2000;16:37–44.
126. Peek SF, Semrad SD, Perkins GA. Clostridial myonecrosis in horses (37 cases 1985-2000). Equine Vet J 2003;35:86–92.
127. Adam EN, Southwood LL. Surgical and traumatic wound infections, cellulitis, and myositis in horses. Vet Clin North Am Equine Pract 2006;22:335–61.
128. Vengust M, Arroyo LG, Weese JS, et al. Preliminary evidence for dormant clostridial spores in equine skeletal muscle. Equine Vet J 2003;35:514–6.
129. Sacco SC, Ortega J, Navarro MA, et al. *Clostridium sordellii*-associated gas gangrene in 8 horses, 1998–2019. J Vet Diagn Invest 2020;32:246–51.
130. McCue PM, Wilson WD. Equine mastitis: a review of 28 cases. Equine Vet J 1989;21:351–3.
131. Motta RG, Nardi Junior G, Perrotti IBM, et al. Infectious mastitis in mare: an overview of disease. Arq Inst Biol 2011;78:629–35.
132. Perkins NR, Threlfall WR. Mastitis in the mare. Equine Vet Educ 1993;5:192–5.
133. Motta RG, Ribeiro MG, Langoni H, et al. Study of routine diagnosis methods of mastitis in mares. Arq Bras Med Vet Zootec 2011;63:1028–32.
134. Langoni H, Prestes NC, Silva AV, et al. Microbial aetiology and sensitivity profile of equine mastitis. Semina (Londrina) 1998;19:17–20.
135. Walker RL, Johnson BJ, Jones KL, et al. *Coccidioides immitis* mastitis in a mare. J Vet Diagn Invest 1993;5:446–8.
136. Donaldson MT, Palmer JE. Prevalence of *Clostridium perfringens* enterotoxin and *Clostridium difficile* toxin A in feces of horses with diarrhea and colic. J Am Vet Med Assoc 1999;215:358–61.
137. Jones RL. Clostridial enterocolitis. Vet Clin North Am Equine Pract 2000;16:471–85.
138. Baverud V, Gustafsson A, Franklin A, et al. *Clostridium difficile* associated with acute colitis in mature horses treated with antibiotics. Equine Vet J 1997;29:279–84.
139. Diab SS, Songer G, Uzal FA. *Clostridium difficile* infection in horses: a review. Vet Microbiol 2013;167:42–9.

140. House JK, Mainar Jaime RC, Smith BP, et al. Risk factors for nosocomial *Salmonella* infection among hospitalized horses. J Am Vet Med Assoc 1999;214: 1511–6.

141. Madigan J, Pusterla N. Life cycle of Potomac Horse Fever - implications for diagnosis, treatment, and control: a review. Lexington: American Association of Equine Practitioners (AAEP); 2005. p. 158–62.

142. Palmer JE. Potomac horse fever. In Infectious Diseases of Livestock. Oxford: Oxford University Press; 2004. p. 583–91.

143. Wilson JH, Pusterla N, Bengfort JM, et al. Incrimination of mayflies as a vector of Potomac horse fever in an outbreak in Minnesota. Lexington: Proceedings of the 52nd Annual Convention of the American Association of Equine Practitioners (AAEP); 2006. p. 324–8.

144. Berryhill EH, Magdesian KG, Aleman M, et al. Clinical presentation, diagnostic findings, and outcome of adult horses with equine coronavirus infection at a veterinary teaching hospital: 33 cases (2012-2018). Vet J 2019;248:95–100.

145. Bertin FR, Reising A, Slovis NM, et al. Clinical and clinicopathological factors associated with survival in 44 horses with equine neorickettsiosis (Potomac horse Fever). J Vet Intern Med 2013;27:1528–34.

146. Frazer ML. *Lawsonia intracellularis* infection in horses: 2005-2007. J Vet Intern Med 2008;22:1243–8.

147. Page AE, Slovis NM, Horohov DW. *Lawsonia intracellularis* and equine proliferative enteropathy. Vet Clin North Am Equine Pract 2014;30:641–58.

148. Pusterla N, Gebhart CJ. Equine proliferative enteropathy: a review of recent developments. Equine Vet J 2013;45:403–9.

149. Pereira CER, Resende TP, Vasquez E, et al. In vitro antimicrobial activity against equine *Lawsonia intracellularis* strains. Equine Vet J 2019;51:665–8.

150. Toth B, Aleman M, Nogradi N, et al. Meningitis and meningoencephalomyelitis in horses: 28 cases (1985-2010). J Am Vet Med Assoc 2012;240:580–7.

151. Smith JJ, Provost PJ, Paradis MR. Bacterial meningitis and brain abscesses secondary to infectious disease processes involving the head in horses: seven cases (1980-2001). J Am Vet Med Assoc 2004;224:739–42.

152. Pellegrini-Masini A, Livesey LC. Meningitis and encephalomyelitis in horses. Vet Clin North Am Equine Pract 2006;22:553–89.

153. Bach FS, Bodo G, Kuemmerle JM, et al. Bacterial meningitis after sinus surgery in five adult horses. Vet Surg 2014;43:697–703.

Emergency Management for Donkeys and Mules

Debra C. Archer, BVMS, PhD[a],*, Rebekah J.E. Sullivan, BVSc[b],
Karen Rickards, BVSc, PhD[b]

KEYWORDS

- Dullness • Hyperlipemia • Respiratory disease • Colic • Laminitis

KEY POINTS

- Emergency management of donkeys and mules follows the same key principles as horses (and ponies) with some variations in presenting clinical signs, approach to handling, physiology, pharmacology, and local anatomy.
- Donkeys and mules show less overt signs of clinical disease, and dullness or lack of normal behavior may indicate potentially severe underlying disease.
- Hyperlipemia is a common secondary consequence of illness or stress and must be monitored and treated at an early stage.
- Pet/companion donkeys are more likely to present with obesity-associated and geriatric disease conditions, and emergency presentations may be acute exacerbations of chronic underlying disease.
- Working donkeys and mules may present with a wide variety of emergency presentations, and economic and social factors need to be considered when deciding on treatment options.

INTRODUCTION

Emergency management of donkeys and mules follows the same key principles as the approach to emergencies in horses (and ponies). However, it is important to be aware of their normal stoical behavior and key differences in approach to handling, clinical presentation of various disorders, physiology, pharmacology, and specific anatomic variations compared with horses.[1] In the developed world, donkeys and mules are frequently kept as pets or companions. Some may be used as working pack animals or may be kept as farmed animals in some countries for meat or milk production.[2] Pet/companion donkeys or mules have a longer life span and are more prone to obesity than their working counterparts, making geriatric and obesity-related disease

[a] Department of Equine Clinical Studies, University of Liverpool, Leahurst Campus, Neston, Wirral CH64 7TE, UK; [b] Veterinary Department, The Donkey Sanctuary, Brookfield Farm, Offwell, Honiton, Devon EX14 9SU, UK
* Corresponding author.
E-mail address: darcher@liverpool.ac.uk

Vet Clin Equine 37 (2021) 495–513
https://doi.org/10.1016/j.cveq.2021.04.013
0749-0739/21/© 2021 Elsevier Inc. All rights reserved.

common in this population.[3] Donkeys and mules may be checked and handled less frequently and may receive little preventive care, for example, dental checks and vaccinations, and subtle signs of disease or changes in behavior may be missed by owners. Emergency presentations may be due to acute exacerbation of chronic underlying disease. Owner education is vital including careful monitoring of behavior, health and quality of life (QOL) (wherein chronic disease is present), good management and appropriate preventive health care. Donkeys in the production industry are more likely to present with reproductive and neonatal emergencies as jennies will be part of a breeding program. Donkeys and mules in the developing world are more likely to be used as working animals, and those presented for emergency care are usually younger. Common emergency presentations include wounds/traumatic injuries, gastrointestinal disease due to ingestion of foreign bodies or parasitism, exhaustion due to overwork/malnutrition, hyperthermia, respiratory disease, tetanus, rabies, and other infectious diseases. The working donkey or mule may be the only source of income for a family, so relatively simple conditions that may not constitute an emergency in the developed world can have a potentially disastrous impact on a family, complicating and potentially compromising treatment options. Appropriate communication and consideration of social and economic factors is important in these populations.

KEY DIFFERENCES IN DONKEYS AND MULES

The general approach to assessment and management of emergencies in donkeys and mules is similar to that in horses. Key considerations are as follows:

- Thorough history taking to identify chronic disease and determine tetanus prophylaxis, vaccination, and deworming status.
- Detailed clinical examination including careful palpation to detect subtle pathology and to assess the body condition score. This is important in individuals with thick coats because considerable weight loss can go undetected.
- Donkeys and, to a lesser extent, mules may not express the true severity of pain they are experiencing, and dullness or absence of normal behavior may be the only presenting sign. Donkeys and mules with overt changes in behavior or signs of disease may be more systemically compromised than they appear externally. Pain scoring systems developed specifically for donkeys may be helpful for assessment and monitoring of treatment.[4]
- Donkeys and mules may be handled less than horses and owned by less physically capable handlers. This, in combination with their natural behavior, can present challenges during clinical examination and drug administration. Mules and working donkeys may be wary of human contact and can be unpredictable in their movements. Even with a leg held up, they can kick accurately and effectively. Patience and consistent, firm, but considerate, handling are paramount.
- As a species, donkeys have evolved to fight, rather than run away from an attack, and their so-called stubbornness is more likely an expression of their natural tendency to display caution when unsure of a situation.[5] Donkeys are usually easy to restrain once a head-collar has been fitted. Mules can be much more challenging to deal with and behave more unpredictably and violently, making human safety important, for example, wearing of head protection. Ear twitching is not recommended because it elicits an aversive response presumably as a result of pain, but some donkeys and mules may tolerate and respond well to careful application of a nose twitch for a short time. Chemical restraint should be used as an adjunct to manual restraint when needed.

- Donkeys are physiologically and pharmacologically different from horses, and mules will have some features common to both. As a desert-adapted species, the donkey appears better able to tolerate dehydration.[6] Use of the skin tent technique to assess hydration status is unreliable in donkeys.[7]
- **Table 1** lists key clinical parameters and techniques that clinicians dealing with donkeys/mules should be aware of. Key hematological and biochemical parameters in donkeys and mules are summarized in a recent review article.[8]
- Body water compartmentalization differs from the horse, and the volume of distribution may vary for many drugs.[6] Metabolism of many drugs is generally quicker in the donkey, such that standard equine dosages are used, but dosing intervals may be more frequent.
- Dosages of commonly administered medications are given in **Table 2**. Few drugs are licensed for use in donkeys, and drugs should be administered in accordance with relevant national legislation and based on weight and consideration of body condition scores (for a more comprehensive review, see the study by Mendoza and colleagues[9]).
- Donkeys may show fewer clinical signs for some transboundary diseases, for example, African horse sickness, which should be considered wherein unusual disease presentations are seen in association with recent import of them or in-contact equids from other countries/regions.
- Donkeys have a propensity to develop hyperlipemia, and situations that result in development of negative energy balance must be avoided. Any ill or stressed donkey must be monitored for hyperlipemia and treated early because the condition can progress rapidly resulting in a high mortality rate. Hyperlipemia complicates treatment of any primary disease and worsens the prognosis.
- Most pet donkeys will have a bonded companion, and they should be kept in sight of each other (irrespective of species) wherever possible during treatment, to reduce stress.

Emergency Sedation and Anesthetic Protocols

An excellent review of anesthesia, sedation, and pain management is detailed in a recent tutorial article;[10] anesthetic protocols are also available from The Donkey sanctuary (https://www.thedonkeysanctuary.org.uk/). In general, the initial dose of sedative, premedication, and induction agents is the same for donkeys as for horses. The major difference is the faster metabolism of many drugs requiring more frequent top-up dosing intervals. Importantly, mules may require up to 50% higher initial doses than horses, which may initially need to be given intramuscularly if temperament dictates. Oral detomidine gel, where available, can be useful for donkeys and mules that are more tolerant of being handled around the head than for injections. However, the effects can be less precise than intravenous administration of sedatives. Incorporating acepromazine into the sedation regime may also be of benefit for mules. A multimodal drug combination (eg, detomidine, acepromazine, and butorphanol mixed in a syringe and administered intramuscularly) has been described in fractious horses and has proven successful in many mules.[1] Use of sedation and local anesthetic nerve blocks (same as in the horse) may avoid the need for general anesthesia. Care should be taken to avoid administration of standard volumes used in horses, which may result in toxic limits of local anesthetics, occurring where multiple blocks are used, for example, enucleation. Therefore, the volume used at each site and the maximum total volume should take into consideration their weight. For longer procedures, additional sedation needs to be administered more frequently, or consideration could be given to

Table 1
Common parameters/procedures and donkey/mule-specific notes

Parameter/Procedure/Terminology	Normal Value or Range/Notes
Terminology	Jenny: female donkey; jackass: male donkey Mule: product of mare bred to a jackass; hinny: product of a jenny bred to a stallion
Rectal temperature	Adult donkey: 36.5–37.8°C/97.2–100.0°F (average: 37.1°C/98.8°F)
Heart rate	Adult donkey: 36–52 beats per minute (average: 44 beats per minute)
Respiratory rate	12–28 breaths per minute (average: 20 breaths per minute) In working equids, resting respiratory rates may normally be up to 59 breaths per minute to maintain normal body temperature in hot climates.
Weight	90–400 kg (average: 180 kg); miniatures ~100 kg, mammoth: 350–400 kg. Horse and pony weigh tapes are not suitable for estimating the weight of donkeys—see donkey weight estimator tool (www.thedonkeysanctuary.org.uk).
Intramuscular injection	Use neck or gluteal muscles—do not use the pectoral region. Adults: 18 G 1.5-inch needle, smaller donkeys/foals: 19 G/21 G 1-inch needle Donkeys have thicker skin and tolerate pushing the needle slowly through the skin better than the slap technique used in horses.
Intravenous injection/catheterization	Owing to the thick coat of donkeys, clipping is always advisable to allow clear visibility of the jugular vein. The prominent cutaneous colli muscle can particularly conceal the middle third of the jugular groove, and the angle of needle introduction is typically steeper than in the horse or pony. A small volume of intradermal local anesthetic and a small skin incision facilitate intravenous catheter placement. A 14 G catheter is suitable for most donkeys.
Epidural anesthesia	2nd intercoccygeal space (the 2nd is wider than the 1st intercoccygeal space)—easier to palpate than in horses Use a 30° angle from the horizontal for needle entry Various analgesic combinations are described: 2% lidocaine hydrochloride at 0.22 mg/kg bwt diluted with sterile 0.9% sodium chloride solution to a volume of 0.2 mL/kg total volume is shown to be effective in donkeys.
Emergency field anesthesia	Various protocols in veterinary anesthesia texts and articles. Injectable anesthetics may need more frequent administration of boluses owing to more rapid drug metabolism in donkeys. Example emergency protocol using ketamine:

(continued on next page)

Table 1 *(continued)*	
Parameter/Procedure/Terminology	**Normal Value or Range/Notes**
	Premedication: • Similar doses as for horses—alpha-2 agonist/opioid Induction: • Ketamine 2.2–2.8 mg/kg & diazepam 0.1 mg/kg IV Maintenance: • One-third induction dose of ketamine administered every 10 min • One-third to half the initial induction dose of alpha-2 agonist given after 15 min if xylazine is used; after 30 min if detomidine is used; after 60 min if romifidine is used
Endotracheal intubation	Can be performed blindly but can be more difficult compared with horses owing to differences in regional anatomy in donkeys. Consider use of a laryngoscope/use of a flexible endoscope if difficult to perform; abnormal conformation/tracheal hypoplasia is more common in dwarf donkeys. Adults: 14–18mm (internal diameter) endotracheal tube; foals: 12-mm internal diameter endotracheal tube
Nasogastric intubation and administration of fluid	Donkeys have relatively narrower nasal passages than horses; use a small-diameter (13 mm) pony- or foal-sized stomach tube to avoid trauma and epistaxis. The recommended volume of fluids that can be administered for a standard donkey of 150–200 kg is 2–3 L; volumes greater than this cause excessive gastric distention and pain.
Rectal examination	Can be performed safely depending on the size of the donkey or mule, and rectal tears are rare if performed carefully. Butylscopolamine (0.3 mg/kg IV) use can facilitate safer examination.
Abdominocentesis	Large ventral subcutaneous fat deposits (up to 10–14 cm) can make abdominocentesis challenging. Ultrasound-guided needle placement and use of a catheter/spinal needle may be required in obese individuals.

Data adapted from Evans and Crane (2018)[1] and Matthews et al. (2019).[10]

use of continuous rate infusions using similar protocols as described for horses, adjusted as per effect.[10]

Administration of Medications and Stall Rest

Oral medications can be hidden in treats such as jam sandwiches, or paste formulation medications can be given sandwiched between ginger biscuits. Administration of medications via nasogastric tubes can be carried out as for horses, but consideration should be given to the size of the tube used and the potential for stress created by

Table 2
Commonly used medications in donkeys and specific notes of key differences from horses

Drug Generic Name	Dose	Dosing Interval/ Duration of Action	Route	Comments on Use in Donkeys
NSAIDs				
Flunixin	1.1 mg/kg	q 12 h	IV	
Phenylbutazone	2.2–4.4 mg/kg	q 12 h – standard q 8 h – miniatures	IV, PO	Cleared more rapidly in horses and in miniature donkeys than in standard donkeys
Carprofen	0.7–1.3 mg/kg	q 24 h	IV, PO	Give IV as a single dose Metabolized more slowly in donkeys
Firocoxib	0.1mg/kg	Shorter than in horses and ponies	PO	Good oral availability (more data required)
Meloxicam	0.6mg/kg		IV	Not recommended for use in donkeys owing to a very short half-life
Sedative/anesthetic drugs				
Detomidine	0.01–0.04 mg/kg 0.04–0.08 mg/kg 0.04 mg/kg	20–40 min, longer for sublingual	IV IM PO (oral gel)*	Alpha-2 agonists should be given in donkeys at similar dosage to horses; for mules, higher dosages should be used (approximately 50% higher dose recommended; no current data for optimal dosage for oral detomidine gel in mules).
Romifidine	0.05–0.1 mg/kg	30–60 min	IV	
Xylazine	0.4–1.5 mg/kg	15–20 min	IV	Usually combined with an opioid to increase the degree of sedation and analgesia.
Acepromazine	0.02–0.05 mg/kg	30 min–2h	IV, IM, sublingual	
Butorphanol	0.02–0.05 mg/kg	30–60 min	IV, IM	
Buprenorphine	5–10 μg/kg	q 8 h	IV	
Ketamine	2.2–2.8 mg/kg		IV	Cleared more rapidly in donkeys especially miniatures; more frequent top-ups required

Guaifenesin	To effect – 50–110 mg/kg for induction			
Antimicrobials				
Na Penicillin G	20,000 IU/kg	q 4–6h	IV	Shorter dosing intervals required in donkeys for beta-lactam antimicrobials
Gentamicin	6.6 mg/kg	q 24 h	IV	Care in mammoth asses – lower volume of distribution, take care to avoid toxicity
Oxytetracycline	5–10 mg/kg	q 12–24 h	Slow IV	Shorter elimination half-life: dosing interval half of that recommended for horses
Trimethoprim sulfamethoxazole	30 mg/kg	q 12 h	PO	Optimal dose not currently known for donkeys
Other				
Dexamethasone	0.05–0.2 mg/kg	q 24 h	IV, IM, PO	Contraindicated if hyperlipemia is evident
Heparin sodium	100–200 IU/kg	q 8–12h	IV	May be used in hyperlipemia; check clotting factors first

Abbreviations: IM, intramuscular; IV, intravenous; PO, per os; SL, sublingual.
Adapted from Evans & Crane (2018)[1] and Mendoza et al. (2019).[9]

repeated administration, increasing the risk of hyperlipemia. If there is requirement for a donkey to be on stall rest, it is essential that owners/carers monitor for signs of inappetence and changes in behavior. Any bonded companion will have to be kept on stall rest too in order to minimize stress. If a patient is receiving intravenous fluid therapy, both the patient and companion will require constant monitoring to prevent chewing or dislodging of the venous catheter. Where this is impractical, companions have been separated but kept in full view of each other through methods such as using gates or hurdles to divide a stall.

It is important to reduce risk factors for impaction colic and hyperlipemia. Consideration should be given to bedding the patient(s) on alternative to straw, such as wood shavings, ensuring constant access to fresh water and enriching the environment to reduce stress and boredom (https://www.thedonkeysanctuary.org.uk/what-we-do/knowledge-and-advice/for-owners/environment-enrichment).

METABOLIC AND HEPATIC EMERGENCIES
Hyperlipemia

When dealing with any sick donkey or mule, it is essential to consider the potential for development of hyperlipemia, particularly in individuals at higher risk. Dyslipidemias including hyperlipemia are more frequent in donkeys than in other equids. The incidence in mules is unknown but is assumed to be higher than in horses.[11] In addition to investigating and treating any underlying disease process, it is essential to diagnose hyperlipemia at an early stage and restore a metabolic positive energy balance as soon as possible to improve survival. Development of hyperlipemia will complicate the treatment and prognosis of any donkey or mule presented as an emergency case, and it is essential to measure blood triglyceride (TG) levels as part of routine investigation, monitoring, and prognostication.

Risk factors for hyperlipemia in donkeys include increased age, obesity, female sex, pregnancy and lactation, feeding of concentrates, concurrent disease, recent weight loss or inappetence, dental disease, recent change of premises, and cardboard bedding.[12,13] Hyperlipemia is most commonly secondary to some form of stress or other illness; 72% of donkeys with hyperlipemia had concurrent disease in one study.[12] Mortality is high in donkeys, varying from 41% to 76%, and is directly correlated with blood TG levels[12] (**Table 3**).

Clinical signs include change in behavior (dullness), anorexia, sham eating, reduced fecal output and mucus-covered feces, halitosis, and reduced borborygmi and ileus. Diagnosis is based on history, clinical signs, and confirmation of elevated levels of

Table 3	
Prognosis associated with different triglyceride levels in aged donkeys with hyperlipemia	
Plasma Triglyceride Concentration (mmol/L)	**Treatment/Prognosis in Donkeys with Hyperlipemia**
<10	Good prognosis with rapid intervention and reversal of negative energy balance using enteric support
10–15	Fair prognosis with aggressive fluid therapy including parenteral nutrition
>15	Poor prognosis even with aggressive therapy—total parenteral nutrition will be required.

Data from The Donkey Sanctuary. Clinical Companion of the Donkey. Available at: https://www.thedonkeysanctuary.org.uk/what-we-do/for-professionals/resources/clinical-companion

serum TG. Concurrent evaluation of any underlying disease process is vital, including identification of dental disease or gastrointestinal pathology. Care should be taken when performing rectal examination because the rectal mucosa may also be friable.

Treatment includes management or treatment of any underlying cause of disease or stress, reversal of the negative energy balance, analgesia, and potential use of gastroprotectants. A recent review article provides an in-depth review of the pathophysiology and treatment.[11] Donkeys/mules should be encouraged to eat by offering a variety of palatable feedstuffs. Appetite stimulants include feeding of bramble cuttings, fresh grass, addition of peppermint cordial and/or fruit juices to feed and giving treats such as apples, carrots, bananas and ginger biscuits. It is essential to minimize stress and keep donkeys with their bonded companion at all times during treatment. If they will not voluntarily eat, nasogastric intubation of the following may be used: 2 to 3 L of warm water (estimated total volume for a 150- to 200-kg donkey), with added electrolyte powders/tablets, dextrose powder (approximately 1 g/kg bodyweight (bwt) but will need to tailor depending on glucose content of electrolyte powders), and 250 to 500 g of ground instant oat breakfast cereal, which should be added just prior to administration and stirred well to prevent blockage of the tube (see the study by Evans and Crane[1] for further details).

If repeat administration is not efficacious, ileus is present, or repeated intubation is causing further distress, then intravenous fluid therapy should be considered. Where hospitalization is not an option, administration of fluid boluses outside of the clinic setting is a practical option. Duphalyte 100 mL/50 kg bwt (B-vitamin, electrolyte, amino acid and dextrose solution) and dextrose 1–2 mL/kg 5% solution can be added to a 3-L bag of lactated Ringer's solution. Partial or total parenteral nutrition combined with insulin therapy may be required in severe cases,[1,14] but this requires hospitalization for careful monitoring of glucose status and can be expensive. Cost and prognosis should be discussed with the owner, alongside the risk of further stress of transportation to hospital facilities.

Acute Hepatic Disease

Chronic hepatic disease is common in nonworking donkey populations, and emergency presentation of a donkey or mule with severe signs of liver disease is most likely to be due to acute exacerbation of chronic hepatic disease.[7] Clinical signs are similar to those seen in horses, including dullness, blindness, neurologic signs (aimless wandering, head pressing), and abdominal pain, but these clinical signs are likely to be less overtly displayed. Some cases may present with pyrexia; in those cases, it is important to establish whether this is due to an underlying inflammatory process only or whether an infectious agent may be responsible (Sullivan, personal observation). Acute hepatic disease is likely to be complicated by development of secondary hyperlipemia.

Serum biochemistry will aid the diagnosis and assessment of severity of disease, and ultrasonographic examination of the liver and biopsy can provide additional diagnostic and prognostic information;[7] at present, there is no specific donkey histopathology scoring system, so the scoring system devised in horses is used.[15] If biopsy results can be obtained quickly, this can aid to decision-making regarding continuing with treatment. However, the potential benefit of biopsy results must be weighed up against the risks of causing further stress and hyperlipemia.

Hyperthermia/Hypothermia

Hyperthermia (heat stress) can occur in working donkeys in hot/humid climates pushed beyond their normal levels of fitness, where underlying disease is present or where they are not acclimatized to the environmental conditions.[16] Hypothermia is more likely to occur in donkeys than in horses owing to their larger body surface area relative to volume allowing for greater heat loss. This can develop in donkeys during periods of extreme cold during winter months in certain geographic regions.[17] It should be noted that use of rugs can be helpful to conserve body heat, but a significant amount of heat loss occurs through the ears.

ORAL AND GASTROINTESTINAL EMERGENCIES
Colic

Donkeys are less likely to display the overt signs of colic seen in horses and are more likely to present as dull and/or inappetant.[7] Owners should be aware of the importance of anorexia, sham eating, and reduced fecal and urinary output as key potential signs of colic. The underlying etiology will vary depending on use, signalment, and geographic location. Gastrointestinal obstruction is a common cause of colic in the donkey; in a working donkey, it is most likely the result of severe dehydration or foreign body obstruction, whereas in the pet donkey, increased risk for impaction is associated with underlying dental disease, diet, and increasing age.[18] Donkeys have a propensity to browse and are highly inquisitive, so it is important to remove any objects within reach of donkey patients or their companion. Although most foreign objects will not be swallowed, ingestion of plastic bags and other objects is a common issue in working equids scavenging for food.

Investigation of the colic case is similar to that in the horse (an in-depth review on managing the colic patient in the field can be found elsewhere in this issue). Hematology and biochemistry is important to rule out hyperlipemia as the primary underlying cause to assess overall systemic status and to monitor for secondary development of hyperlipemia. Peritoneal and blood lactate levels may be measured to assist with prognosis if facilities are available. There are no published data relating to normal lactate reference ranges in donkeys, but work performed at The Donkey Sanctuary indicates that levels may be comparable with those from horses.

It is safe to perform rectal examination in most adult donkeys and mules, except those in miniature breeds or those that are very small. Care must be taken to avoid personnel injury, particularly when performing rectal examination of mules. Outside of a clinic setting, stocks are unlikely to be available, so well-placed hay bales can be placed between the hindquarters and the examiner. Short-acting chemical restraints, such as xylazine and or use of butylscopolamine, at standard equine doses can facilitate examination. See **Table 1** for practical tips on performing nasogastric intubation and abdominocentesis. Transcutaneous ultrasonographic examination of the abdomen can provide useful additional diagnostic information. Donkeys usually have heavy coats and will require clipping and skin preparation to increase the likelihood of obtaining diagnostic images. Ultrasonography can be useful to locate a suitable site for abdominocentesis and determine the quantity of ventral abdominal fat because this can be significant in donkeys, particularly those that are obese.

Treatment of colic in donkeys and mules is similar to that in horses. The key aims are (1) correction of the underlying problem (including the potential need for surgical intervention), (2) provision of analgesia, (3) maintenance or restoration of normovolemia, (4) monitoring for development of hyperlipemia, and (5) identification and management of underlying disease/etiological factors (eg, unidentified dental pathology or high levels of gastrointestinal parasites). To prevent development of hyperlipemia, starvation of donkey patients with colic is not recommended. Small volumes of easily digestible feedstuffs and walking in hand to pasture, if manageable for the patient, are important. Intravenous fluid therapy types and administration rates can be extrapolated from horse data.

If a surgical lesion is suspected, early discussion with the referral center is important. Given the ability of donkeys to mask pain, they may have already developed significant systemic compromise by the time veterinary advice is sought by owners. If patients are to be transported, provision must be made for their bonded companion(s) to accompany them. The companion will also require monitoring during any hospital stay because the process of transportation and stress is a risk factor for hyperlipemia. Provision should be made for appropriate-sized hospital accommodation—if stable doors cannot be lowered, then a gate or hurdle may need to be used to enable donkey patients to see out of their stall.

Colitis

Colitis in the donkey may be a life-threatening condition that is challenging to diagnose.[7] The etiologies are assumed to be similar to the horse, with cyathostominosis, *Clostridial spp.*, *Salmonella spp.*, and other infectious or toxic ingested agents identified in a UK population. Dullness, fever and occasionally diarrhea (this is often not evident in colitis cases in donkeys) are the key presenting signs, and treatment is similar as for horses. The authors have used smectite as an intestinal adsorbent at standard equine dosages, but note that the frequent nasogastric intubation needed may present additional unwanted stress to the patient. The donkey's gut microbiome differs from that of the horse,[19] so the efficacy of standard equine probiotics is questionable.

Other

A number of other gastrointestinal diseases have been identified in donkeys and are detailed in a recent review article.[7] The presentation and treatment of esophageal obstruction choke is similar to that in the horse. It is paramount that any donkey presenting with choke has a full dental examination once the obstruction has resolved because, particularly in geriatric donkeys, dental pathology is an important risk factor. Gastric impaction has also been reported as a cause of colic in UK donkeys, and there is sparse literature detailing diagnosis and management. Ileus, pain after nasogastric intubation and enteral fluid administration, and evidence of gastric distention on transabdominal ultrasound justify use of gastroscopy to confirm a diagnosis. Rectal prolapse is seen more commonly in working donkeys associated with exhaustion and/or parasitism.[20] Treatment is the same as for that in the horse. Pancreatitis may be suspected in donkeys or mules with nonspecific abdominal pain and raised amylase and lipase levels, but definitive diagnosis is rare. It may also develop secondary to hyperlipemia.

RESPIRATORY EMERGENCIES
Asthma

In pet donkeys, crises associated with acute exacerbation of chronic equine asthma are seen frequently.[21] The specific challenge with donkeys is suitable provision of a clean air environment and dust-free feedstuffs suitable for the patient and companion. Although unlimited pasture access may enhance respiratory health, this can result in unwanted weight gain and obesity-related disease. Turnout onto bare pasture is ideal if weight gain is or becomes an issue or use of a grazing muzzle can be implemented. As with horses, soaking hay and feeding of straw may reduce dust and calorific content. There are commercial dust-free donkey-specific short chop products available in some countries, if dental disease prevents the feeding of long fibers. If long fibers are soaked, a ration balancer containing vitamins and minerals should be provided to prevent micronutrient deficiencies.

Pulmonary Fibrosis

In the population of donkeys at The Donkey Sanctuary, respiratory emergencies have also been presented that are not the result of asthma but are instead due to the underlying pulmonary fibrosis, with a prevalence of 35% identified in one study.[22] This condition can be very difficult to diagnose until an advanced stage, assumed to be due to the sedentary nature of companion/pet donkeys masking signs of progressive, slow respiratory compromise. Acute deterioration of respiratory function is likely a result of secondary bacterial infection and/or after acute exposure to allergens, for example, during removal of manure from the stall and placement of fresh bedding material (Sullivan, personal observation). Secondary tracheal collapse may also be seen. Reduced lung sounds may be evident on thoracic auscultation, and ultrasonographic evaluation of the pleural surface may reveal comet tail reverberation artifacts and areas of consolidation of the lung tissue, which is consistent with fibrosis (**Fig. 1**). The pathology of pulmonary fibrosis appears to be different in donkeys compared with horses, beginning in the subpleural tissues then extending diffusely into the parenchyma as interstitial fibrosis. Asinine herpesvirus (AHV)-4 and AHV-5 have been isolated in a case series of donkeys with interstitial pneumonia,[23] suggesting that herpesvirus may have a role in the etiology of donkey pulmonary fibrosis. Dyspnea as a result of acute exacerbation of pulmonary fibrosis does not resolve with administration of smooth muscle relaxants or systemic B-2 agonists. Treatment is currently confined to symptomatic treatment and clean air management, but the prognosis for severely dyspneic cases is extremely poor. TG levels should be checked in any dyspneic donkey or mule because development of hyperlipemia will worsen the prognosis further.

Tracheal Collapse

Tracheal collapse is more common in geriatric donkeys, likely owing to age-related tracheal cartilage degeneration.[21] It can also develop secondary to other respiratory pathology including pulmonary fibrosis. Acute cases may present with moderate to severe dyspnea, flaring of nostrils, and efforts to mouth breathe. Treatment is symptomatic including immediate movement to a clean air environment, if possible, without

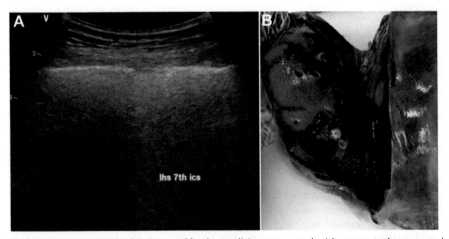

Fig. 1. An 11-year-old donkey in good body condition presented with severe tachypnea and dyspnea. Thoracic ultrasonographic examination revealed extensive pleural surface irregularities and altered echogenicity (*A*). Postmortem examination confirmed extensive chronic, diffuse, severe fibrosing interstitial pneumonia (*B*).

further exacerbating the degree of stress. Long-term, affected donkeys and their companion should be kept in dust-free environments, and their weight should be monitored carefully to prevent obesity.

Infectious Respiratory Disease

Many donkeys are not vaccinated against equine herpesviruses (EHVs) and/or equine influenza, and pet donkeys may not mix with others very often. Donkeys infected with equine influenza virus are likely to be more severely affected than horses and to develop secondary bronchopneumonia (not so in mules). Early treatment with antimicrobials and careful monitoring is important. Avian influenza has been shown to infect donkeys and should be considered as a potential cause of respiratory disease in groups of donkeys in affected areas during disease outbreaks.[24]

In working equids, respiratory disease is a common clinical presentation, with varying severity of disease being evident.[25] It is not uncommon for different groups of donkeys to mix at locations such as markets, making disease spread a significant problem. Coughing, nasal discharge, submandibular swellings, and pyrexia are frequent signs of strangles (caused by *Streptococcus equi. var equi*), which can develop into an emergency situation if large numbers of animals in close contact are affected and unable to work, in addition to individual cases of dyspnea due to lymph node enlargement. Education regarding strangles and appropriate biosecurity should be part of any community engagement initiative.

MUSCULOSKELETAL EMERGENCIES

Foot abscesses and laminitis are common causes of acute lameness in donkeys and mules.[26] Usually, pathology is at a more advanced stage when clinical signs of overt lameness are seen owing to their stoic nature. If recumbent, feed intake may have been reduced, and thus, it is essential to check for evidence of hyperlipemia and ensure good nursing care to make sure they are eating and drinking. Hoof testers are also less useful for detecting response to foot pain compared with horses, particularly in hot climates, wherein the hoof capsule can be extremely hard. Treatment is similar to horses: paring the sole to establish drainage, remove any necrotic or undermined sole, soaking the foot, and/or application of a poultice.

The radiographic anatomy of the foot of the donkey is slightly different to that of the horse,[27] and the differences are less marked in mules. Generally, in donkeys, the foot has a more upright anatomy, and the distal phalanx is positioned more distally within the hoof capsule. The extensor process in donkeys is not normally in line with the coronary band (**Fig. 2**).

Laminitis

Episodes of laminitis in pet/companion donkeys kept on soft ground may go unnoticed by owners. Donkeys will not develop the classic stance seen in horses/ponies unless on hard ground, and the only clinical signs may be slow weight shifting or placing hind legs further under the abdomen, lying down for longer periods, or reduced physical activity. The key radiographic signs are similar to those in horses with increased angular deviation between the dorsal aspect of the distal phalanx and dorsum of the hoof wall and increased distal displacement of the distal phalanx.[27] Owing to the position of the distal phalanx in relation to the frog in donkeys compared with horses, traditional frog supports are not advised because they may act as a fulcrum rather than providing mechanical support. In the immediate presentation of the emergency case, thick cotton wool pads or Styrofoam blocks for heavier donkeys

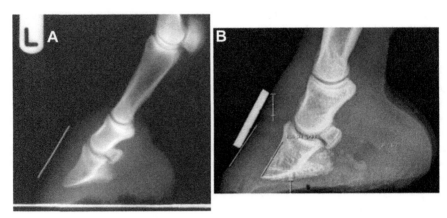

Fig. 2. Lateromedial radiographs of a normal donkey hoof (*A*) and a donkey with laminitis (*B*).

may be used. Once the condition is stabilized, acrylic resin can be used to create a custom shoe with or without a gel insert for solar support.[1] Providing a deeply bedded stall can also be helpful to reduce discomfort. Use of Non-steroidal anti-inflammatories (NSAIDs) to provide analgesia is also important (see **Table 2**).

WOUNDS AND OTHER INTEGUMENTARY EMERGENCIES

Wounds, severe abrasions, and bite injuries are more common in working equids. The potential for rabies should be considered in endemic areas where a bite injury has occurred. Tetanus prophylaxis should also be administered in any donkey or mule that sustains a wound and is not currently on tetanus prophylaxis. Working equids' clinical evaluation should also include a general assessment of systemic health including underlying acute issues such as dehydration and pain and chronic issues such as low body condition scores. Malnourishment and use of ill-fitting harnesses and inappropriate tack such as bits is likely to be a significant problem in many working equids' wound presentations. Preventive care should focus on education regarding appropriate harness/bit use and care and maintaining donkeys in as good general health and weight as possible.

NEUROLOGIC EMERGENCIES

Donkeys can develop neurologic signs secondary to EHV and AHV (AHV-3, now known as EHV-8).[28] Testing is available in some specific centers using PCR.

REPRODUCTIVE AND URINARY EMERGENCIES

Covering dates may be unknown, so it can be difficult to assess readiness for birth and prematurity. Gestation is approximately 12 months (331–421 days) in the donkey, and owing to the greater density of microcotyledons in the donkey chorioallantois, jennies are more likely to deliver live twins than mares.[29] Dystocia is managed in the same way as for mares, but the narrow, tortuous lumen of the cervix predisposes to cervical lacerations during dystocia. Donkeys are also more likely to develop necrotic vaginitis after prolonged dystocia, and topical antimicrobial and steroid cream can be used to prevent cervical and vaginal adhesions.[29] Management of retained fetal membranes is the same as for the mare, with additional need to monitor for development of hyperlipemia.

Male donkeys have relatively larger reproductive organs than the horse and, in particular, have a very large testicular artery. This increases the risk of postcastration hemorrhage unless the testicular artery is ligated directly or indirectly via placement of a transfixing ligature around the vaginal tunic. This will depend on age of the donkey and technique used. They commonly have large quantities of scrotal fat, which also can make ligation more difficult and which can prolapse from the castration site.[1]

OPHTHALMIC EMERGENCIES

Ocular pathology is commonly seen in geriatric donkeys, and ophthalmic examination should form part of routine/annual assessment. In comparison with horses, the donkey's orbital socket is usually deeper, and the globe is positioned in a more sunken position.[30] The corneal surface is large, and corneal ulcers are common ocular pathology, although donkeys are generally less prone to traumatic injuries, presumed to be due to the fact that they are less flighty than horses. The conjunctival sac is large, and the distal nasolacrimal duct opening can be found on the dorsolateral aspect of the nares, not ventrally as in horses.

In the case of an acutely painful eye, examination should include assessment to check for foreign bodies. Donkeys often bury their heads in hay/straw and have a thick coat and periorbital hair, particularly in the winter, increasing the risk of organic foreign bodies becoming lodged in and around the eye. The donkey's inherent stoical behavior can mask ocular lesions until disease is advanced or pain is severe, and both eyes must be checked for the presence of subtle underlying chronic pathology.

NEONATAL EMERGENCIES

Donkey and mule foals require around 250 mL of colostrum per hour for the first 6 hours of life, and failure of passive transfer (FPT) can by assessed using commercial equine snap tests to assess IgG status.[1] Equines' hyperimmune serum can also be administered in donkey foals with FPT. This is used as a standard at The Donkey Sanctuary, and no adverse reactions have been observed. Commercial foal milk replacer can also be used in orphan foals. Owing to their small size and narrower nasal passages compared with horses/ponies, suitable-sized equipment must be used. An equine male urinary catheter can be useful for nasogastric intubation, and 20 to 22G catheters are used for intravenous fluid therapy. Neonatal isoerythrolysis is more common in mules than in horse foals. The principles of treatment are the same as for foals (see article on this issue: *Emergency Management of Equid Foals in the Field* by Dr. Elsbeth A. Swain O'Fallon).

CARDIOVASCULAR EMERGENCIES

Where severe hemorrhage has occurred requiring blood transfusion, ideally blood should be obtained from a donor donkey, and crossmatching should be performed as for horses. Where this is not possible, horse blood can be administered safely to donkeys. Importantly, donkey/mule blood cannot be administered to horses owing to the presence of RBC antigens (donkey factor) that cause transfusion reactions in horses.

PREVENTIVE CARE

Education of owners/handlers working with donkeys or mules is critical regardless of whether they are kept as pets, production animals, or working animals. They should be aware of the normal behaviors and be alert to even subtle changes in behavior or lack of normal behavior as indicators of underlying pain or disease. For those working with working equids in developing countries, this can be a difficult balance because owners/handlers themselves may have severe health challenges or be facing extreme poverty. Treatment of donkeys/mules in these situations has to take into account the economic and behavioral drivers and the need to understand the practical challenges including barriers to veterinary treatment/rest and challenges around communication.

Routine health-care checks should include assessment of general management, vaccination, and deworming status, regular dental checks, and monitoring of weight and body condition scores. Where donkeys/mules have ongoing medical issues, owners should be advised of the need to consider QOL issues.

QUALITY OF LIFE ASSESSMENT

Acute exacerbation of chronic disease conditions is common in pet/companion donkeys, and consideration of QOL can assist decision-making regarding whether it is appropriate to attempt treatment for an emergency condition or not. This may need to be done immediately, or over the ensuing days, depending on the severity of the presenting condition. Owners may struggle to come to terms with advice to euthanize a pet donkey or mule who, to a lay person, has not been ill prior to this point. It is crucial to take a holistic standpoint, taking into account the history and general assessment of the donkey/mule. Gradual weight loss, severe dental disease, reluctance to move, hair rubs, or even superficial wounds over carpi and hocks may all be indicative of underlying pathology, which is relevant to decision-making in any emergency situation, particularly in geriatric donkeys/mules. There are numerous tools and guidelines available for owners and vets to use together to assess individual animals (eg, https://www.thedonkeysanctuary.org.uk/what-we-do/knowledge-and-advice/for-owners/monitoring-your-donkeys-quality-of-life).

EUTHANASIA

The same techniques for euthanasia of horses and ponies are applicable to donkeys and mules (see article on this issue: *When All Else Fails: Alternative Methods of Euthanasia* by Dr. Tracy A. Turner). These primarily involve use of chemical agents and use of a free bullet or captive bolt, followed by pithing/exsanguination. The landmark for placement of the gun or captive bolt is 1 to 2 cm above the intersection of lines drawn from the base of the ear to the contralateral lateral canthus (**Fig. 3**). Owing to the strong bonds that form between donkeys, a remaining bonded donkey companion should have the opportunity to spend time with the body prior to removal. Companions should also be monitored closely because they will be at increased risk of developing hyperlipemia. Use of chemical agents is the same as for those licensed for use in the horse.

One of the challenges in performing euthanasia of equids in the developing world may be the lack of suitable drugs or availability of firearms. Options for disposal of the carcass, which may be eaten by scavengers, may also preclude use of chemical agents such as barbiturates. Aortic severance per rectum may be an acceptable technique to use where no other option is available. The donkey or mule must be anesthetized or heavily sedated in recumbent patients before this is performed for welfare and personnel safety.

SUMMARY

Donkeys and mules may present with a variety of emergency conditions that follow the same basic principles of diagnosis and management as in horses, with some key

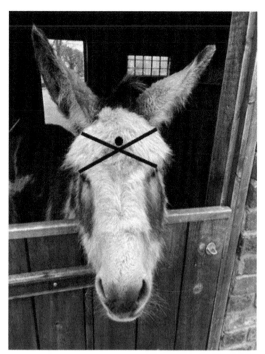

Fig. 3. Landmark for free bullet/captive bolt placement; this is slightly higher than in the horse/pony and should be 1 to 2 cm dorsal to the intersection of a line drawn between the base of the ear and the contralateral lateral canthus.

differences in diagnosis and management. It is important to be aware of important differences in donkey and mule behavior, and few overt clinical signs may be demonstrated unless severe pain or advanced disease is present. Different emergency conditions are more likely to present in companion/pet donkeys and mules than in working donkeys and mules or those used for production purposes. Stress and illness frequently result in development of secondary hyperlipemia in donkeys, which must be monitored and treated early.

CLINICS CARE POINTS

- Keep companions close by when examining/treating a donkey to reduce stress and improve patient compliance.

- Take a blood sample early in the physical examination and allow the samples to settle whilst carrying out the rest of the patient assessment. This allows a crude visual assessment of the clarity of the serum/plasma to be made in order to rapidly assess triglyceride concentrations.

- Early intervention to provide energy even before a diagnosis of hyperlipaemia is made can improve patient outcomes.

- Be aware of lack of routine preventive care such as vaccination against tetanus/influenza and dental treatment – client education is important for inexperienced donkey / mule carers.

- Stoicism will mask deteriorating clinical signs so thorough and regular examinations are required to monitor progress and reassess prognosis. Ensure adequate analgesia is being provided.
- Colitis cases often do not present with diarrhea.

DISCLOSURE

The authors have nothing to disclose.

REFERENCES

1. Evans L, Crane M. The Clinical Companion of The Donkey *Produced by The Donkey Sanctuary.* 2018. Available at: www.thedonkeysanctuary.org.uk. Accessed August 3, 2020.
2. Davis E. Donkey and mule welfare. Vet Clin North Am Equine Pract 2019;35(3): 481–91.
3. Barrio E, Rickards KJ, Thiemann AK. Clinical evaluation and preventative care in donkeys. Vet Clin North Am Equine Pract 2019;35(3):545–60.
4. van Dierendonck MC, van Loon JPAM, Burden FA, et al. Monitoring acute pain in donkeys with the equine utrecht university scale for donkeys composite pain assessment (Equus-donkey-compass) and the equine utrecht university scale for donkey facial assessment of pain (equus-donkey-fap). Animals 2020. https://doi.org/10.3390/ani10020354.
5. McLean AK, Navas González FJ, Canisso IF. Donkey and mule behavior. Vet Clin North Am Equine Pract 2019;35(3):575–88.
6. Grosenbaugh DA, Reinemeyer CR, Figueiredo MD. Pharmacology and therapeutics in donkeys. Equine Vet Educ 2011. https://doi.org/10.1111/j.2042-3292.2011.00291.x.
7. Thiemann AK, Sullivan RJE. Gastrointestinal disorders of donkeys and mules. Vet Clin North Am Equine Pract 2019;35(3):419–32.
8. Goodrich EL, Behling-Kelly E. Clinical pathology of donkeys and mules. Vet Clin North Am Equine Pract 2019;35(3):433–55.
9. Mendoza FJ, Perez-Ecija A, Toribio RE. Clinical pharmacology in donkeys and mules. Vet Clin North Am Equine Pract 2019;35(3):589–606.
10. Matthews N, van Loon JPAM. Anesthesia, sedation, and pain management of donkeys and mules. Vet Clin North Am Equine Pract 2019;35(3):515–27.
11. Mendoza FJ, Toribio RE, Perez-Ecija A. Metabolic and endocrine disorders in donkeys. Vet Clin North Am Equine Pract 2019;35(3):399–417.
12. Burden FA, Du Toit N, Hazell-Smith E, et al. Hyperlipemia in a population of aged donkeys: description, prevalence, and potential risk factors. J Vet Intern Med 2011. https://doi.org/10.1111/j.1939-1676.2011.00798.x.
13. Reid SW, Mohammed HO. Survival analysis approach to risk factors associated with hyperlipemia in donkeys. J Am Vet Med Assoc 1996;209(8):1449–52. Available at: http://europepmc.org/abstract/MED/8870744.
14. Durham AE, Thiemann AK. Nutritional management of hyperlipaemia. Equine Vet Educ 2015. https://doi.org/10.1111/eve.12366.
15. Durham AE, Smith KC, Newton JR, et al. Development and application of a scoring system for prognostic evaluation of equine liver biopsies. Equine Vet J 2003. https://doi.org/10.2746/042516403775467171.
16. Dey S, Dwivedi SK, Malik P, et al. Mortality associated with heat stress in donkeys in India. Vet Rec 2010. https://doi.org/10.1136/vr.c504.

17. Stephen JO, Baptiste KE, Townsend HG. Clinical and pathologic findings in donkeys with hypothermia: 10 cases (1988-1998). J Am Vet Med Assoc 2000;216(5): 725–9.
18. Cox R, Proudman CJ, Trawford AF, et al. Epidemiology of impaction colic in donkeys in the UK. BMC Vet Res 2007. https://doi.org/10.1186/1746-6148-3-1.
19. Edwards JE, Shetty SA, van den Berg P, et al. Multi-kingdom characterization of the core equine fecal microbiota based on multiple equine (sub)species. Anim Microbiome 2020. https://doi.org/10.1186/s42523-020-0023-1.
20. Getachew AM, Innocent G, Trawford AF, et al. Gasterophilosis: a major cause of rectal prolapse in working donkeys in Ethiopia. Trop Anim Health Prod 2012; 44(4):757–62.
21. Rickards KJ, Thiemann AK. Respiratory disorders of the donkey. Vet Clin North Am Equine Pract 2019;35(3):561–73.
22. Miele A, Dhaliwal K, Du Toit N, et al. Chronic pleuropulmonary fibrosis and elastosis of aged donkeys: similarities to human pleuroparenchymal fibroelastosis. Chest 2014. https://doi.org/10.1378/chest.13-1306.
23. Kleiboeker SB, Schommer SK, Johnson PJ, et al. Association of two newly recognized herpesviruses with interstitial pneumonia in donkeys (Equus asinus). J Vet Diagn Invest 2002;14(4):273–80.
24. Abdel-Moneim AS, Abdel-Ghany AE, Shany SAS. Isolation and characterization of highly pathogenic avian influenza virus subtype H5N1 from donkeys. J Biomed Sci 2010;17(1):25.
25. Stringer A, Christley R, Bell C, et al. Owner reported diseases of working equids in central Ethiopia. Equine Vet J 2016;49. https://doi.org/10.1111/evj.12633.
26. Thiemann AK, Poore LA. Hoof disorders and farriery in the donkey. Vet Clin North Am Equine Pract 2019;35(3):643–58.
27. Collins SN, Dyson SJ, Murray RC, et al. Radiological anatomy of the donkey's foot: objective characterisation of the normal and laminitic donkey foot. Equine Vet J 2011;43(4):478–86.
28. Garvey M, Suárez N, Kerr K, et al. Equid herpesvirus 8: complete genome sequence and association with abortion in mares. PLoS One 2018;13:e0192301.
29. Canisso IF, Panzani D, Miró J, et al. Key aspects of donkey and mule reproduction. Vet Clin North Am Equine Pract 2019;35(3):607–42.
30. Mendoza FJ, Toribio RE. Perez-Ecija Donkey internal medicine – Part II: Cardiovascular, Respiratory, Neurologic, Urinary, Ophthalmic, Dermatology, and Musculoskeletal disorders. J Eq Vet Sci 2018;65:86–97.

When All Else Fails
Alternative Methods of Euthanasia

Tracy A. Turner, DVM, MS

KEYWORDS

- Euthanasia • Barbiturates • Potassium chloride • Magnesium Chloride

INTRODUCTION

The term euthanasia is derived from the Greek and means good death. The term is usually used to describe ending the life of an individual animal in a way that minimizes or eliminates pain and distress. A good death is tantamount to humane termination of an animal's life. In the context of AVMA Guidelines, the veterinarian's duty in performing euthanasia includes, but is not limited to, his or her ability to induce death in a manner that is in accord with an animal's interest and/or because it is a matter of welfare and the use of humane techniques to induce the most rapid, painless, and distress-free death possible. These conditions, although separate, are not mutually exclusive and are codependent.

In regard to horses, overdose of intravenous barbiturate has been the most commonly used method for equine euthanasia.[1] Unfortunately, barbiturates present several problems; disposal of remains must be carried out promptly through commercial rendering, on-farm burial, incineration or cremation, direct haul to a solid waste landfill, or biodigestion. This will help prevent exposure of wildlife and domestic animals to potentially toxic barbiturate residues. Disposal of remains must be conducted in accordance with all federal, state, and local regulations. Recently, rendering facilities have refused equine carcasses owing to barbiturate use. The same is true for landfills and even composting owing to the worry of soil and water contamination by barbiturates. These drugs invoke legal responsibilities for veterinarians and animal owners to properly dispose of animal remains after death. Animal remains containing pentobarbital are potentially poisonous for scavenging wildlife, including birds (eg, bald and golden eagles, vultures, hawk species, gulls, crows, ravens), carnivorous mammals (eg, bears, martens, fishers, foxes, lynxes, bobcats, cougars), and domestic dogs.[2] Federal laws protecting many of these species apply to secondary poisoning from animal remains containing pentobarbital. The Migratory Bird Treaty Act, the Endangered Species Act, and the Bald and Golden Eagle Protection Act may carry civil and criminal penalties, with fines in civil cases up to $25,000 and in criminal cases up to $500,000 and incarceration for up to 2 years.[2] Serious repercussions may occur when veterinary health professionals who should be well informed about the necessity

Turner Equine Sports Medicine and Surgery, 10777 110th Street N, Stillwater, MN 55082, USA
E-mail address: turner@turnerequinesportsmed.com

Vet Clin Equine 37 (2021) 515–519
https://doi.org/10.1016/j.cveq.2021.04.014
0749-0739/21/© 2021 Elsevier Inc. All rights reserved.

for proper disposal of animal remains fail to provide it, or fail to inform their clients how to provide it, whether there was intent to cause harm or not.[3,4] As such, the use of barbiturates is becoming a less popular method of euthanasia, and the need to use other methods of euthanasia is becoming more common.

ALTERNATIVE METHODS OF EUTHANASIA

Penetrating captive bolt and gunshot are two less commonly used but highly effective and acceptable methods.[1] Penetrating captive bolt and gunshot euthanasia should only be used by well-trained personnel who are regularly monitored to ensure proficiency, and firearms must be well maintained. This procedure requires selection of an appropriate firearm and bullet with sufficient velocity, energy, and size to pass through the skull (enter the brain) and cause massive brain destruction. For horses, a .22-caliber long rifle up to a 9 mm may be required. The muzzle should be within 1 to 2 feet of the animal's forehead and perpendicular to the skull, with the intended path of the bullet roughly in the direction of the foramen magnum. This will reduce the potential for ricochet while directing the bullet toward the cerebrum, midbrain, and medulla. The muzzle should be aimed at a point where a line crosses from the lateral canthi of the eyes to the base of opposite ears (**Fig. 1**). Captive bolt is used in a similar fashion. Appropriate restraint or sedation is required for application of either gunshot or the penetrating captive bolt, and special care should be taken to ensure that personnel are not injured by ricochet from free bullets. Unfortunately, veterinarians are not routinely trained with these two methods.

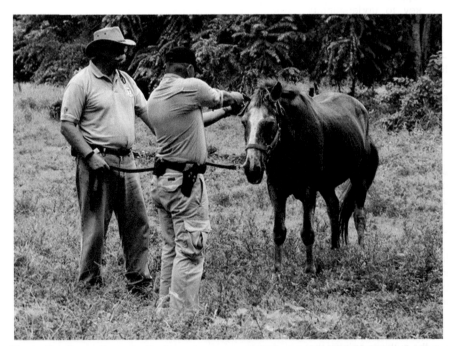

Fig. 1. Gunshot euthanasia: the horse has been sedated, a proper caliber weapon has been selected (.38 caliber), and the muzzle is pointed perpendicular to the forehead, where two lines bisect drawn from the lateral canthus of the eyes to the base of the ear (*red* X).

In order to determine if an alternative method of euthanasia is acceptable, the AVMA considers several factors: (1) ability to induce loss of consciousness and death with a minimum of pain and distress; (2) time required to induce loss of consciousness; (3) reliability; (4) safety of personnel; (5) irreversibility; (6) compatibility with intended animal use and purpose; (7) documented emotional effect on observers or operators; (8) compatibility with subsequent evaluation, examination, or use of tissue; (9) drug availability and human abuse potential; (10) compatibility with species, age, and health status; (11) ability to maintain equipment in proper working order; (12) safety for predators or scavengers should the animal's remains be consumed; (13) legal requirements; and (14) environmental impacts of the method or disposition of the animal's remains.

The AVMA Guidelines classify euthanasia methods as acceptable, acceptable with conditions, and unacceptable.[1] Acceptable methods are those that consistently produce a humane death when used as the sole means of euthanasia. Methods acceptable with conditions are those techniques that may require certain conditions to be met to consistently produce humane death, may have greater potential for operator error or safety hazard, are not well documented in the scientific literature, or may require a secondary method to ensure death. Methods acceptable with conditions are equivalent to acceptable methods when all criteria for application of a method can be met. Unacceptable techniques are those methods deemed inhumane under any conditions or that the Panel on Euthanasia (POE) found to pose a substantial risk to the human applying the technique.

The POE recognizes there will be less-than-perfect situations in which a method of euthanasia that is listed as acceptable or acceptable with conditions may not be possible and a method or agent that is the best under the circumstances will need to be applied.[1]

A key to understanding appropriate euthanasia techniques is understanding conscious versus unconscious. Unconsciousness may be defined as loss of individual awareness that occurs when the brain's ability to integrate information is blocked or disrupted. In humans, the onset of anesthetic-induced unconsciousness has been functionally defined by loss of appropriate response to verbal command; in animals, it is defined by loss of the righting reflex.[5,6] This definition, introduced with the discovery of general anesthesia more than 160 years ago, is still useful because it is an easily observable, integrated whole-animal response.

Anesthetics produce unconsciousness either by preventing integration or by reducing information received by the cerebral cortex or equivalent structure(s). Further, the abrupt loss of consciousness that occurs at a critical concentration of anesthetic implies that the integrated repertoire of neural states underlying consciousness may collapse nonlinearly.[7] Data from different species suggest that memory and awareness are abolished with less than half the concentration required to abolish movement. Thus, an anesthetic state (unconsciousness and amnesia) can be produced at concentrations of the anesthetic that do not prevent physical movements.[6]

There are several adjunctive techniques that are useful under general anesthesia. Injecting a solution of potassium chloride, magnesium chloride, or magnesium sulfate intravenously or intracardially is a simple technique. In addition, exsanguination or pithing may be performed under general anesthesia. A new technique uses lidocaine injected intrathecally to cause death.

Techniques

It is the author's opinion that a simpler, safer, and more esthetic method of euthanasia is to induce anesthesia first with intravenous xylazine (1.1 mg/kg) to induce heavy sedation followed by intravenous ketamine (2.2 mg/kg). This combination in the author's experience reliably provides 10 minutes of anesthesia, which is plenty of time to accomplish any of the following adjunctive measures. In addition, there is evidence that drug residues after use of these drugs are safe.[8]

Potassium chloride may be administered intravenously or intracardiac. The potassium ion is cardiotoxic, and rapid IV or intracardiac administration of 1 to 2 mmol/kg (0.5–0.9 mmol/lb) of body weight (1–2 mEq K+/kg; 75–150 mg/kg [34.1–68.2 mg/lb]) of potassium chloride will cause cardiac arrest.[9] Practically, mix 2 tablespoonfuls of Lite salt into 120 mL of water into solution and administer to effect. Likewise, magnesium salts can be supersaturated into solution and administered intravenously. Magnesium has the advantages that it has an analgesic effect, causes muscle relaxation, and prolongs anesthesia. These would all be beneficial during a euthanasia procedure.

Another advantage of these drugs is that potassium chloride and magnesium salts are not controlled substances and are easily acquired, transported, and mixed in the field.[1] Potassium chloride and magnesium salt solutions, when administered to an unconscious equid, result in the remains that are potentially less toxic for scavengers and predators and may be a good choice in cases where proper disposal of animal remains (eg, rendering, incineration) is impossible or impractical.[10,11]

Disadvantages of these drugs are they may cause muscle spasms shortly after injection, especially potassium chloride because it causes muscle depolarization. Potassium chloride and magnesium salt solutions are not approved by the Federal Drug Administration (FDA) for use as euthanasia agents. Saturated solutions are required to obtain suitable concentrations for rapid injection into equids, and failure to use saturated solutions can cause the procedure to go poorly.

A recently described technique is the use of intrathecal lidocaine during intravenous anesthesia.

After induction of anesthesia, an area over the atlanto-occipital space would be prepared enough (clipped) to allow identification of landmarks. The horse's head is flexed to open the atlanto-occipital space. A 6-inch 18 gauge needle is inserted just on a line along the cranial edge of the atlas and on the midline. The needle is directed toward the lower jaw and advanced until the dura is penetrated. Sixty milliliters of cerebrospinal fluid is removed, and 60 mL of 2% lidocaine hydrochloride is administered within 30 seconds.[12]

The main advantage of this technique is all drugs are readily available and relatively inexpensive. The animal remains of this technique would be less toxic to the environment than using barbiturates.

The main disadvantage of this technique is it requires specific skills. Also, the technique is slightly slower in causing cessation of respiratory, cardiovascular, and neurologic function than barbiturate euthanasia.

A variation of this technique is to pith the horse after induction of anesthesia. The operator manipulates the pithing tool through the atlanto-occipital space to substantially destroy both brainstem and spinal cord tissue.[1]

The final technique involves exsanguination.[1] Because anxiety is associated with extreme hypovolemia, this should be performed only under general anesthesia. Exsanguination can be performed by opening the throat; however, this is not esthetic. As a result, a per-rectal technique may be more appealing. A knife or scalpel is introduced per rectum. The caudal aorta is identified and cut.

SUMMARY

Acceptable methods of equine euthanasia have problems. Barbiturates create environmental issues and disposal problems. Gunshot and the use of penetrating captive bolt require special training. Adjunctive techniques performed after inducing anesthesia offer a simple alternative that require skills more typical of veterinary training and pose a lower risk of environmental toxicity.

DISCLOSURE

The author has no conflicts of interest and no funding sources. The author is a member of the AVMA Panel on Euthanasia.

REFERENCES

1. AVMA Panel on Euthanasia. AVMA guidelines for the euthanasia of animals (2013 Edition). American Veterinary Medical Assn; 2013.
2. Krueger BW, Krueger KA. US Fish and Wildlife Service fact sheet: secondary pentobarbital poisoning in wildlife. Available at: cpharm.vetmed.vt.edu/USFWS/. Accessed Mar 7, 2011.
3. O'Rourke K. Euthanatized animals can poison wildlife: veterinarians receive fines. J Am Vet Med Assoc 2002;220:146–7.
4. Otten DR. Advisory on proper disposal of euthanatized animals. J Am Vet Med Assoc 2001;219:1677–8.
5. Hendrickx JF, Eger EI II, Sonner JM, et al. Is synergy the rule? A review of anesthetic interactions producing hypnosis and immobility. Anesth Analg 2008;107: 494–506.
6. Antognini JF, Barter L, Carstens E. Overview: movement as an index of anesthetic depth in humans and experimental animals. Comp Med 2005;55:413–8.
7. Alkire MT, Hudetz AG, Tononi G. Consciousness and anesthesia. Science 2008; 322:876–80.
8. Aleman M, Davis E, Knych H, et al. Drug Residues after Intravenous Anesthesia and Intrathecal Lidocaine Hydrochloride Euthanasia in Horses. J Vet Intern Med 2016;30(4):1322–6.
9. Saxena K. Death from potassium chloride overdose. Postgrad Med 1988; 84(97–98):101–2.
10. Lumb WV. Euthanasia by noninhalant pharmacologic agents. J Am Vet Med Assoc 1974;165:851–2.
11. Ciganovich E. Barbiturates. In: Field manual of wildlife diseases. General field procedures and diseases of birds. Biological Resources Division information and technology report 1999–001. Washington, DC: US Department of the Interior and US Geological Survey; 1999. p. 349–51.
12. Aleman M, Davis E, Williams DC, et al. Electrophysiologic study of a method of euthanasia using intrathecal lidocaine hydrochloride administered during intravenous anesthesia in horses. J Vet Intern Med 2015;29(6):1676–82.

Moving?

Make sure your subscription moves with you!

To notify us of your new address, find your **Clinics Account Number** (located on your mailing label above your name), and contact customer service at:

Email: journalscustomerservice-usa@elsevier.com

800-654-2452 (subscribers in the U.S. & Canada)
314-447-8871 (subscribers outside of the U.S. & Canada)

Fax number: 314-447-8029

Elsevier Health Sciences Division
Subscription Customer Service
3251 Riverport Lane
Maryland Heights, MO 63043

*To ensure uninterrupted delivery of your subscription, please notify us at least 4 weeks in advance of move.

ELSEVIER